HUMANIZING
MADNESS:

PSYCHIATRY AND
THE COGNITIVE
NEUROSCIENCES

By Niall McLaren, M.D.

An application of the philosophy of science to psychiatry

Library of Congress Cataloging-in-Publication Data

McLaren, Niall, 1947-
  Humanizing madness : psychiatry and the cognitive neurosciences : an application of the philosophy of science to psychiatry / by Niall McLaren.
    p. ; cm.
  Includes bibliographical references and index.
  ISBN-13: 978-1-932690-39-2 (trade paper : alk. paper)
  ISBN-10: 1-932690-39-5 (trade paper : alk. paper)
  ISBN-13: 978-1-932690-40-8 (hardcover : alk. paper)
  ISBN-10: 1-932690-40-9 (hardcover : alk. paper)
  1. Psychiatry--Philosophy. I. Title.
  [DNLM: 1. Psychiatry. 2. Mind-Body Relations (Metaphysics) 3. Philosophy, Medical. 4. Psychological Theory. 5. Psychophysiology. WM 100 M4786h 2007]
  RC437.5.M43 2007
  616.89'001--dc22

               2007016021

Distributed by: Baker & Taylor, Ingram Book Group, Quality Books
Future Psychiatry Press is an imprint of
Loving Healing Press
5145 Pontiac Trail
Ann Arbor, MI 48105
USA

http://www.LovingHealing.com or
info@LovingHealing.com
Fax +1 734 663 6861

Future Psychiatry Press

Table of Contents

TO SEE ILLUSTRATIVE CASES AND OTHER CLINICAL MATERIAL, VISIT WWW.FUTUREPSYCHIATRY.COM.

Introduction

"A change to a new type of music is something to beware of as a hazard to all our fortunes. For the modes of music are never disturbed without an unsettling of the most fundamental political and social conventions."
—Plato

I–1. Personal Preliminaries

The purpose of this book is to show what a scientific theory of psychiatry should look like. Unfortunately, a lot of psychiatrists think this to be a rather silly objective, pointing to what they believe are several perfectly adequate theories already available. My response is that the mere existence of a number of different theories confirms what the cynics have long known: the more theories there are, the less likely any of them is right. Cynical or not, my view is that all the theories used in psychiatry in the late 20th Century are wrong.

In the 1970s, when I trained, psychiatry in Australia was somewhat different from what was on offer overseas. Rather than adopt the hard-line Freudian view of American psychiatry, the very biological approach common in Britain and Scandinavia, or the ascetic behaviorist line, Australians tried melding all the available schools into a benign and non-doctrinaire 'eclectic psychiatry. Eclecticism, which means picking the best bits of a range of offerings, was seen as, if not morally superior (Australians don't like extremism), then certainly a vastly more practical notion. Good eclectic psychiatrists could do more for their patients by adopting whatever approach seemed likely to give the best results.

Thus, depressed people were diagnosed as suffering a biological disorder and given tricyclic antidepressant drugs and Electro-Convulsive Therapy (ECT). Adolescents were awarded complex Freudian formulations which lent themselves to long-winded courses of psychotherapy. Middle-aged housewives with their phobias and obsessions were seen as suffering learned disorders and were treated by behaviorist methods. Schizophrenia and manic-depressive psychosis, of course, were seen as biological disorders, while people with personality disorders were preferably not seen at all.

Unfortunately, the psychiatry in which I trained was neither intellectually demanding for the trainee nor, I suggest, very helpful for the patients. Yet it was clearly an improvement on what had gone before. The old mental hospitals were still there, still full, their walls gone but the bars still on the windows. In many places, the patients still wore uniforms while the staff, also in uniform, bore heavy, jangling key rings and defensively custodial attitudes.

Yet it was a time of ferment, of change too rapid for the orthodoxy to manage. In a few short years after, say, 1970, a strongly humanist and anti-institutional influence spread, mainly from the USA but also from centers in Britain. The revolutionary idea that, merely by being caught up in the mental hospital system, people could be, if not driven mad, then certainly kept mad, quickly gained a following. Polemical writers such as Thomas Szasz in the US and Ronald Laing in Britain were widely read, and not just by people working in the mental health field. Anybody with intellectual pretensions had to be familiar with these writers. While this was going on, the psychiatric establishment seemed to have nothing new to say in response. In 1973, when *Science* published the startling paper *On Being Sane in Insane Places*, the establishment was enraged but not pensive. Down on ground level, as I then was, it seemed that the orthodoxy had overnight been rendered irrelevant, all their rigid theories of illness turned into yesterday's news by the simple idea of looking at the mentally-ill just as ordinary folk with a few problems.

It all seemed so very clear, so very superior, that learning the old theories would soon turn out to be a waste of time. And that, I suppose, is what adolescence is all about, whether it be in a family or in a profession. People entering a profession need that particular sense that the millennium is just around the corner. If they didn't have the roseate myopia that goes with it, if they knew just how hard the work would be, then they would probably all take up surfing or play guitars under trees.

On my first morning in psychiatry, my registrar (now a senior professor) took me to his office and, for about two hours, talked about psychoanalytic theory. At the end, I reeled out, stunned by his vast and effortless scholarship, by his untroubled familiarity with the arcane Freudian labyrinth. I wandered off to have cup of tea, asking myself: "How can anybody know all of that?" What I meant was not: "How could anybody know that much?" because, after studying medicine for six years, I knew that vast scholarship cost just a few more years' study. Instead, I had in mind the rather deeper question of: "How can anybody know that all that stuff is true? He believes it, but can he prove it?"

For anybody trained in philosophy, that is hardly a revolutionary question but, for a junior doctor trained during the materialist sixties, it was a bit radical. Everybody knew that if it was science, it had to be right, and Freudians invariably claimed that theirs was the only true science of mental life. So there could be no argument. Several times over the next few weeks, I essayed questions of this type but was quickly put in my place by my registrar's confident manner. He could answer any and every objection I raised, and I couldn't argue with his ever-ready answers. Freud surely was the man for all questions.

But at the same time, I was also very interested in the biology of mental life, if there is such a thing. In those days, there definitely seemed such a thing. To anybody studying biology after Watson and Crick, it seemed just a matter of time before the True Theory of Mind rolled off the scientific production line. Compounding this confidence, I had arrived at psychiatry via the unusual path of first wanting to study neurosurgery. Unfortunately, neurosurgery wasn't as interesting as I had hoped, but a term in psychiatry seemed to offer the chance of intense intellectual stimulation combined with getting to know people as people.

Consequently, I had to balance Freud on the one hand with reductionist, materialist biology on the other. In 1970s eclectic Australia, being able to jump from Freud to brain transmitters in the same sentence was seen as a virtue. But it soon became clear to me that something was wrong. In talking of mental disorders, my seniors would often talk about brain structure and function in outmoded terms. Or they might talk about neurotransmitters in mental illness when I knew perfectly well that nobody knew enough about them in health to say what they would be doing in illness.

This was a worry. In the burns unit or the cardiology department, when the consultant said this or that, then it was not going to be wrong. But in psychiatry, people could talk in terms which I knew intuitively were unprovable or just plain wrong, and nobody said anything. Indeed, the more outrageous the claim, the more awed people seemed and the less inclined they were to argue. I recall one professor confidently saying that a middle-aged man was depressed because he had had a gastrectomy and could no longer absorb Vitamin B6. But I had already spoken to the man and knew he'd had a vagotomy and pyloroplasty, not a gastrectomy; his vitamin levels were all normal; and he was a most offensively obsessional man whose family had finally tired of his demanding and domineering ways, hence his depression. And, despite the professor's sublime confidence in his own assessment, gastrectomy causes low VitB12, not B6. So much for academic psychiatry.

However, the first project in psychiatric training is to tackle the vast reading lists, which tends to subdue even the most fractious of trainees. For me and my peculiar quest for certainty, it made things worse. How can one talk of narrowing the search for the faulty neurotransmitters in schizophrenia, and at the same time have people writing purely psychological accounts of the disorder—and even have others saying that it doesn't exist, that it is invented by psychiatrists to keep mental hospitals full? They couldn't all be right. But my registrar had an answer for this, too. He announced that the essence of a good psychiatrist is to be able to tolerate ambiguity. That shut me up for a good week, I recall, until I realized that it licensed the very opposite of scientific certainty, it made a virtue of being too weak-willed to take a stand.

Perhaps the easiest solution seemed to be what most psychiatrists did, which was to ignore, politely but always firmly, what one didn't believe in. Except there was another problem: if psychiatry is a science, it isn't possible to jump from one theory to another. At best, only one theory can be right and all others are necessarily wrong. In my own puritanical way, belief couldn't and didn't enter the debate. I would accept what the facts dictated, not what faith or fantasy demanded.

Before long, I had decided that if anybody in psychiatry genuinely knew what he was talking about, I certainly hadn't met him. By April, 1975, twelve months after starting my training, my original plans to become a psychoanalyst had been abandoned. From my reading and from intuition, I knew that nobody could ever know what Freudians routinely claimed to know. I was also deterred more than a little by their habit of quoting from the master, analyzing the quote, then winding up with another quote which proved it all again—just like Christians and Marxists.

At the end of that year, I was warned by A Very Senior Psychiatrist that unless I straightened my ideas, I didn't have a future in psychiatry and, just to emphasize the point, was told not to apply for another post with his hospital. That was quite shocking: what are ideas for, if not to tear to bits? In due course, I passed my psychiatry finals and was let loose upon the unsuspecting public. Within a week of my last exam, I had decided to spend a little time clearing up the point of what constitutes the scientific theory of psychiatry.

That was nearly thirty years ago, and what follows is my preliminary outline of what is wrong with the state of theorizing in modern psychiatry.

My style of writing has been constrained by two pressures. On the one hand, I like to present things briefly but people sometimes object that the work isn't clear. However, spelling everything out in detail tends to sound polemical. Confusion or polemics, there's a conflict I haven't resolved. As a matter of style, I don't adopt the spurious objectivity of modern scientific writing. I use the first person personal pronoun in two ways. Firstly, I use it to distinguish very clearly between my views and other people's. I never use expressions like "It is suggested…" when I mean "I suggest…" Secondly, I use the philosophical I, which means that if I can experience or do something, so can every other living human of reasonable intellect. It means: "This is common to human experience and doesn't need to be argued." These different uses should be quite clear.

I-2. What Is Psychiatry?

Before we start, it will help to describe what psychiatry is. Firstly, psychiatry is a medical specialty. You cannot call yourself a psychiatrist in Australia unless you have the degree of Fellowship of the Royal Australian and New Zealand College of Psychiatrists (RANZCP) or its equivalent. To become a psychiatrist, you will have to pass a medical course (normally six years in this country) and then work several years as a medical officer in a teaching hospital before applying to join one of the psychiatry training programs. All training programs in Australia are organized by the RANZCP. Once you're accepted into training, and assuming all goes well, you will get your specialist degree after a heap of exams spread over another five years. This means about thirteen years of study since leaving school, sometimes more.

Psychiatrists believe that people have minds in their heads, and that disordered minds produce disordered behavior. By talking to people, asking them questions about how they think and feel, and by watching them, psychiatrists decide what's wrong in the head and prescribe treatments of various sorts. Because psychiatry is a medical specialty, and because medicine is based in biology, so the orthodox psychiatric concept of the mind and its disorders also has its foundations in biology. It is now standard psychiatric theory in most countries that the mind becomes disordered because the brain is disordered. Most psychiatrists accept that mental disease just is brain disease, that mental symptoms are nothing more than brain illnesses manifest in a particular way.

Consequently, the proper way of relieving these peculiar symptoms is to correct the underlying disturbance of brain function using physical treatments such as drugs, ECT or, in extreme cases, brain surgery. Thus, a depressed person who sees a psychiatrist will almost certainly be told: "You have a chemical imbalance of the brain, and these antidepressant tablets will cure you." If the depression doesn't get better, the patient (not client) may well be admitted to hospital for a course of ECT. It is all very rational and intellectually not very demanding but, as I will argue, it is all very wrong.

One thing has to be understood: psychiatry is not a branch of psychology. Psychology is a completely different subject. It is a university course, often part of the Arts Faculty, and has a totally different orientation from psychiatry. Whereas psychiatry is a very practical field, much more concerned with results than theories, psychology had its beginnings in philosophy departments over a hundred years ago and still has an intensely academic orientation. I don't think that will ever change. Psychiatry is about getting mentally-ill people better, and whatever works will be used. Psychology is essentially a research program aimed at working out the principals and mechanisms of normal mental life. Its practical aspects are secondary. If psychiatrists know anything about normal mental life, it is largely accidental. Psychologists, on the other hand, start with theories about normal behavior and work from there.

Psychiatrists work mainly in general hospitals, in mental hospitals, in university departments attached to hospitals, and in private practice. The sorts of disorders seen in psychiatric practice include every sort of mental disturbance, with the emphasis on the more severe types. Typically, psychiatrists see psychotic people, people with severe anxiety or depressive states, and the huge, blurred borderland between general medicine and mental life.

Years ago, it would have been said that mental hospitals treated mad people ("psychotics") against their will using physical methods of treatment based in a biological theory of insanity while private psychiatrists mostly treated miserable or frightened people ("neurotics") by talking to them. General hospitals did a bit of everything, especially if they had a university department of psychiatry, in which case they would probably use a lot of what are called behaviorist methods (as well as ECT). The theory of behaviorism argues that abnormal behavior is learned by the same principles as normal behavior, and can just as readily be unlearned ("cured"). It is (or was) a central theory in psychology, and psychiatrists simply borrowed it because it promised results. Also, it didn't clash with the biological theories of mental illness, which made life easier. Nowadays, that very simple division of labor has broken down.

I-3. Theoretical Preliminaries

This book is about theories. Why theories? Without theories, the practice of psychiatry drifts. Treatment becomes a mish-mash, heavily influenced by the latest charismatic writer (and psychiatry has plenty) and passing fads. A rational form of treatment should flow from the theory so that it becomes a rule-governed process, rather than hit-and-miss. Too often, existing theories have done little more than obstruct the proper development of ideas. In Part I, my intention is to show that they have long-outlived their usefulness. Bad theories waste resources by dictating the wrong research programs. Theories stand or fall on their content, and my conclusion is that each of them is so flawed as to be beyond salvation.

Part II consists of the much more interesting task of writing the "design specifications" of a new theory of human mental function for psychiatry. This approach is completely different from the way most of our theories have arisen, which is by elaboration on a chance discovery. We have to start at the beginning, with no preconceived ideas, using just the observable behavior and experiences of Citizen Joe Blow. If our definition of science excludes certain essential aspects of human life (as the behaviorists tried to do), then we have to change our model of science. All of this is explained along the way, every step is set out clearly with no hidden premises, so readers can see why I have taken a particular path and can agree or disagree with the move. However, there will be errors in this section but at least they should be more obvious than the errors buried in the old theories. The essence of Part II is this: No hidden premises. If there are any, I would like to hear of them.

Finally, Part III models the theory to the area of human mental disorder. This is the interesting bit, as my theory is meant to dictate treatment, not the other way around. I appreciate that, until now, available treatments have always dictated the theory, but it will bring us into line with the rest of medicine.

I–4. Summary of Part I: Psychiatry in Crisis: Intellectual Failure in the Science of Mental Disorder

It is a hallmark of a mature science that there is an agreed theoretical basis which gives rise to an accepted research program. Psychiatry is not such a science. While there is a measure of agreement as to the subject matter of psychiatry and what psychiatrists are allowed to do, that's about the limit of it. Of course, that limit does no more than define a technology. On the theoretical basis of psychiatry, there is no agreement. Granted, the dominant approach to mental disorder today is what is termed biological psychiatry but it merely dominates the research program and, anyway, that's just what is happening today. Tomorrow could see yet another of the vertiginous swings which have characterized psychiatry for the past one hundred years. These types of swings have led some perfectly sensible people to ask why they should take psychiatry seriously.

Given the array of theories available to every practitioner in psychiatry, we need some sort of standard to assess them. The process of abstractly comparing theories against an independent standard is known as meta-analysis. In the older, more formal sense, meta-analysis means the dispassionate comparison of the form of different theories which, for want of a better term, means philosophy, the love of knowledge. If we are comparing scientific theories or talking about what constitutes a science, we are talking about the philosophy of science. A large part of the philosophy of science consists of the derivation of different standards by which we can decide whether to take a theory seriously or not. As Joan Robinson didn't quite say, "The purpose of studying theory in psychiatry is to learn how to avoid being deceived by psychiatrists."

In the main, errors made by psychiatric theorists are fairly obvious because, all too often, ordinary common sense was lacking when the theory was written. The authors thought they were on to a good thing and their audiences were desperate for anything that sounded convincing. I am absolutely convinced that modern psychiatry is dying from the head up. Whether my work remains convincing after reading is up to you, the reader.

I-5. Summary Of Part II: The Working Mind

Since the beginning of recorded history, three questions seem to have occupied as much of our time as any others: How did we get here? Where are we going? How do we do it? No, that's probably an exaggeration. There are more pressing questions, such as: Where's our next meal coming from? How can we clobber our neighbors? Who's going to sleep with me tonight? Food, shelter and sex always take priority, but as soon as there was a relative degree of security and comfort, people's minds turned to questions of the mind. I also imagine that, as soon as people could start to think about minds in abstract, they started to think about madness.

In an ideal world, a theory of mental disorder would flow directly from a theory of mind. That is, a theory of mind is logically prior to a theory of disturbed mind, although anybody looking objectively at modern psychiatry would have no reason to suspect this. In my training in the 1970s, we were not given any instruction in concepts of mind. I remember enquiring about this once. The lecturer looked at me blankly and asked: "Why?"

Why indeed.

Should psychiatrists have any concept of mind? The gloomy survey in Part I implies that there might be some advantage in it. Part II starts the process of deriving a theory of mind suitable for psychiatry.

I-6. Summary Of Part III: Toward The Future Of Psychiatry

In the final chapters, I want to use the model derived in Part II to understand the crucial questions of mental disorder. That is, I want to develop a rational explanatory model of mental disorder. Since 1980, when the American DSM-III was published, psychiatry has not had an explanatory model of mental disorder, rational or otherwise. The entire nosology is avowedly atheoretical, meaning it assumes nothing about mental disorder but simply clumps it into separate categories. It should be understood that this amounts to an admission that psychiatry has no scientific basis. If there were a proper scientific theory for psychiatry, then it would necessarily be the basis of the nosology; it wouldn't be possible to have an agreed theory and not use it. If there isn't a proper theory, then the nosology can be no more than a prelude to science, an introductory clearing of the decks, as it were. Psychiatrists can't have it both ways. They can't claim on the one hand to be functioning within a scientific framework yet, on the other, also claim that their diagnostic system is atheoretical. There is no such thing as a non-theoretical science as a science is necessarily committed to a theory; science just is the process of explicating and testing a theory.

In any event, there are two objections to the notion that there can be an atheoretical nosology. Firstly, it isn't atheoretical at all, because if a researcher assumes the different sorts of mental disorder are categorically distinct, then he has made a major theoretical assumption. This needs to be proved, not simply accepted *ex vacuo*.

Secondly, there is an important principle in science which the DSM, with its endlessly proliferating categories of mental disorder, cheerfully breaches. This is the principle of parsimony or Occam's razor, named after Bishop William of Ockham who died in 1347. The principle, which has a number of variants (and may well have antedated him), states that the number of explanatory entities must not expand beyond the minimum necessary. Because the DSM system is based upon superficial appearances only, and says nothing about possible underlying mental mechanisms, it is not an explanatory system. Purists could therefore argue that the Razor doesn't apply, but the counter-objection is simple: why bother? If the huge numbers of separate diagnoses don't have some deeper significance, who needs them? This is especially the case when the different diagnoses can only be treated with the same small range of drugs. Orthodox psychiatry has become a sort of modern Scholasticism where researchers pore feverishly over the data, trying to find every conceivable point on which reality can be fractured into hundreds of entities with no significance beyond their names.

This section moves beyond mere description. I intend to look beyond the surface appearances, using the hidden mechanisms of mental life to explain the appearances rather than simply leaving them as isolated curiosities for biochemists to pick over. This will necessarily involve readjusting the borders so laboriously (and, at times, bitterly) drawn by the huge DSM committees but, if we want to move from "mere description" to an explanatory account of mental disorder, it is inevitable. It would be akin to the move from a structural classification of diseases (say, all lung diseases vs. all renal diseases) to an etiological system (all infectious diseases vs. all neoplastic diseases). Change inevitably breeds resistance, as the philosopher, Thomas Kuhn, warned.

In this context, the views of Air Chief Marshall Sir Hugh Dowding, victor of the Battle of Britain, are of particular interest. In his memoirs, *Twelve Legions of Angels* (1946), he wondered why, when they entered military service, some of the best brains in Britain "seem to lose their critical faculty." In a chapter entitled *Why are senior officers so stupid?* he noted: "If a junior officer puts forward a suggestion, the implication is that a senior officer might have thought of it, ought to have thought of it, and didn't think of it ... After being squashed a sufficient number of times, according to his tenacity, the junior officer ceases to put forward unwelcome suggestions...."

Replacing the word *officer* with *psychiatrist* indicates a universal application to Dowding's opinion which resonates with Kuhn's hypothesis. People who have spent thirty or forty years looking at mental disorder through a descriptive lens are not suddenly going to throw it out for another, because that would imply their model was never any good but they said nothing. That's asking a bit much of ordinary people and, after all, most psychiatrists are very ordinary, very conventional people.

My intention in the final Part is simply to sketch an outline of how a rational theory of psychiatry should be derived from a definitive model of mind. By answering the question, *What causes mental disorder?* I will show that a non-biological account of the major psychiatric syndromes is neither fanciful not counter-intuitive. Rather, it shows how to integrate the normal and the abnormal, how an understanding of the pathological flows directly from a detailed model of normal function.

Accordingly, I will not be giving many references in Part III as the argument should be self-evident. If it isn't, then all the references in the world won't save it.

—Niall McLaren
www.FuturePsychiatry.com

Darwin, Australia,
February, 2007.

Part I: Psychiatry in Crisis: Intellectual Failure in the Science of Mental Disorder

<table>
<tr><td>1</td><td># Brain Disease, Mental Disease And The Limits To Biological Psychiatry</td></tr>
</table>

1-1. Introduction

There is an ancient and universal notion that there is something we can add to or subtract from the diet that will cure all sorts of mental woes. In a sense, this is what biological psychiatry is all about, because underlying this particular belief is the concept that, even if there is an immortal and immaterial human soul that separates us from the beasts of the field, it has a very touchy stomach. Ultimately, they say, a man is what he eats. Generations of grandmothers have believed that constipation causes an accumulation of toxins in the bloodstream, which in turn affect the mind, causing all sorts of niggly behavior—but only in children. While grandmothers may become niggly themselves, it is always for good reason.

The principle is simple. Whatever the mind is, it can get sick just like everything else on earth. Despite thousands of years of religious indoctrination, there has always been a fifth column of old women frightening children with the idea that the mind sickens if they can't produce a good bowel action each day. But in biological psychiatry, this notion is extended to cover the complete state of the body as the final determinant of the mental state.

Now this is not Descartes' concept of the mind immaterial and unextended, the ethereal mental captain of the physical ship, as it were, but it is a widespread and very powerful notion. In every culture, people take drugs to feel or think better or to arouse or still various passions. In this context, "drug" means any physical agent introduced to the human body with the purpose of inducing a change. Drugs are therefore not the same as talismans or spells, which effect changes by supernatural means. Folk medicine as practiced by grandmothers is very largely built upon the concepts underlying modern biological psychiatry. So what are they?

Unfortunately, and despite the vast sums of money being spent on the biological research program in psychiatry, I am not aware that the principles underlying biological psychiatry have ever been explicated by its practitioners. In the main, biological psychiatrists have accepted as true all the materialist concepts that form the basis of general medicine. Central to these is the idea of reductionism, the belief that higher or more complex functions or entities can be reduced to or explained away as the outcome of activity or processes at less complex levels. This notion is certainly not new, and underlies all of the more orthodox sciences such as physics, chemistry and biology. Thus, we say that a towel dries in the sun, not because the sun spirit sucks the water out of it, but because water molecules trapped in its fibers acquire energy from the sun and, as explained by the kinetic theory of heat, break free of their mutual attraction and drift off. Cars move because of chemical energy in petrol, antibiotics safely destroy bacteria in the body, 'sunrise" is the impression given by the earth's rotation, and so on. What we see is the outcome of unseen processes among invisible particles. Reductionism "explains away" the appearances.

So too with the mind: biological reductionism argues that all thoughts, all mental activity or events of all kinds, result directly from certain neurophysiological events, and that a perfect understanding of all human affairs will automatically follow from a perfect understanding of the brain. Over the past hundred or more years, people have increasingly tended to accept that reductionism will explain human affairs just as it explains, say, ape affairs or cabbage affairs. I believe that this confidence has been misplaced (even in apes), but the set of beliefs and attitudes known as biological psychiatry depend very closely on reductionist concepts.

1-2. Biological Psychiatry in Practice

So what is biological psychiatry? Moving from the restricted to the general, three themes are seen in the literature:

1. "Biological psychiatry investigates possible pathophysiological bases to mental disorder" [1].

2. "Mental disorder is brain disorder" [2].

3. "All mental events are brain events" [3].

Since each of these themes defines a field of study and limits the means of investigation, they constitute research programs. In each case, the field of study is mental disorder, which is to be viewed and investigated from the standpoint of the established biological sciences. Unfortunately, the field of mental disorder is rather difficult to define, especially at its edges (e.g. separating normality from personality disorder), but mainstream mental illness is sufficiently well-defined to leave no doubt. Similarly, there is general agreement as to the nature of questions that can be asked in biological research, the form in which they must be cast, and the methods of investigation.

With few exceptions, research in all areas of biological psychiatry adheres closely to accepted methodologies. Techniques are borrowed from other, successful disciplines, adapted as necessary to human research, and then applied in a standard form. Necessarily, psychiatry lags a little behind the latest research in biology, as it takes time to understand the significance of recent developments and somewhat longer to apply these to questions in psychiatry (as well as the inevitable delays in funding). But while these aspects of research in the biology of psychiatry may be unexceptionable, there is another, more problematic, element, namely the nature and form of the questions being asked. Unlike a field with an agreed scientific methodology, there is no formal means of deciding whether questions in psychiatry are of a form suitable for this type of research. They derive informally from the researcher's overall view of the subject matter, meaning his apprehension or ontology of the nature of mental disorder. Unfortunately, my apprehension may well seem a misapprehension to you.

1–2(A). Restricted Biological Psychiatry

The references quoted above represent three quite divergent views on the nature of mental disorder. The first reference, by Berger and Brodie, is taken from a large, respected textbook of psychiatry. It is based on the empirical evidence that some sorts of brain disease can result in recognized syndromes of mental illness. The different contributors to that section of the handbook carefully avoided any particular theoretical commitments, as the conclusion to the section on schizophrenia shows: "...studies of the biology of schizophrenia have produced many findings of CNS dysfunction, none specific for this disease and none shared by everyone with the diagnosis ... Direct evidence for a specific neurotransmitter or receptor abnormality is not yet available. One hopes that as knowledge of normal CNS anatomy and physiology expands and new methods for exploring aberrations from normal become available, new insights into the cause or causes of this very devastating illness will be possible" [1, p 449].

This is a commendably cautious stance in an area fraught with conceptual and methodological difficulties. Only a person who denies that disturbances of brain function can affect mental function (hardly a tenable position) could take exception to this attempt to map out an area of research. As they noted, the results of this research program have been remarkably slow coming.

1–2(B). Unrestricted Biological Psychiatry

The second reference, from a textbook by the British psychiatrist Michael Trimble, represents a very much harder line on the nature of mental disorder, as his opening quote shows: "Mental disorders are neither more nor less than nervous diseases in which mental symptoms predominate, and their entire separation from other nervous diseases has been a sad hindrance to progress" (attributed to Henry Maudsley, 1870). Later, he quoted the German psychiatrist Griesinger as "...reflecting the essential nature of biological psychiatry ... 'Insanity being a disease, and that disease being an affection of the brain...'" (p11).

Trimble quickly dismissed the possibility that psychological factors can cause mental illness. He approvingly quoted Maudsley's acerbic dismissal of metaphysics (p21-3), immediately labeling psychoanalysis (and all psychodynamic theories) as metaphysics. He continued: "The distractions of psychoanalysis for present-day psychiatry cannot be over-emphasized. To base theories of etiology, pathogenesis and treatment on ideas that were dominant nearly a hundred years ago makes little sense ... Psychiatry ... tenaciously accepts so much of the old dogma, and so reluctantly embraces the new." Psychiatry, he insisted, is "...concerned with behavior in its widest sense, and has continually searched for knowledge of brain-behavior relationships and somatic underpinnings of psychopathology."

We can conclude from this that Trimble's position is as follows:
1. All mental disorder is brain disorder;
2. Psychiatry is essentially a biological discipline;
3. Psychodynamics is outmoded and empty metaphysics.

These are fairly blunt statements of intent, but they are certainly not un-usual. These ideas dominate psychiatry in the late twentieth century, especially in Britain, Scandinavia and, more recently, the United States. In fact, one of the doyens of American psychiatry, Samuel Guze, recently asked whether there is any other kind of psychiatry besides the biological, adding: "...there is no such thing as a psychiatry which is too biological" [4, p315]. Stated as baldly as this, we can see why some people have started to worry about "hegemonistic biologism" in psychiatry [5].

The greater part of Trimble's text consists of detailed accounts of biological research in a wide variety of mental disorders. Oddly enough, and in clear contrast with the moderate stance seen in Berger and Brodie, neither the book itself nor any of its chapters contains a summary, almost as though the author believed that the research material spoke for itself. To my mind, this is a serious omission, one which makes sense only if its readers accept the basic premises of his case as outlined above. In Trimble's schema, all pathological mind-body interaction goes but one way, from the body to the mind, a view most psychiatrists would reject. The concept of psychosomatics rests on the notion that the mind can influence the body.

The unanswered question in Trimble's approach to psychiatry is clear: Is it a fact that all mental disorder is brain disease? This is certainly not trivial as the whole objective of clinical and theoretical psychiatry is to understand the nature of the phenomena of mental disorder. However, regardless of how many professors line up behind the biological banners, the matter cannot be resolved by fiat. In this type of question, mere weight of opinion counts for nothing. Unfortunately, Trimble shows no awareness that there may be an issue at stake here. Mental disorder is brain disorder; therefore, as hollow metaphysics, all other considerations lie outside the purview of psychiatry and, by intimation, of rational thought. But Maudsley's nineteenth century dictum is the critical issue here, and the following argument will show some of its weaknesses.

Consider Maudsley's proposition:

Proposition P1: All mental disorder is (just a special form of) brain disorder.

In the first place, there is no logical way of proving this assertion true as it is not a necessary truth. At best, it could be an empirical truth, inductively true but thereby open to refutation by finding a single case of psychologically-determined mental disorder. This point is important. If Trimble asserts that it is impossible for mental disorder to be caused by anything other than brain disease, then he is making the same type of wild and unsupported statement of which he finds psychoanalysts guilty. But if he allows that there may be cases of mental disorder that do not result from brain disease, then he had no grounds for making his assertion in the first place.

Nonetheless, we can disprove P1 by considering the truth value of its negation, as follows:

P2: No cases of mental disorder are not also cases of brain disease.

This sounds a little clumsy, so it can be rephrased as follows:

P2a: There are no cases of psychologically-determined mental disorder.

But, as the diagnostic category of Post-Traumatic Stress Disorder explicitly recognizes, Proposition P2a is empirically false so Trimble's basic proposition, P1, is false. Despite his assertion, not all mental disorder is due to brain disease. A complete list of all brain diseases (known and unknown: we're talking hypothetically here) would not account for all mental disorders. There will always be some left over as examples of pure psychological disorder. He is therefore unwarranted in his remaining assertions, that psychodynamics is outmoded and empty metaphysics, and that psychiatry is essentially a biological discipline.

Returning to P1, there is another way of tackling Trimble's metaphysical stance on mental disorder, which is to look at the nature of the "human machine." In any complex machine (i.e. one that controls its own output by means of its information-processing capabilities), the disordered output resulting from an unseen physical disturbance of one sort or another can always be mimicked by a programming error. For people, what this means is that any and all disturbed behavior can in principle have either physical or psychological causes. Every psychiatrist keeps this critical point in mind all day: "Is what I am seeing a genuine psychological disorder, or is it really a physical illness such as a tumor, or is it just clever acting?" For anybody who takes the job seriously, this question is a ceaseless worry because there is no reliable rule of thumb.

For these two reasons, I assert that Trimble's case for biological psychiatry must fail. It seems to me that Trimble could only have overlooked these quite elementary considerations if he had assumed a more general position with respect to the mind. His basic proposition, P1, would become valid under the following, specific condition. Assume that:

P3: All mental events are brain events.

Given this very broad assumption, it would then follow that, as a subset of the universal set of mental events, all abnormal mental events (the stuff of mental disorder) will necessarily be brain events. Assuming that one is justified in judging brain events normal or abnormal according to whether their associated mental events are normal or not (and I don't believe this assumption is justified), it would therefore follow that:

P1: All mental disorder is brain disorder.

Accepting this argument would validate Trimble's thesis, but P3 is part of a much larger question, namely, metaphysics. At its most basic level, a successful account of mental disorder depends on a successful account of mind. Were Maudsley, or Trimble, or Guze, or any other biological psychiatrist ever aware of that? It seems to me that psychiatrists simply assumed that whatever worked in biology would automatically work in human psychology.

This principle was never questioned. It was accepted as part of the worldview, the ontology, on which reductionist biology depends, as Guze noted: "Most of us who adhere to the medical model believe that the fullest understanding of human health and illness, including psychiatric conditions, will depend increasingly on growing knowledge in biology ... this explains the redefinition of many personal and social problems into concerns of medicine" [6, p7]. This implies that a complete understanding of human biology will give a complete understanding of personal and social problems. I see no evidence to support this extreme position.

I asked whether we are justified in judging brain events normal or abnormal according to whether their associated mental events are normal or not. If, for the purposes of the argument, we accept that mental events just are brain events, how then should we judge the brain events if we decide that the mental event is abnormal? The question is simple: can a normal brain event still constitute an abnormal mental event. I would say yes, it can. Consider the example of grief. When we experience a massive loss of one sort or other, we typically go through a particular response known as the grief reaction. This is sufficiently common in its incidence and form to be regarded as a normal event. But grief, as we all know, is horrible; life would be far easier if we didn't have to feel it. So is grief normal or abnormal, and how should we classify the brain events underlying it? It depends on how you look at it, which is, of course, no basis for determining brain events abnormal.

It is perfectly legitimate to allow that abnormal mental events could be the outcome of normal mental events, because nobody has ever proven a strict one-to-one relationship between mental events and their (assumed) underlying brain events. People tend to use the analogy of computers to explain the difference between normal and abnormal mental and brain events. The machinery of a computer (its hardware) may be perfectly normal yet it persists in producing an abnormal output. We explain this by saying that its programs (software) are defective. By analogy, people argue that while the brain's physical machinery (its "wetware") may be perfectly normal, its programs (belief systems and information) may be disorganized, thereby producing an incoherent output (weird behavior). This is an interesting analogy, but there is nothing to say that brains and computers run by the same principles.

Putting all this aside for the moment, and taking Trimble's book at face value, it can fairly be said that he has not proven that a single mental disorder is due to physical disease of the brain. All he did was to indicate that for each major mental disorder, certain laboratory findings are somewhat suggestive of the thesis that some of the classic mental disorders might be due to physical disease of the brain.

1–2(C). Unlimited Biologism: Extreme Reductionism

Turning to reference [3], from J-P Changeux' *Neuronal Man*, we find Trimble's unspoken assumption stated quite explicitly: "There is no justification for a split between mental and neuronal activity. What is the point of speaking of 'mind' or 'spirit'? It is only that there are two 'aspects' of a single event ... It seems quite legitimate to consider that mental states and physiological or physicochemical states of the brain are identical." Oddly enough, one must wait almost to the end of the book to read this clear statement of Changeux' beliefs. At the beginning, he announced: "It is not my intention to identify the brain with a clock, to treat the nerve cells as cogwheels, or even to make the organization of neuronal networks resemble at all costs the circuits of a computer or any other artificial mechanism" (p38). However, having said that, he repeatedly referred to the "cerebral machinery" and, on p58, spoke approvingly of "the metaphor of the brain as a computer."

There are numerous examples of this quirk, which occur at points of tension in his work. He wants to say that humans are unique creatures with singular mental gifts, yet these gifts are also entirely explicable in reductionist terms: "A global activity can thus be reduced to physico-chemical properties and can be described in the same terms as those employed by the physicist or the chemist" (p95). The clear implication is that it really isn't so singular after all. But whereas he argues at length that science can encompass spiritual qualities, spiritual entities are specifically and repeatedly dismissed as fanciful.

Like Trimble, Changeux bluntly dismisses suggestions that the mind cannot be investigated by objective science, arguing at length that the neurosciences have progressed grandly towards a materialist vision: "Animal spirits could now be identified as movements of atoms and molecules. The science of the nervous system had become molecular" (p34-36). Later, he said: "Man no longer has need for 'Spirit': it is enough for him to be Neuronal Man" (p169). But in taking this extreme position, he has made a major mistake, that of believing that any 'spiritual" entity is necessarily self-delusory mysticism, whereas desirable "human" (spiritual?) attributes are always reducible to neurology. This is too arbitrary to be science. He would have been better to have stated his central idea at the outset instead of letting it emerge by degrees, because the empirical evidence he adduces in support of his case is irrelevant to his metaphysical assertion that mental states are brain states. This question cannot be answered empirically.

To demonstrate this point, a great deal of the evidence Changeux quoted as favorable to his materialist position was used years before by Eccles [7] in support of precisely the opposite conclusion, namely, that the human mind exists as an immaterial entity with supernatural powers. Both authors made the same mistake, of believing that empirical evidence could decide a metaphysical question. These types of questions must be argued from first principles, as they are of a form on which no empirical evidence can be brought to bear. The evidence is true, but in each case, it is quite beside the point, as irrelevant as last year's telephone book. Its truth or falsity does not determine the truth of the metaphysical question.

As mentioned, all that counts in Changeux' work is the notion that mental states are brain states, a well-known question in philosophy. Can "modern biological and genetic science" explain, as Guze believed [4, p322], such matters as social environment and culture? If so, psychiatry's claims to be a separate discipline would dissolve. Psychiatry would become just a branch of clinical neuroscience, just as has been advocated from time to time [8].

I have already argued that mental illness cannot be identified with brain disease, but we need to look at the broader proposition (P3). It can be rephrased to read:

P3a: Mental events are identical with brain events.

This is one of a range of theories developed by philosophers arguing the materialist case. Materialism states that there is nothing in the Universe above or beyond matter and energy and their interaction. With few exceptions, it explicitly denies emergent phenomena, i.e. those that cannot ultimately be reduced to matters of particles and energy. While materialism has been outstandingly successful in fields such as particle physics, molecular biology and astronomy, it has never been able to give an adequate account of the persistent notion that minds exist as immaterial entities with causal significance in the material realm.

1-3. Biological Psychiatry and Mind-Brain Identity Theory

One approach to this problem has been the concept of Epiphenomenalism, the view that minds may well exist but they are no more significant causally than the cloud of steam over a factory (attributed to TH Huxley, Charles Darwin's cousin). This concept, however, does not stand up to close examination. One can readily devise little experiments to show that something with all the properties of a mind can be causally significant. Thus, materialists have tried another approach, now known as Mind-Brain Identity Theory (MBIT). Taking as their starting point an uncompromising materialism, Smart [9], Armstrong [10], Place [11] and others have argued that mental events certainly occur but, as a matter of contingent fact, they are nothing more than brain events. The question of causal significance loses some of its impact in this formulation as there is no problem over the junction of mind and body.

In Smart's opinion, "...it seems that even the behavior of man himself will one day be explicable in mechanistic terms ... (there is) ... nothing in the world but increasingly complex arrangements of physical constituents" [9]. Armstrong agreed: "...the sole cause of mind-betokening behavior in man and the higher animals is the physico-chemical workings of the CNS" [10]. Sensations and all other mental events, he insisted, are brain events as a case of strict identity.

In my view, it is no coincidence that, albeit unwittingly, biological psychiatrists have adopted MBIT. As psychiatrists, we are concerned with disorders of the mind (insofar as they can be distinguished from disorders of the CNS, the field of neurology), yet biology closes some of the available options for accounting for the readily observable properties of mind. Firstly, as a materialist discipline, biology denies that immaterial minds can exist, and secondly, as reductionist empiricism, it rejects the possibility that minds may be emergent phenomena. The biological psychiatrist is thus forced to see minds as real, causally significant and yet capable of a complete reductionist analysis. Only MBIT can satisfy these very restrictive requirements.

Unfortunately, powerful arguments have been erected against MBIT. Over fifty years ago, Norman Malcolm countered the central notions of MBIT [12]. Firstly, he argued that as an empirical fact, MBIT would be unintelligible as it is irrefutable. The only convincing test of whether thoughts and brain events are identical would be to identify thoughts positively, i.e. independently of the subject's reports of them. Clearly, that would be impossible.

Secondly, Malcolm demonstrated that there are emergent (i.e. irreducible) laws and properties. Examples include the rule that hearsay evidence is inadmissible, the annualized national current account deficit, or the doctrinal beliefs underlying Holy Communion. These matters govern human behavior yet they cannot be reduced simply to matters of molecules or fundamental particles. Explanations of these, and a host of similar notions, always rely on the concept of an Intelligent Observer to render the account plausible.

This criticism is very important because, as will be discussed in Chapter 3 (Behaviorism), a key element in the reductionist program is to eradicate all abstract notions, replacing them with accounts of "mere particles in action." When you or I talk in "mentalese" (the language of "folk psychology") of "wanting to do this" or "fearing to see that", we are relying on the concept of ourselves as sentient, intelligent beings. That is, we see ourselves as beings with a mind of some sort, with free will and abstract reasoning, who are at least one step above mere beasts. Now because wishes, wants, hopes and plans etc. can't be measured in any way, orthodox science doesn't admit them as proper objects of study. Reductionist biology therefore had to get rid of them, and one of the most far-reaching attempts to do so was seen in Skinner's Radical Behaviorism (see Ch.3).

Skinner was satisfied that he had dealt Mentalism a death blow, that he had shown a way of explaining all human behavior without invoking unobservables. The philosopher, Daniel Dennett, criticized Skinner's work incisively, showing that the Intelligent Observer hadn't been eradicated, just hidden better. In attempting to assemble his non-mentalist psychology, Skinner had argued that there is no such thing as a causally-significant "intelligence". He believed that all human behavior could be explained without resorting to mentalist notions such as intelligence, motivation, ambition, etc.. But Dennett showed that Skinner had not removed the notion of intelligence from his explanations of behavior at all, but had merely moved it around in the environment. He termed this "taking out a loan on intelligence," a remarkably apt expression because it entails a settling of logical accounts. This Skinner never did. Crudely, all he managed to do was fiddle with the environment so that it only seemed as though rats and pigeons were dim-witted. By putting the poor creatures in a sterile environment that could play tricks on them, Skinner earned them an entirely undeserved reputation for stupidity (i.e. for functioning at a reflex, non-intellectual level). But it takes intelligence to set up such an environment: intelligence is needed to prevent the subjects showing their native cunning, as it were.

The Intelligent Observer lives on; unobservables such as intelligence and motivation cannot be reduced to matters of particles and energy or, at least, it would take a highly intelligent and strongly motivated person to do it. Thus, a critical element of the MBIT program fails.

Thirdly, Malcolm argued that even if, as MBIT asserts, it is true that thoughts and brain events are one and the same thing, it is not true to extend the argument by saying that explaining the brain event necessarily explains the thought. More generally, this means that explaining a computation does not depend on explaining the mechanism by which the computation was achieved, be it by human brains, computers or extra-terrestrials. This is because the computation is encoded in the physical substrate but exists independently of its medium, and unless one knows the code (which requires intelligence), one cannot comprehend the computation. As an everyday example, try "reading" your CDs with a magnifying glass, and then comparing them with your vinyl LPs. You will not be able to tell head-bangers from baroque.

The example of computation is interesting, as it shows the inadequacy of MBIT from another point of view. The number of arithmetical computations (sums) the human brain can compute is infinite, whereas the number of neurons involved is definitely not infinite. It is not possible to establish a relationship of identity between the elements of a finite series (the neurons) and those of an infinite series (the sums). It could be argued that while there can be no relationship of identity between sums and neurons, there is potentially one between the approximately infinite combinations of some thirty billion neurons. However, this attempt at a solution runs into the same sort of problem. Is there a fixed relationship between a particular combination of neurons and a particular sum? If so, how does the brain "know" just when to send a sum to that special set of neurons? Or, were these neurons determined genetically? There isn't enough genetic material in the human genome for this purpose. These sorts of objections spell the end of the line for MBIT.

Using different arguments, Popper [13] reached the same conclusions as Malcom, and quoted a number of authors of similar opinion. Churchland [14] has outlined arguments for and against Identity Theory, concluding that it has failed to live up to the bold claims made for it in the heroic post-war era.

MBIT was devised to overcome the problem of codes (language, mental events, etc.) simply by eradicating it, by declaring it a "non-problem." The central problem for naive materialism (of which biological psychiatry is an example) is that when coded systems interact in a suitable substrate, they are not constrained by the ordinary laws governing the interaction of matter and energy. They have their own laws, formalized as the logic of that particular system. The logical is independent of the biological, which MBIT states is impossible. In order to be able to claim success, its proponents must be able to map the higher order human functions such as language, mathematics, music, etc. directly to a lower order material element.

In the case of humans, those code-users par excellence, mental events such as wanting to be a poet or planning genocide cannot be reduced to a simple, unadorned matter of neurons firing in our skulls. All these events, and all that we regard as distinctively human, involve choices, and choices are arrived at by manipulating symbols. Symbols, however, are quite independent of the material base they are coded in. At the level of meaning, there is a disjunction between a symbol and its material substrate. There has to be. That's what 'symbol" means: something that stands for or represents another thing without being that thing itself. Reductionism cannot bridge that gap, because the gap represents the leap from the material realm to the immaterial. These are substantively different and necessarily so. We could never *imagine* what a brain would look like if there were not an epistemological gap between information and its substrate.

1–4. Reductionism as the Logic of Biomedicine

Medicine is a technology tempered by humanist considerations, but the scientific basis of general medicine lies firmly within the boundaries of reductive materialism. As an ontological choice, classic materialism states that there is nothing in the universe beyond matter and energy and their interactions, i.e. it positively excludes supernatural elements. More recently, this definition has been extended to take account of the concept of information as a controlling influence, so the definition now reads: Materialism declares there is nothing in the universe beyond matter-energy interactions and any informational states that control them. This still excludes the supernatural since informational states are rule-bound whereas the supernatural realm is not.

All the sciences in which modern medicine is based are indisputably reductive in nature. In philosophy, reduction is a particular form of explanation, where explanation is the act or process of making an event intelligible or comprehensible by showing how or why it occurred [15]. Specifically, reduction is the nomological process whereby "concepts or statements that apply to one type of entity are redefined in terms of concepts, or analyzed in terms of statements, of another kind ... more elementary or epistemologically more basic". Berry had no doubts about the place of reduction in science: "Reduction is seldom an uncontentious activity, and to list some of the many varieties of reductionism is to list a series of controversies" [15, p530].

In biology, which is taken to be part of the deterministic system, "how" and "why" are essentially the same. For example, there is a banyan tree growing in a split in a rock in my back yard. It grows there because, years ago, a seed of *Ficus virens* landed in a small crack that had enough soil and water and sun and air to allow the seed to germinate and grow. That one statement explains both how the tree grew, and why it was a banyan and not a duck, i.e., given each set of events, the succeeding events could not be otherwise. The molecular theory of genetics explains how the characteristics of the parent are reliably transferred to the offspring; plant physiology explains how seeds germinate and grow by converting carbon dioxide to complex chemicals by means of photosynthesis, and so on.

So, by a rule-driven process, the observable event of a tree "reduces" ultimately to "mere chemistry," i.e. to (relatively) mundane matters of genes controlling enzymes that convert chemicals that facilitate special processes to produce particular structures which, ultimately, become the spreading wonder of a huge fig tree.

This example illustrates three important points of philosophical reduction: that there are observations to explain, a lower order explanatory theory in which to recast the observations, and what are termed "bridge laws" or "identity statements" connecting the two in a formal relationship [16, p679]. For example, given the common observation that some things are hot, and assuming the (lower order) atomic theory of matter, the bridging law is that temperature just is mean translational kinetic energy, i.e. an identity relationship. In reality, this relationship holds only for ideal gases under highly specified circumstances; for anything else, temperature seems to be far more complex. Thus, the suggestion that, without further iteration, an identity relationship can be defined for the most complex thing in the universe betrays a serious lack of understanding of the principles involved. Nonetheless, while "real world" reduction is sometimes just notional, there must always be the potential for connecting the observations and the theory in a formal, causative relationship. This principle is specifically designed to exclude the supernatural.

When an observation is to be explained by reduction, there must already be a reducing theory capable of resolving the questions posed by the observation. The theory cannot be derived from the observation itself, as that would beg the question. This was one of the major problems with psychoanalysis.

In ordinary use, we can distinguish two forms of reductionism, ontological and explanatory [17]. Ontological reductionism states that, despite outward appearances, all higher order entities are composed of a limited number of lower order elements. Thus, the myriad chemical compositions seen on the earth's surface can be reduced to combinations of the ninety or so naturally occurring elements. For example, diamonds, graphite and soot all reduce to the element carbon.

Explanatory reductionism is the view that any explanation of the behavior of higher order entities will derive nomologically from the behavior of the lower order elements that compose the higher orders. Complete explanatory reductionism says that all behavioral states of the higher order elements ultimately have a physico-chemical explanation [18]. Partial or limited explanatory reductionism states that anything that can be explained will be shown to have a physico-chemical explanation. Clearly, this leaves a potential explanatory gap, which some people prefer to bridge by supernatural factors.

Within the animal kingdom, the question "why" assumes a different significance. Why did the dingo stalk the young kangaroo? Because, we would say, it wanted to eat, and it knew meat is more satisfying than grass, and joeys are easier to catch than older animals ... This introduces a factor not present in the example of the banyan tree, the notion of intention. We now agree that plants do not grow "for" any purpose; they just grow when conditions are right. The nature of the biological machines we call plants is that, all things being equal, they could not do otherwise than follow their innate plans. Tree trunks go up and roots go down; explanations of these matters are wholly physico-chemical and do not involve or require the tree to "know" anything, in any sense of the word.

Even though slugs can move, there is no reason to assume they function at levels much more complex than plants but, for higher animals, it becomes harder to dismiss the claim that they know what they want and can work out how to get it. As their behavioral flexibility increases, so they seem to be able to choose goals and work toward them in a directed manner not available to plants. The question why something happened can therefore be differentiated from how it happened, because it now includes the notion of purpose, i.e. that the behavior is directed toward achieving a future goal. Mechanism is supplemented by purpose. This immediately raises the question: can purpose be reduced to mere mechanism?

For many years, under the influence of behaviorism, biologists assumed that observable behavior itself constitutes the raw data of reductionism but this is incorrect. The reason is that the same behavior in different species, or within different individuals of the same species, or even an individual at different times, can have an indefinite range of causes (as purposes). Reducing the behavior itself to "mundane matters of genes controlling enzymes that convert chemicals that facilitate special processes to produce particular structures" will overlook the animal's unique reason for doing it. Therefore, any attempt to reduce the behavior of higher animals to "mere brain activity" must first propose some form of guiding or self-controlling inner state (a theory of mind, in human terms) amenable to reductive analysis. That is, the mental life constitutes the observations from which, after suitable analysis, the bridging laws will yield an explanation in terms of the lower order theory (in this case, neurophysiology). For anything that smacks of mental life in any species, there is currently no such theory.

Given this handicap, is there a program for psychiatry in this ontology? If psychiatry is seen as no more than a branch of orthodox biomedicine [5], then its research program is ready-made: mental disorder reduces to a matter of physical brain disorder, i.e. mental disorder is wholly a matter of biological disturbances of the brain. Physical pathology of the brain is not only necessary and sufficient for mental illness, but tells us everything there is to know about mental illness. This is now the dominant research paradigm in psychiatry. However, despite the enormous advances of the core neurosciences, and notwithstanding the very large sums of money spent on the biology of mental disorder, psychiatry's biological program has yielded no convincing empirical support for Maudsley's optimism. Was this impasse predictable? That depends on whether mental illness reduces to brain illness because, otherwise, the entire program is misconceived.

Oddly enough, biological psychiatrists have hardly bothered to investigate this crucial point. The view of Samuel Guze, one of the doyens of biological psychiatry, that "there cannot be a psychiatry which is too biological" [4,6], is accepted as a proven fact. Indeed, there appears to be no awareness that the biological approach to psychiatry is simply an opinion, a choice that trainees make very early in their careers, long before they know enough psychiatry (or philosophy) to be making such major decisions [19]. The rest of this chapter looks at the question of whether reductive biologism is an appropriate research program for psychiatry.

1-5. Mental Illness in the Reductionist Biomedical Framework

I start from the point that mental disorder is a reality, i.e. there are and always have been people who, all other things being equal, are so distressed or disorganized that they cannot consistently perform at the level of their peers. Because their difficulties appear to lie wholly within the mental sphere, we say they are mentally ill. Biological psychiatry states that, while their problems are manifest in the mental sphere, the actual cause of mental troubles consists of disturbances at the neurobiological level, the mental disorder is driven by the biological disturbance. Since mental symptoms reduce directly to brain pathology, it is at this point that treatment should be directed. Apart from ordinary courtesy, human considerations do not enter the equation.

It is, however, one thing to believe that mental states reduce to brain states, something else again to show just what this means in real life. By saying that mental disease just is brain disease, Maudsley was arguing that the relationship of the observation to the reducing theory was a special case of bridging law, an identity statement. This is an extreme position, so it is worthwhile exploring more moderate stances.

One view says that, even though we cannot specify the nature of mind or its relation to brain, their relationship is so close that specific brain disorders produce characteristic disturbances of mental function. The exploration of these disorders is entirely empirical and does not presuppose knowledge of normal mental function. There are certainly plenty of precedents for this view, e.g., GPI, dementia, intoxications, metabolic disturbances, etc.. These types of conditions produce their effects by acting directly upon vital brain centers, so that reversing the causative element (where possible) effects a cure. One doesn't need to know what brain centers are affected by alcohol to realize that abstinence cures intoxication. Historically, the field of psychiatry has contracted as the causes of these disorders were uncovered and the patients referred to other specialists.

It should be understood that this approach applies only to abnormal mental states. It says that, whatever its nature, normal mental life is sufficiently anchored in the material universe for brain disturbances to have profound mental effects. It might be countered that, while neurological illnesses do lead to disturbances of mental life, they are so profoundly different from what we term psychiatric disorders that they tell us nothing. The heartland of psychiatry, anxiety, depression and the major psychoses stubbornly resists reductive analysis. For these conditions, the crude biological model outlined above must be rendered more precise.

One commonly held opinion is that the causative lesions of the standard psychiatric syndromes are subtle, transient disturbances of neurochemical function that are currently beyond our technology. Essentially, this is only a modification of the concept behind intoxication. In this type of model, the simplest explanation of mental disorder is that normal brain function is subverted by a functional excess or deficiency of a particular chemical. The imbalance disrupts a crucial point of mental function and is manifest as one or other of the psychiatric syndromes. While the specific site may be tiny, its effect may be pervasive, to the extent of disrupting the rest of the person's daily life. Apart from a localized chemical "lesion," the brain is probably quite healthy.

For example, since anxiety is a part of normal life, and the anxiety system (whatever that is) is activated by daily vicissitudes, all the biological psychiatrist needs propose is that the dedicated circuits subserving the anxiety response are set too finely, as it were. Under genetic influences, certain neurons release too much of a stimulating transmitter, or others react to unusually low levels, perhaps via a lack of inhibition. As a result, the sufferer reacts biologically to neutral environmental stimuli as though they were a threat. The primary, treatable condition is a small biochemical lesion in an as yet uncharted part of the brain. Reversing that lesion may involve drugs, brain surgery and so on but it will not involve talking. Why not? Because the neurochemical lesion is primary, and will no more be reversed by talk than a drunken man can be talked to his senses again. In intoxications, causation is unidirectional.

This model can be extended to include the notion that certain brain systems may produce or be sensitive to abnormal chemicals that cause the mental symptoms. Either the chemicals act directly upon neuronal systems to produce symptoms, or they interfere with normal neurotransmission. An important point of this type of model is that the patient's symptoms are of no further significance. Once the chemical defect is reversed, they will disappear.

This hypothesis is wholly empirical but lacks any firm evidence. Despite massive expenditure over many years, nobody has found a single case of formal mental illness that fits this model, nor any likely chemicals. The history of schizophrenia is littered with theories which went nowhere: somebody once fed serum from patients to spiders and reported their webs were disorganized. In about 1938, a British psychiatrist, Ian Skottowe, suggested the disorder was due to defects in glucose metabolism in cortical neurons, but this was based in the belief that insulin coma was an effective treatment. In the 1950s, following the discovery of LSD, it again seemed schizophrenia might be revealed as a case of metabolic poisoning but nothing came of it.

Theorizing in biological psychiatry is powered by technology; the latest theories are always based in the latest machines. As new machines appear, so the theories change but, for the uncommitted, there are good reasons to remain cautious.

1-6. Objections to Biological Reductionism in Psychiatry

1-6. (a). Where does ontological reductionism stop? If we say mental disorder can be reduced to brain disorder, at what level of brain function should we stop the process? Some people attribute mental function to whole brain systems, others want to assign it to the level of neurons, still others invoke quantum levels. Yet the definition of reductionism is that functions at any level can always be further reduced to less complex levels. Nobody can say where it ought to stop because that would deny the central tenet of reductionism itself. So we just keep going but, strictly speaking, since the ultimate particles of matter are nowhere in sight, reductionism is an infinite regress and is therefore non-scientific. Biological psychiatrists need to bear in mind that their central thesis has limits. It is a guiding principle, not a natural law, one to be applied wisely, not indiscriminately.

1-6. (b). Complete biological reduction denies the possibility that the brain may have emergent properties. Oddly enough, biological psychiatrists take this as a virtue of their system. They see the null hypothesis as: "There are no emergent properties" but they have misplaced the onus of proof. The proper approach is to oblige reductionists to prove their point, by using the following formulation: "Not everything is capable of reductionist analysis." The proof is as follows.

Any nomological process is bidirectional but the process opposite to reductionism is absurd. Complete explanatory reductionism states that all behavioral states of the higher order elements ultimately have a physico-chemical explanation. This means that ultimately, all human products, such as symphonies, the rules of chess, monotheistic religions, conspiracies, geometry, jokes and prawn cocktails, etc., derive logically from the rules governing, say, electrons. I say this is meaningless; the burden of proving that it is genuinely meaningful rests with its advocates. Nothing about the laws of subatomic particles can be taken to predict sonnets. Electrons do not determine, *qua* order or ordain, they merely set limits: the offside rule in soccer does not flow inexorably from the laws governing atomic nuclei. Some things cannot be reduced just because there cannot be a bidirectional bridging law linking the observation and a lower level of organization. As a corollary, if all human laws derive from physics, then we wouldn't be able to change any of them.

1-6. (c). Reductionism licenses the mereological fallacy [17]. Mereology is the study of the relationship between a whole and its parts. Reductionism encourages people to assign mental properties to different parts of the brain after the manner of the phrenologists. Attributing functions of the intact human being to parts of the body, including the brain, is fallacious. One cannot say: "I have a mind *and* I have a brain," because that implies there is a third entity beside these two (historically called the Self, I, pure consciousness, the spirit, etc.).

1-6. (d). Three hundred years ago, Locke stated: "It is past controversy, that we have in us *something* that thinks." Reductionism tries to define the mind out of existence. Biological psychiatry attempts to sidestep crucial questions on the nature of mind by redefining them in physical terms, as though the act of redefinition amounted to an explanation:

"Daddy, how do we add up?"

"Don't worry, dear, your brain does it for you."

"Oh goodie, that means I don't have to practice."

It leads to absurdities like people trying to "learn" in their sleep, or using special diets, music, exercises, drugs or massage to improve their intellect or personality, and so on.

While there will be no dispute that any human behavior generated by natural laws (perhaps events such as sleep, childbirth, hunger, etc.) is reducible, the crucial point surely is to decide just which behaviors are nomologically determined and whether the rest require another model. Naive reductionism, including biological psychiatry, begs this question. Roughly speaking, the really interesting human behavior, anything that reliably distinguishes us from chimps, is non-nomological and therefore not amenable to a reductive materialist analysis.

An additional difficulty for reductionists is this: they can never tell when their program is failing. If a particular behavior does not prove amenable to reductivist analysis, they have to keep looking for the nomological law that will satisfy their need. If, however, the behavior is non-nomological, they are chasing the end of a rainbow but, by giving up, they would admit their model has failed.

1-6. (e). Mental disease and brain disease are not identical:

1-6. (e) (i). Despite Maudsley's dictum, it is manifestly clear that mental disease is *not* the same as brain disease. Mental disorders have properties which brain disorders do not have, and *vice versa,* so any bridging law cannot be an identity statement. Depression is a sustained mood of sadness and despair associated with ideas of guilt and worthlessness; chemicals must somehow be involved in generating these moods but chemicals are not themselves moods. They are the mechanism of the mood, but not the cause. Asserting otherwise is an example of the mereological fallacy. The only possible meaning to Maudsley's claim is that brain disease is both necessary and sufficient for mental disorder, which is completely different but patently false (see below).

1-6. (e) (ii). Maudsley's axiom could only be true as a subset of the larger, Mind-Brain Identity Theory, which asserts that all mental events are brain events. As outlined above, this theory fails to account for symbolic mental events and is no longer taken seriously.

1-6. (e) (iii). If all cases of mental disorder must reduce directly to brain disorder, biological psychiatry positively excludes the possibility of psychological causation of mental disorder. Anybody who believes that mental disorder just is brain disorder must also believe that psychological factors can never contribute to a mental breakdown. Allowing a single case of a psychologically-determined mental disorder (such as the post-traumatic states) destroys the case for strict reductive biological causation of mental disorder. Furthermore, if an instance of mental disorder has a prior mental cause, then that too could have a mental cause, as could all its contributing causes, *ad infinitum*. That is, any psychological matter could have caused the mental disorder so there could never be a direct relationship between the psychological event and the subsequent mental disorder. The nature of the mental disorder would not identify the particular precipitating psychological event.

The larger case of mind-brain identity theory also implies that no mental event can be caused by a prior mental event, which is absurd. At most, the classic biological model could apply to part but not all human mental disorder.

1-6. (f). The intoxication model disproves itself. We know that chemicals interfere with normal mental function, that's one of the problems with being human, but it doesn't prove that all or any mental disorders are due to intoxications. Nobody seriously believes that we are so different from the rest of the animal world as to be immune to hypoxia, chemicals, fevers, sleep deprivation and the myriad physical states that can disturb mental life, but these produce confusional states, and the classic mental disorders are not confusional states. However, while it may over-stretch credibility to suggest that the major mental disorders are due to tiny, transient chemical changes in highly specific areas of the brain with no relation to the external world or the individual's past, it is not logically impossible, and my case is that reductionist biological psychiatry is not just inappropriate but is logically impossible.

Consider one of the most common of all mental disorders, anxiety. An anxious person suffers from an excess of anxiety, meaning that, when we assess his surroundings objectively, he feels anxious too often and too intensely. The intoxication model says that, somewhere in a crucial choke-point in the neuronal circuits subserving the anxiety response, there is an excess of an excitatory chemical, or lack of an inhibitory one (I don't take the idea of naturally-occurring toxic chemicals seriously).

Let's assume our anxious subject is terrified of frogs. Strict reductionism says that exposure to a frog has nothing to do with his panic, it is generated biologically. Immediately, there is a problem for the model, because people with a true phobia will panic not only at the sight of a frog, but also when they think they are in a place where frogs are likely to be found. His belief that he is likely to see a frog cannot reduce to a physically determined brain state because there has been no physical event to cause it. As Skinner was fond of saying, an event that hasn't happened can't control behavior. So thoughts clearly can trigger panic, even though biological psychiatry insists they can not. MBIT will not save them but, for the purposes of argument, we will allow that, just at the moment the person imagines he might come face to face with a frog, his "fear center" receives a pathological stimulus and switches on an emotion of unreasoning panic.

Unless we agree to an infinite series of fantastic coincidences, the problem I see for biological psychiatry is just this: by what stronger reason should that pathological stimulus be regarded as a primary biological phenomenon (i.e. not related to his mental state), and not itself be the result of a prior psychological event? In the final analysis, biological psychiatry cannot tell whether a chemical dysfunction at the sub-microscopic level is an independent biological event or whether it is psychologically determined. This is partly because biological psychiatry denies psychological causation but also because it couldn't recognize it anyway, just because it has no conceptual tools for the task. That's what the word "biological" means.

1-6. (g). Humans are subject to certain natural laws, but they are the same laws as apply to the other great apes. Behaviorally, all the higher primates cluster in social groupings with very obvious dominance hierarchies. The laws that draw us together are balanced by our innate fear of strangers, so our primary social groups are tribal. The need to dominate, coupled with our territorial and other possessive urges, leads to friction at the borders of the tribes, and so on.

Characteristics such as xenophobia, territoriality, curiosity and the sense of play, etc., are well-developed even in baboons. What we sometimes call "human nature" is really just "higher primate nature." Is the concept of beauty a natural law? Children don't need to be told that flowers are pretty or to avoid foul-smelling things, that a growling dog is scary or a whimpering puppy can be cuddled. While these notions are correctly the province of a reductionist psychology, there is little reason to believe that, dominance apart, they contribute significantly to the causation of mental illness. Even though we share something like 97% of our genetic material with *Pan troglodytes,* we are more that just "naked apes." What really counts in human affairs is unique to us. Attempts to reduce mental disorder to matters of primate ethology will remain unproductive just because we humans are more than mere chimps jumping around in trees.

1-7. Conclusion

The impetus behind the biological psychiatry program is the view that because reductionism has been so successful elsewhere, it should also be successful in psychiatry. Its supporters never question this point, but simply proceed as though its truth is self-evident. It most certainly is not self-evident nor, as I have argued, is it true. Epistemologically, biological psychiatry should be but a small part of a larger research program in which human mentality takes priority. That this is not the case is consistent with the argument for psychiatry being prescientific, a case I will develop later. At best, the naive reductionist view diverts resources toward pointless research [19] but, at worst, it leads to a smugness that stops the very engine of scientific progress, self-criticism.

Most of the behavior that distinguishes us from our closest relatives is governed by laws we determine ourselves, i.e., they are emergent properties. We are the only animals that do this to any extent: without our rules, we can't even talk to each other. Before we can be *Homo sapiens,* we must be *Homo nomothetikos,* the law-giver. That is, a small part of our behavior is nomological but the great bulk, and all that is really interesting, is controlled by rules set by convention. These include all the rules of society such as language, mathematics, science, industry, sport, commerce, agriculture, etc. Even humor gets its laughs just because it breaks rules: no rules, no laughs. There is a discontinuity at the level of symbolic language: symbols cannot be reduced to their substrate.

Thus, Mind-Brain Identity Theory fails in its major ambition, which is to show that our linguistic symbols have a relationship of identity with their material bases. Human symbolic behavior cannot be reduced to matters of neurons alone. I conclude that there is no means of saving the broad and ambitious programs mapped out for biological psychiatry by Trimble, Changeux, Guze and by so many others. There is certainly no way a rigid biological approach can explain the whole of human experience and, I have argued, no way it can form the basis of a general theory of psychiatry. It therefore cannot claim to be any better than the other theories currently used in our discipline.

Perhaps the most interesting question remaining is why biological psychiatrists have tried to over-reach themselves in this way. Was it necessary to claim that all mental disorder is necessarily produced by organic factors? Surely the answer is a matter of common sense—some disorders are the outcome of brain disorder, and some are pure psychological disorders occurring in the setting of a perfectly healthy brain. There is no contradiction inherent in this statement. What is contradictory is when one side in the brain vs. psychology debate attempts to subvert the scientific ethos by declaring the outcome of the debate a win for their side. When religious leaders do that sort of thing, we scientists profess to be scandalized.

<table>
<tr><td>**2**</td><td># Behaviorism from the Psychiatric Perspective</td></tr>
</table>

2-1. Introduction

Biological psychiatry says there is a mind but, as a matter of contingent fact, it is reducible and ultimately identical with the brain. The very large group of theories lumped together as psychodynamics takes an opposing view. They say there is a causally significant mind that cannot be reduced to its material substrate yet, even though it is unobservable, we can still talk meaningfully about it. From the psychodynamic point of view, the nature of mind may be a metaphysical dilemma, but talking about the mind in action is not meaningless.

The simplest type of psychodynamic theory is what Dennett has called "folk psychology." This is what you or I understood about the mind before we became sophisticates, or what our grandparents believed all their lives. Simply, it means a model of mind in which the non-stop, three-ring circus inside my head, where I can "see," "feel" and "hear" all manner of delights and horrors, this internal video set is where I really live, where I experience and decide all that counts in my life. You might see my body, but you can't see the real me. I have an accountable public life and a private, inner life where I can get away with all sorts of things up to and including the odd murder. "I" am an insubstantial creature inside my head.

But I am not just a passive observer of my body getting on with its business, I actually run my body. I decide things, I put my plans into action or change my mind, decide to be good or bad, do what feels good or (less often) what is honorable, work out what I should have said, plot vengeance, and so on. Actually, I have quite a full life here inside my head and even though I can't see inside yours, I'm sure you do, too.

Unfortunately, what seems clear in daily life isn't quite enough in the more extreme cases. Do we believe the man who says he didn't know the gun was loaded? Or if he knew it was loaded, that he meant no harm? What should we say to the fellow who insists that Martians talk to him telepathically or the chap who goes to water every time he sees a cockroach? While we struggle with these and many similar cases, attempts to render my inner experience into a rational, non-question-begging account of "minds in general" quickly run into enormous difficulties. It soon becomes apparent that, as long as we talk in metaphor or in vague generalities, we can limp along, fairly sure that we understand each other, but anything more precise becomes mired in qualifications and counter-examples.

In the mid-nineteenth century, empirical enquiries into the nature and function of mind consisted mainly of introspection, attempts to sneak up on the mind and catch it in the process of "minding", as it were. Highly intelligent people sat around, trying to apprehend the nature of the experience called "seeing an orange patch" or "hearing middle C". After this had been going on for quite some time, it became apparent that "armchair philosophizing" (actually armchair psychologizing) wasn't going anywhere, and a few radicals started to look for something more reliable. They decided it was necessary to abandon all talk of minds as mere froth and bubble, as relics of the age of superstition whose only function is to distract serious researchers from their proper paths. This stern approach dominated psychology for the greater part of the twentieth century, only recently slipping into history. The principle underlying this approach is quite simple: Science is about observables. Any theory that goes beyond the directly observable has to be firmly anchored in careful, replicable measurements. But since the mind is unmeasurable in principle, then it is by definition excluded from the realm of scientific enquiry.

2-2. Early Behaviorism

Reliability was first claimed by Wilhelm Wundt, a nineteenth century German philosopher who is credited with laying the foundations of psychology as a separate, empirical discipline. Wundt first graduated in medicine but soon gravitated to physiology, studying and later lecturing under the great Helmholtz. From there, he became a professor of philosophy, which led to his interest in what became psychology. As a philosopher, he accepted that the immediate contents of consciousness comprised the subject matter of psychology but as a physiologist, he had a radically different approach to its study. Abandoning introspectionism, Wundt applied the conventional methods of physiology, as Helmholtz devised them, to the study of mental processes. This was strikingly original and he was largely responsible for establishing experimental psychology as a specialty in its own right. Later in his career, he published extensive researches into what are now called cognitive psychology and social psychology. In fact, Wundt was probably the first to use the term "folk psychology."

Of course, Wundt did not live in an intellectual vacuum. By the mid-1870s, empirical psychology was waiting to happen. The physical and biological sciences were racing ahead and it was only a matter of time before the ethos that permitted them, and which they in turn validated, spread to encompass all rational enquiries. Schools of psychology were soon flourishing in major academic centers in the Western world. In Britain, under the influence of Francis Galton, a nephew of Charles Darwin, psychology was very mathematical, focusing on intellectual assessment, the genetics of personality and such like. In the United States, a similar revolution took place, profoundly influenced by Wundt's students and later by the experimentalist John B. Watson, who publicized the work of the Russian researcher, Ivan Pavlov. But until Watson, consciousness was still very much the proper domain of psychology.

Watson objected very strongly to the mentalist element in the evolving German tradition. He was unrepentant on the direction he expected the new psychology to take: "I can state my position here no better than by saying that I should like to bring my students up in the same ignorance of (the mind-body problem) as one finds among the students of other branches of science" [1, p166]. All considerations of mind and mental contents, of consciousness and introspection, were impediments to progress that "bound (psychology) hand

and foot". Observable behavior was all that counted; all talk of unobservable intervening variables, such as minds, was doomed to sterility. Very early, he adopted a rigid biologism: "The findings of psychology become the functional correlates of structure and lend themselves to explanation in physico-chemical terms." And the goal of all this was "...to learn general and particular methods by which I may control behavior." He believed it would be possible to write such a psychology in just a few years.

Watson had a particularly confident, even abrasive, style of writing which, coupled with the confused results of fifty years of introspectionist psychology, had a strong appeal in the newly assertive scientific atmosphere after the First World War. Introspectionist psychology abruptly collapsed, to be replaced by an aggressively objective, anti-mentalist science of behavior. Psychologists saw themselves as flag-bearers in the continuing scientific revolution aimed at dragging Man from his special seat just a little below the angels. They were content to use the mind to investigate behavior, much as chemists used it to investigate materials, but never to investigate itself. Consciousness, they believed, was a red herring, even a deadly trap, and all mention of it was soon swept away.

Watson was not entirely an intellectual Vandal; he knew that if he wanted to demolish a well-established academic field, he had to offer something else in its place. What he had in mind was building a new, general psychology based on Pavlov's concept of the conditioned reflex. Whether this was his intention, or whether he conceived of conditioning as simply an investigatory method isn't entirely clear but others certainly tried. Their efforts were not appreciated by the great Pavlov himself who argued against this ambition. Interestingly, just like Watson, Pavlov was an early and fervid supporter of Mind-Brain Identity Theory: "...uniting or identifying the physiological with the psychological, the subjective with the objective, which I am convinced comprises the most important present-day scientific undertaking" [2].

Twenty-five years into the new century, psychology had become behaviorism, the study of observable behavior, an idea that exerted a profound effect upon many areas of human endeavor. For the next sixty years, human studies were dominated by the notion that, if the mind exists, it is rendered irrelevant by the fact that it cannot be studied rationally. Now this opinion isn't entirely correct. Strictly speaking, the early behaviorists were saying: "The mind can't be studied rationally by our methods." This is not the same thing as saying it can't be studied by any methods at all. So for sixty years, human psychology painted itself into an unproductive corner, all the while spreading disdain for anything that did not reach its particular and largely self-proclaimed standards of science.

2-3. Skinner's Radical Behaviorism

The most far-reaching and thorough-going attempt to construct a non-mentalist human psychology was Skinner's Radical Behaviorism. Burrhus Frederic Skinner was an American psychologist raised in the "Brave New World" of early twentieth century scientific psychology. He had an exceptionally long career, published profusely, and was utterly dismissive of anybody's efforts but his own. His disdain for his opponents (and there were many) was so complete that he rarely if ever bothered to answer their objections to his theories. Late in his life, people started to wonder whether he was capable of considering that he could be wrong.

Skinner wrote in a particular, objective style, rigidly eliminating all mentalist references. He spoke of "organisms" that "emit behaviors" which are then "reinforced" by their "environmental consequences." A behavior acting or operating upon the environment is an "operant." Because operants can be reinforced, they can be made to dominate the organism's behavior or eliminated, depending on their effects. Operants can be conditioned by their consequences, so that psychology's ultimate goal of "shaping and maintaining behavior" (i.e. controlling it, in Watson's blunt language) comes within reach.

To take a common example, a baby gurgles and grunts. By their happy responses, the doting parents encourage their infant to use closer and closer approximations of real words. Language is thus acquired without the aid of unseen and unknowable "intervening variables" (minds). Correct use of language is maintained by, essentially, the fact that speaking properly gets us what we want (i.e. it is positively reinforcing). For a radical behaviorist, the reinforcing environment (the verbal community) shapes and maintains language by contingent reinforcement of the organism's verbal operants. A Skinnerian account of speech does not need a mind to learn the language.

Skinner's psychology was profoundly influential, especially in the United States. Generations of psychologists were trained in the theory and practice of radical behaviorism. An enormous research program developed, and Skinnerian methods of behavior management were applied in fields ranging from schools to prisons. However, and despite his vast output, there are problems in pinning down his views as, in his successive publications, Skinner tended to supersede his work rather than to revise it. Thus, he could say at one stage that the mind was irrelevant, later that it existed but couldn't be studied, and later still that it was quite relevant but was nothing special anyway. However, not long before he retired as one of America's most distinguished scientists, he published several works that have to stand as the definitive statements of his position. In *Beyond Freedom and Dignity* [3], he wrote a popularized version of his otherwise fairly opaque theory, and in *About Behaviorism* [4], he outlined his philosophy of behaviorism.

From about the late 1950s onwards, his ideas were subjected to increasingly critical analysis. In 1957, Scriven [5] dissected Skinner's assertion that a true account of human behavior must be essentially (or totally) atheoretical. This was the basis, Scriven argued, for Skinner's intense opposition to Freudian psychoanalysis. Scriven concluded that Skinnerian radical behaviorism was itself definitely not atheoretical: "...Skinner has elevated the relatively atheoretical nature of his approach into a sterile purity that his (own) approach fortunately lacks" (p94). An essential element in the Skinnerian program had failed. Radical behaviorism was therefore open to attack on theoretical grounds, which Skinner had previously denied (and, typically, he continued to deny).

A more telling critique of the radical behaviorist program followed publication of Skinner's *Verbal Behavior* in 1957. The psycholinguist and philosopher, Noam Chomsky [6], reviewed the psychologist's account of language acquisition, including the claim that human verbal behavior can be predicted and controlled "by observing and manipulating the physical environment of the speaker" (p 26). "(Skinner) confidently and repeatedly voices his claim to have demonstrated that the contribution of the speaker is quite trivial and elementary, and that precise prediction of verbal behavior involves only specification of the few external factors that he has isolated experimentally with lower organisms" (p 27-28).

Chomsky's critique was brief (about thirty pages to review Skinner's book of nearly 500 pages), precisely targeted and devastating. In a series of carefully-marshaled points, he showed that all the basic premises of the radical behaviorist approach to language were devoid of scientific content. One by one, he took Skinner's major concepts, showing that "...if we take his terms in their literal meaning, the description covers almost no aspect of verbal behavior, and if we take them metaphorically, the description offers no improvement over various traditional (folk) formulations" (p 54).

Chomsky argued that the scientific ethos in radical behaviorism was illusory, that terms such as stimulus, response, operant, reinforcement, control, etc., were hollow, merely "...the illusion of a rigorous scientific theory with a very broad scope (p 30) ... Skinner's claim that his system ... permits the practical control of verbal behavior is quite false" (p32). Skinner's every effort failed. He could not define stimulus with any precision, "stimulus control" lacked the sense he claimed for it, his law of reinforcement was tautological, "...the term reinforcement has a purely ritual function" (p38), and so on. This led Chomsky to characterize the psychologist's work as "hopelessly premature," "empty", etc. He concluded: "If it were true in any deep sense that the basic processes in language are well-understood and free of species restrictions, it would be extremely odd that language is limited to man" (p30).

His review was a small masterpiece; forty years on, nobody has improved on it and nor, for that matter, did Skinner. He never revised his book to take account of Chomsky's objections. Since then, and despite intense efforts, the Skinnerian research program on "verbal behavior" has largely faded from view. Towards the end of the 1970s, a number of critiques of radical behaviorism appeared, including those by a psychological methodologist, Brian MacKenzie, and by a philosopher, Daniel Dennett.

MacKenzie's work [7] was another small wonder, a precisely detailed analysis of psychological epistemology. After an exhaustive and demanding review, he concluded that behaviorism had given us only "...some portion of the tools appropriate for building a science—but not the science itself ..." (p 170). It would not be possible to summarize his work beyond this, his last sentence, but Skinnerian radical behaviorism was particularly criticized for its "systematic pretensions" (p 163) and its total failure to deliver on any of its promises. After the intellectual edifices (of Skinner's psychology) had crumbled, all that was left was a set of skills that were not unique to radical behaviorism. Simply speaking, Skinnerians described and controlled animal behavior somewhat better than other psychologists and lion tamers, but not differently, and certainly not radically so.

Dennett's criticism of Skinnerian radical behaviorism [8] is articulate and equally incisive. In his opinion, Skinner made several substantial mistakes in his theory. Firstly, he mistakenly supposed that all mentalism is necessarily supernatural and thus no better than superstition. He (Skinner) therefore determined to sweep all mentalist explanations from his theory, but on this crucial first step, he failed. We cannot translate mentalist accounts of human behavior into non-mentalist statements. Skinner's work is in fact a good source of failed attempts to do this. Dennett was able to show that a non-magical account of that most mentalist of concepts, intelligence, was indeed possible, meaning that a major plank in the rationale for radical behaviorism collapsed.

Secondly, Dennett argued that Skinner made a mistake in generalizing the results of his laboratory experiments on rats and pigeons to humans. It is one thing to place lower animals with limited means of dealing with the environment in a highly restricted environment, and then announce that their behavior is necessarily under the control of a few very simple principles. It is something else again to assume that those principles necessarily govern all human behavior under all possible circumstances: "Since all the explanations he has so far come up with have been of the unmasking variety (pigeons, it turns out, do not have either freedom or dignity), Skinner might be forgiven for supposing that all explanations in psychology, including all explanations of human behavior, must be similarly unmasking ... Pigeons do not exhibit very interesting or novel behavior, but human beings do" [8, p 66-7]. Dennett's argument can be summarized as saying that genuinely intelligent creatures can always mimic the behavior of less-endowed animals. Therefore, the necessary first step for the Skinnerian program was to prove that humans don't have genuine intelligence, rather than simply assuming it to be the case.

This leads to a well-known contradiction for behaviorists, which is that if they argue that humans don't have intelligence, or creativity, or motives, then they must also believe it of themselves. The philosopher Alfred Ayer once said that to be a behaviorist is to pretend to be anesthetized from the neck up. If, as Skinner argued, scientific creativity is just a matter of being in the right environment, why did he accept all his honors and awards? Kline [9] has summarized this criticism pungently: "If we only do what we have been reinforced to do, then presumably Skinner, also being subject to schedules of reinforcement, writes what he writes simply because he has been so reinforced. There is thus no reason to think that (Skinnerian psychology) is true, or ... that Skinner believes it to be true. Hence, why should we bother to examine it?" A genuinely non-mentalist theory of behavior cannot come to grips with such quintessentially mentalist concepts as truth and falsity. Only thinking creatures can appreciate errors—and falsehoods.

This leads to another of Dennett's criticisms, which is the notion of the "undischarged homunculus" in Skinner's theory. Skinner claimed he had eradicated the need for mentalist explanations but, as a matter of logic, he had not. All he had done was shift them around, from an homunculus or "little man" in the head to another man hidden in the environment. This led him to argue [3] that there is no such thing as a creative artist. What we think of as a creative artist, he insisted, is merely an artist skilled at arranging a "creativity-inducing environment." But who decides what constitutes a creativity-inducing environment? The artist, presumably, so Skinner merely shifted the problem from one of explaining creativity to one of explaining how people decide what will induce creativity (presumably a fairly creative exercise in its own right).

There is an "undischarged mentalist debt" or homunculus lurking in every one of Skinner's allegedly neutral environments. In another context, Scriven noted the same "covert and unjustifiable substantive implications" buried in an avowedly non-mentalist behaviorism: "I remember the glee with which I discovered that nobody actually produces operational definitions, even when they say they do. (Cordell L.) Hull's work is replete with examples of allegedly operational definitions. Within three lines of many of these, he will insert an ontological addendum but still insist that the defined term has no meaning except as an intervening variable" [7, p145].

As mentioned, Dennett is of the view that, at the beginning of his career, Skinner made a profound and far-reaching mistake by equating mentalism with the supernatural. The psychologist was determined to eradicate from his "science of general psychology" all mentalist concepts, and therefore never looked seriously at the age-old questions of whether a non-mentalist psychology is possible or, crucially, whether mentalism is genuinely beyond analysis. Thus, there was a great deal of circularity, even question-begging, in Skinner's psychology, i.e. he frequently assumed the truth of that which required proof. For example, it is typical of humans that we "plan ahead," which means just what everybody thinks it means. But Skinner didn't allow any mentalist concepts, and planning ahead is entirely mentalist. Behavior is under the control of the environment, he believed, but since future events haven't yet happened, they can't control behavior. What appears to be a case of people planning ahead is actually a matter of their past history of reinforcing contingencies controlling their behavior. Given a detailed account of everything that has happened to them, we would be able to say just what compels them to act in a particular way right now such that, lo and behold, a few days or weeks down the track, they get whatever it is they said they wanted in the first place.

Unfortunately, in discarding mentalism as non-science, Skinner adopted another bit of non-science. As every psychologist knows, keeping track of the history of reinforcing contingencies of even a laboratory animal is difficult; working out what happened to a human years before, when no records were kept, is impossible. What he called a "proper behavioral analysis" is just magical thinking. Skinner was led to this error by his major assumptions:

1. Mentalism is necessarily supernatural;
2. Therefore, behavior must be under environmental control;
3. But future events can't control behavior because they haven't yet happened;
4. Therefore, the controlling element must lie in the past history of environmental contingencies.

The real question here is whether we can derive a natural or non-question-begging means by which future events can control behavior (equivalent to the mentalist or folk explanation, "If you want to pass your exams, you'd better study now"). I believe we can, and an everyday example will demonstrate the point. I ride my bicycle to the university, locking it in the rack before attending a lecture. After the lecture, I decide not to go straight home as I want to go to the library to collect a book the lecturer has mentioned. In order to get to the library, I need my bicycle but, for the life of me, I can't recall where I left it. I stand for a few moments, carefully "tracing" my movements since leaving home and then experience that flash of recollection that says: "It's outside the gymnasium."

It is true that I don't have any sort of "real" picture of all the university's bike racks in my head, nor is there a physical model of my pushbike rattling around in my head. In order to recall where I left my machine, I need to have a means of representing it in my head, and of coding that information in a system of memory. Since rats can easily recall how to get back into a house, and pigeons never forget where they have placed the first two sticks for a new nest, we can't argue that memory is not a natural mechanism. The whole process may in fact be biological for all that it matters. But if manipulating the internal representation can successfully locate my bicycle even when I can't see it, then I would say that, on first principles, the same or a similar mechanism should also be able to cope with organizing to go the library to collect a book I have never seen. There is no substantive difference between my behavior being controlled by a bicycle I can't see and a book I can't see. Both matters involve the manipulation of information coded in my head. If there is nothing supernatural about using this type of mechanism to explain the effect of past events on my behavior, then there is nothing supernatural about using it to plan ahead.

As it happened, the book didn't control my behavior as it was on loan. It was the (mental) expectation that I would find it that counted.

Strictly speaking, of course, my wish to borrow the book was a past event as soon as I had formulated it and, in that sense, Skinner couldn't object to it controlling my behavior. Collecting the book wasn't part of the wish, and that is true of all future events. I simply set up a behavioral program that should have ended with my leaving the library with a particular book under my arm. If future events genuinely controlled human behavior, then we would never make mistakes. In his fanatical opposition to the notion of internal control of behavior, Skinner was forced to confront the idea that future events could control behavior. His "reflex" rejection of that possibility led him to miss the point that current internal representations aren't in the future.

Why didn't Skinner think of these obvious objections? The answer is that only a full-blown, anti-mentalist Skinnerian system requires the abolition of plans as mental events and, almost certainly, he didn't believe there was any chance of error in his system. What seeps through his later works in particular is a profound satisfaction with his ideas. Everything he described seemed to fit his notions remarkably well, and he devoted a lot of space in *Beyond Freedom and Dignity* to showing just this point. I suggest the reason human behavior fitted his flawed theories so very well was because he didn't offer an explanation of human behavior at all, just a redescription from a novel point of view. Explanations can easily be proven wrong but descriptions, even in new languages, can never be wrong. Intellectually, descriptions take no chances and radical behaviorism fell straight into this trap.

In our old, poetic ways, we say that a if slave driver wants a slave to work harder, he will give him a good whipping to teach him a lesson; in turn, the slave quickly works out that, by appearing to be busy, he can avoid the lash. This is a fairly humdrum, mentalist "explanation" that involves motives, hopes, fears and other unobservables. Skinner rewrote this to read: "Thus, a slave driver induces a slave to work by whipping him when he stops; by resuming work, the slave escapes from the whipping (and incidentally reinforces the slave driver's behavior in using the whip)" [3, p26]. All traces of mentalism have been removed; we are left with a bare, environmentalist account (not quite: I think the word "induce" has a covert mentalist element). But the quote says no more than that which it was designed to replace; it can't say more, as it is just another way of saying the same thing, and it doesn't say less as it hides the mentalism in the environment. As an attempt to explain human behavior, radical behaviorism is mere description masquerading as explanation. This is not to suggest that mentalism itself is anything more than description because, until we have an explanatory account of mind-body interaction, mentalism is just another pseudo-explanation. Just like radical behaviorism.

Skinner believed that he had found the non-mentalist key to controlling and predicting behavior, and argued that all human behavior fitted his concepts. Now this is true, all human behavior can indeed be made to fit his devastatingly simple concepts. The real question is: should we do this? The history of ideas is littered with failed theories where somebody tried to reduce all human activity to the outcome of one or two fundamental principles. Thus, Skinner needed to show why our understanding of ourselves would necessarily be improved by his particular stance, how a non-mentalist theory (or description, as it really was) was an improvement over the mentalist. For him, of course, there was a very simple answer: by eradicating superstition, our self-understanding would automatically be improved. Is this true? Or can there be a naturalistic account of mentalism? It was one of the more maddening features of behaviorists that they never addressed this question, but simply assumed the answer to be in their favor. The fact that nobody had ever derived a natural theory of mentalism was enough to convince them that it could never happen, with the result that eschewing mentalism was the only rational path to follow.

In *Beyond Freedom and Dignity*, Skinner did not argue this point but outlined his new way of looking at age-old questions. Throughout this book, he insists that we while we have long looked at human behavior through mentalist spectacles, we can in fact also look at it from an environmentalist stance. He simply translates the mentalist concepts used in ordinary language, rewriting them in terms that have the effect of showing humans as marionettes dangling from environmental threads. All behavior, he argues, can be seen as the outcome of a previous history of contingent reinforcement of essentially random actions or operants. So it can, but should it? Or does the effort destroy something vital of our understanding of behavior?

Skinner never proved that his view was the only one available, nor did he show that his had greater predictive value or any of the other features that distinguish science from faith. He simply said: "We can look at all human behavior from this point of view," as though the reason for doing so was self-evident. Despite the unwavering conviction that sustained him for the better part of sixty years, he did not explain human behavior just because he failed to address these critical questions. He never wrote his technology of behavioral control, because he didn't have one.

2-4. Pavlov's Conditioning Model

Skinner was not the only psychologist in the behaviorists' century. In Europe, the dominant behaviorist theory was based in the work of the Russian psychologist, Ivan Pavlov (1849-1936). Every first year psychology student knows that Pavlov discovered the process of conditioning by observing dogs salivating in response to the dinner bell. At the time of his momentous discovery, Pavlov was studying digestion and had exteriorized the salivary flow in dogs so that their response to different stimuli could be precisely measured. He found that putting meat powder into their mouths caused a copious flow of saliva but before long, the dogs started to salivate almost as much when they heard the bell announcing lunch.

Pavlov's legendary formulation of this event was to regard the meat powder as the unconditioned stimulus and the salivary flow it stimulated as the unconditioned response. During the process of conditioning, the lunch bell became the conditioned stimulus, and the secondary salivary flow the conditioned response. In due course, Pavlov extended his concept to cover all forms of human learning until conditioning became the atomic building block of human behavior. This is what all basic psychology textbooks state; it's what all psychology students believe. Such a pity, then, that like most legends, there's hardly a word of truth in it.

Some parts of this comfortable little story are true. Ivan Pavlov was indeed a Russian scientist who worked with salivating dogs, but that's about all. He was a physiologist and, to his death, denied that he was a psychologist. It is true that he was studying the process of digestion in dogs when he discovered something about saliva and lunch bells, but he never claimed to have discovered a universal process called conditioning. As far as he was concerned, the concept of artificially-controlled physiological responses was simply a means of laboratory investigation and probably nothing more. He never believed that it was the (or even a) basic building block of human behavior and was antagonistic to the hope held by many psychologists of using it to build a general psychology.

In one of the last papers of his very long career, which was also his first paper in the psychological literature, Pavlov [2] attacked many of the concepts on which behaviorist psychology was based: "The psychologist takes conditioning as the principle of learning, and accepting this principle as not subject to further analysis, not requiring ultimate investigation, he endeavors to apply it to everything and explains all the individual features of learning as one and the same process ... (the psychologist) takes one physiological fact and ... gives it a specific meaning in ... the learning process (but) does not seek an (empirical) confirmation of that meaning" (p 91). Psychologists, he insisted, were still too much influenced by their historical origins as philosophers to understand the scientific process. They were not empirical researchers, but theorists who ignored scientific facts as it suited them: "...a whole mass of concrete facts remain without the slightest attention on (the psychologist's) part" (p 100).

Pavlov did not trust psychologists. Despite their protestations of scientific determinism (which, in any case, he believed to be false), they simply "...disguised by various scientifically decent synonyms" the same "dualism and animism" in which ordinary people believed. At no stage was he sympathetic to the idea that a behavioral analysis will allow control and prediction of behavior: "The variety and number of these (cortical) stimuli are countless, even in an animal like a dog." All his research indicated that the cerebrum was more, not less, complex than anybody had previously thought. Simple reductionism in any form was anathema to him: "I reject point blank and have a strong dislike for any theory which claims a complete inclusion of all that makes up our subjective world" (p 122; bear in mind that he did not take psychology's anti-mentalism seriously). Physiology would eventually explain what reductionist psychology couldn't: "...it is clear to me that many psychologists jealously ... guard the behavior of animals and man from such physiological explanations, constantly ignoring (established physiological processes) and not attempting to apply any of them to any extent" (p 123).

This would seem to be a fairly clear and authoritative rejection of behaviorist psychology's attempts to found a general psychology in the theories of Ivan Pavlov. On the other hand, of course, it could be that the great man was wrong, that psychologists correctly saw more in his work than he did himself. This is not the case: Pavlov was right and the psychologists were wrong, because there is no process of conditioning. Without conditioning, there is no modern theory of learning, meaning psychology loses a large part of its claim to a separate existence.

The case against the notion of conditioning has been argued by a number of different authors, including Popper [10]. A paper by Efron [11] appeared at a time when behaviorists saw little standing between them and complete domination of the field of human psychology. For example, in the introduction to his textbook, Yates [12] gloated over the impending collapse of psychoanalysis: "It will surely not be long before every Hollywood star has his or her behavior therapist." In fact, Freudian narcissism powers the Hollywood scene today just as it always has done.

In the title to his paper, Efron asserted that the concept of the conditioned reflex was meaningless. He pointed out that, within psychology, different authors use the term "conditioned reflex" in a variety of totally different ways. He cited a dispute between two authors, one of whom argued that worms can be "conditioned" while the other insisted that the first did not know the difference between "true conditioning" and "pseudo-conditioning." Efron made a number of points:

a) that these types of disputes were due to "epistemological chaos" rather that to disagreements over genuine scientific facts;

b) the chaos derives from the assumption that all human behavior can be explained by eliminative materialism, i.e. that all "concepts of consciousness, volition and the causal efficacy of mental processes" can and should be excluded from the field of science;

c) that in attempting to eliminate all mention of conscious mental processes, reductionist biologists (essentially psychologists) have degraded the narrow concept of the reflex by progressively broadening it to the extent that it has long since become meaningless;

d) all attempts to salvage a meaning for conditioning, such as operationalism, are doomed to failure because they necessarily enter an infinite regress.

Efron showed that, 150 years ago, the term "reflex" had a very restricted meaning, essentially that of the automatic response to an external stimulus in an intact, functioning animal: "The definition of 'reflex' action contains, therefore, by implication, reference to a class or classes of action which are non-reflexive ... Behavior which is automatic, innate, involuntary, and independent of consciousness needs to be isolated conceptually (i.e. defined) only because other behavior exists which is voluntary, learned and dependent on conscious activity ... To attempt to use the concept 'reflex' while at the same time denying the validity of the concepts of 'consciousness' and of 'volition' is not logically permissible" (p 491). But this is exactly what reductionist psychology and biology intended to do: deny consciousness. Not explain it, nor show it was necessarily irrelevant or an artifact, but to deny the mentalism of their own minds.

The term "reflex" was seized by late nineteenth century physiologists as part of a broad drive against the notions exemplified by Bergson's *elan vital*. Researchers wished to dispense with the "mysticism" inherent in such concepts as consciousness, intention, mentality, etc. They therefore declared these notions to be non-scientific and wrote a new "science" that did not depend on them. But in so doing, they simply replaced one form of mysticism by another, all the more pernicious by being implicit. The neurophysiologist Karl Lashley explicated the "reductionist's credo": "Our common meeting ground is the faith to which we all subscribe ... I believe, that the phenomena of behavior and mind are ultimately describable in the concepts of the mathematical and physical sciences" (quoted in Efron, p 500). This particular form of mysticism is known as promissory materialism, which has been around a long time without delivering on any of its major promises (that's why it's called "promissory").

In order to eradicate mentalism, psychologists had to broaden the concept of the "unthinking reflex," eventually to the point where it was used to explain thought itself. Their campaign had to be managed this way. It was not possible to eliminate consciousness by reducing it to matters of brain chemistry (i.e. neurophysiology), because that would eliminate them as scientists. Therefore, they had to pursue the alternative approach, which was to squeeze consciousness out of existence by expanding the unconscious, automatic basis of behavior until it included everything that the concept of consciousness had previously encompassed. In their mechanistic world, the basic element of behavior was the reflex (like a thought is the basic element in a mentalist world), but in order for it to subsume all that minds once did, it had to be redefined "...in such a fashion that it no longer rested upon the concept(s) of consciousness and volition" (p 501).

"In sum," Efron continued, "the mechanistic biologist (i.e. psychologist) retained the word reflex because it enabled him to make implicit use of the old concept of the reflex (i.e. involuntary behavior independent of consciousness) without admitting that his 'new science of behavior' still logically rested upon the concepts of consciousness and volition. This epistemological procedure is known, in some scientific circles, as 'having your cake and eating it too'" (p 501).

In Efron's view, and supported by lengthy quotes, Pavlov was one of those responsible for expanding the definition of "reflex" to the point where it became facile. Using it, Pavlov could explain "every activity of man and beast" that, unfortunately, led directly to an infinite regress and even to self-contradiction: "By virtue of (Pavlov's) definition, it is a reflex if a hungry dog salivates in response to a bell which has in the past signaled the appearance of food; it is a reflex if I purchase a painting today which I saw and enjoyed last year; and it is a reflex if a man tries to escape from his tormentors in a concentration camp" (p 506). Of course, the artist and the torturers would also be acting reflexly.

Efron's case against the conditioned reflex is unimpeachable, yet it had remarkably little effect on behaviorist psychology. But it can be extended further. If we look at the term "conditioned reflex" as it stands, it has no meaning. Reflex we understand (or we think we do); but conditioned? What does this mean? We think it has a meaning, but only because we have heard the term so often that we accept it as real, rather in the way American psychiatrists of the fifties and sixties thought they knew what they meant by the term "schizophrenia": there was a tacit agreement not to question each other's understanding of the term.

The original meaning of Pavlov's term emerges through his writings, but certainly not with any great clarity. It would appear that the salivating response his dogs showed to food was originally termed "unconditional," meaning one that appeared without further conditions. The food was a "stimulus to an unconditional response" (shortened to "unconditional stimulus") in that, without any conditions attached, it worked every time (strictly speaking, as Efron has argued, this isn't true). So an "unconditional stimulus" leads to an "unconditional reflex response." The bell, however, has to be associated with the food before it can elicit any sort of response; its efficacy as a stimulus is "conditional" upon its relationship with the (unconditional) food stimulus. This is associationism; there is no "process of conditioning" to be found, but Pavlov's translators always used the term "conditioned reflex," implying something quite different from "conditional reflex". "Conditional" is an adjective, and its meaning is quite clear, but using the word "conditioned," which has the form of a past participle, implies there is a verb "to condition." Today, there is such a verb in English, but its meaning is quite the same as "to associate." Skinner himself admitted this as long ago as 1931: "If we remain at the level of our observations, we must recognize a reflex as a correlation" (quoted in Efron, p 498).

Pavlov was not much fussed which word people used to describe his concept of non-conscious automatism: "Of course," he said, "the terms 'conditioned' and 'unconditioned' could be replaced by others of arguably equal merit... we might retain the term 'inborn reflexes,' and call the new type 'acquired reflexes'; or call the former 'species reflexes' since they are characteristic of the species, and the latter 'individual reflexes' since they vary from animal to animal in a species, and even in the same animal at different times and under different conditions. Or again we might call the former 'conduction reflexes' and the latter 'connection reflexes'" (quoted in [11], p 504). Quite clearly, if he had used any of these other terms, then the concept would not have been reified so quickly or so thoroughly. And if psychology had not had the specious concept of conditioning as its basic building block, its history in the twentieth century would undoubtedly have been very different.

If the conditioned reflex does not exist, and there is no process of conditioning, how was academic psychology able to maintain these fictions for 75 years or more? As with many of the great theoretical movements of the twentieth century, we may never have a precise answer but certain factors contributed.

In the first place, psychologists desperately needed an "atomic element" on which to build their discipline. In the fifty years from its tentative, introspectionist beginnings, psychology made little or no real theoretical progress and was in grave danger of collapsing as a separate body of knowledge. Watson [1] acknowledged this in his 1915 "call to arms" for behaviorism: "I do not wish unduly to criticize psychology. It has failed signally, I believe, during the fifty-odd years of its existence as an experimental discipline to make its place in the world as an undisputed natural science... We have become so enmeshed in speculative questions concerning the elements of mind, the nature of conscious content that I, as an experimental student, feel that something is wrong with our premises and the types of problems which develop from them" (p 163). Unless psychology radically altered its theoretical orientation, he foresaw no chance of progress in the next two hundred years.

Without the reflex theory of behavior, psychology was doomed to wander unprofitably on the edges of other, better-established disciplines such as philosophy or physiology, even to wither and die. Without it, there would be no modern learning theory, no behaviorist revolution and therefore no basis for psychologists to claim a separate existence.

The need for psychology to find something, anything, was profound. A reviewer said of Watson's "Behaviorism" [1924]: "Perhaps this is the most important book ever written. One stands for an instant blinded with a great hope" (quoted in [7]). MacKenzie continued: "Not for an instant, but for fifty years, psychologists were blinded with the great hope that they could make psychology a genuine and successful science..." Their need blinded them to the weaknesses of the "reflex theory" of human behavior and condemned twentieth century psychology to a long and vastly expensive detour.

Secondly, at the time he proclaimed the behaviorist revolution, Watson knew practically nothing of Pavlov's work. He had never met the physiologist, never read any of his publications and had available to him only a few summaries: "...all of the researches have appeared in Russian and in periodicals which are not accessible at present to American students. At least, we have not been able to obtain access to a single research publication. The German and French translations ... give the method only in the barest outline. Bechterew's summary was the only guide we had in our work ..." [13, p 94]. Watson stormed the citadels of introspectionism, his mortal enemy, without realizing his shells had no powder! Fortunately for him, the citadel was ready to collapse. Almost certainly, this easy victory helped convince the early behaviorists they were on to something big.

Finally, Pavlov himself almost certainly contributed to the widespread misunderstanding of his work. In common with many of his more literary compatriots, Pavlov's style of writing was turgid, even opaque, and it is clear that his different translators had difficulty with his novel terminology. He was given to propounding "laws" on the basis of a few observations, but even with the best efforts of his translators, their meaning was not always apparent. For example, in his lecture "A Brief Outline of the Higher Nervous Activity," [14, pp 48-50], he listed a series of "laws" that today are simply quaint. Yet these were dutifully translated and, no doubt, closely studied for their essential meanings. So when Watson, in particular, was championing the concept of "conditioning," he did so with very little exposure to the research on which the notion was based. The jump from a Russian experimental physiology to an American general psychology was blind. Even Watson himself leaves no doubt: he was motivated more by his wish to break with introspectionism than by any certainty that the new "science of behavior" could satisfy the needs psychologists were placing upon it [13, p 105].

In simple terms, Watson's proselytizing for his "truly scientific psychology" was based very largely on his desperate wish to find a means of smashing his intellectual enemies. A forceful and convincing writer, it is perhaps not surprising that when he was forced to resign his chair for conduct unbecoming of a professor (in fact, only adultery), Watson entered the world of advertising and eventually died a very wealthy man. Academically, however, his early works leave no doubt that he had little idea of the foggy concepts with which his distant mentor was grappling. Misled by fragmentary translations of complex gropings towards an inchoate science, Watson thought there was a law-like process connecting stimulus and response, when all the experimental evidence suggested only an ephemeral association. Since then, generations of psychologists have accepted unquestioningly the myth of conditioning.

(As an aside, the two volumes of Pavlov's "Conditioned Reflexes and Psychiatry" [14] are a major cause of much of the confusion that surrounds his scientific beliefs. Without much effort, it is possible to find quotes supporting a range of conflicting theoretical positions. This was not unique to Pavlov. Eysenck himself noted how the Russian proclivity for vague and fluid terminology made testing their hypotheses almost impossible [15, p 247]).

2-5. Eysenck and the Decline of Behaviorism

Regardless of the deficiencies we now find in the classical theory of conditioning, Pavlov was highly influential in Europe. In the former USSR and in Eastern Europe in particular, but also in the West, programs based in his ideas have been widely accepted in the management of a range of mental disorders. In fact, very few disorders have not, at one stage or another, been the subject of research deriving from the Pavlovian or classical behaviorist model. In London, the professor of psychology at the Institute of Psychiatry, Hans Eysenck, was for many years a powerful and partisan publicist for Pavlovian theories and methods.

It would not be possible to summarize briefly Eysenck's vast output, but anybody reading his work will be struck, firstly, by his apparently encyclopedic knowledge of the psychological literature, and secondly, by the calm and pervasive certainty that he knows (which he also radiates strongly in personal appearances). The difficulty lies in divining just what it is he knows. What does Hans Juergen Eysenck believe? This is not such an easy question to answer. If one were to start with one of his earlier books, *The Dynamics of Anxiety and Hysteria*, from 1957 [16], one would be left with the clear impression that behaviorist psychology is about to conquer the world. The little that

Clark L Hull didn't say about psychology, according to Eysenck's fulsome dedication, would shortly be revealed. Unfortunately, even so soon after Hull's death, his psychology had fallen into disrepute.

Peters [17] was scathing in his review, calling Hull's *Principles of Behavior* (1943) an enormity. Far from explaining the entirety of human behavior in atomic terms such as "colorless movements and mere receptor impulses", Peters concluded: "...Hull developed some simple postulates which gave dubious answers to limited questions about particular species of rats. He never asked, let alone tried to answer, any concrete questions about human behavior. He was in love with the idea of a science of behavior; he was not acutely worried about concrete questions of explaining human behavior." In his brief history of psychology, Thomson [18] noted: "We need not concern ourselves with (Hull's) highly idiosyncratic presentation. Nobody else seems to have adopted it..." (p 239).

Eysenck's 1957 book was just a pot-boiler. By 1981, he had withdrawn from his earlier, confident stance to a more moderate position. In his introduction to an anthology he edited [19], he said: "...above all, (this book) is not a model of personality ... The book uses extraversion-introversion (E) as an example to illustrate the way in which a model of personality can be constructed." To anybody who thought psychologists used models of personality in their daily work, this comes as something of a shock. Here, after a hundred years of psychology, we have one of their most influential authors admitting that psychological theorizing on personality is still bogged down in preliminaries.

The concept of E being very much Eysenck's, he wrote the first chapter in the book. It soon becomes clear that he was using the opportunity in a familiar way, not so much as an explication of his ideas as an attack upon his fellow psychologists. This time, however, his approach was different. Far from asserting that his form of behaviorism was necessarily correct and all other psychologies wrong, his stance was, at first glance, more moderate. He stated outright that his theory was "...by no means finished, even in its major outlines" and that, "Like all scientific theories, that linking E to cortical arousal encounters many anomalies..." These small deficiencies caused him no great concern: "Indeed, the existence of anomalies proves that a theory is *in fact* scientific (his emphasis): only unfalsifiable theories are without such anomalies, and unfalsifiable theories are by definition outside the scientific pale. This does not mean that we should be proud of such anomalies, and cherish them forever. We should make every effort to clarify the issues, look at different parameters, and try in every way to see if the apparent anomalies cannot be made to conform to our theories" (p XII).

He then mentioned Popper's work approvingly but with one proviso: despite everything the philosopher had said against verificationism, Eysenck believed the philosopher was wrong. Eysenck also omitted to mention Popper's long-standing antipathy for the doctrine of behaviorism, which he regarded as "totally mistaken" [20, p 503]. If, in fact, Eysenck had ever read Popper, he betrayed no understanding of it in this paper. Most unusually for him, he did not give references to the philosopher's work.

In the body of his chapter, Eysenck expounded his views on the philosophy of science. Science, he believed, proceeds in an orderly fashion from "...fact-collecting on the basis of vague hunches, serendipitous discoveries of unforeseen regularities and inductive generalizations. When sufficient data have been collected along these lines, we are in the position of being able to put forward hypotheses of relatively small compass, and now the emphasis shifts to verification; unless we can verify these hypotheses, at least within the confines of certain parameter values, it is unlikely that they will be pursued further or interest other scientists. Given that this stage is successfully passed, we enter the realm of theory-making proper, and now falsification becomes the most important aspect of our experimental work. When a given theory is firmly established, it becomes a scientific law ... Thus, what constitutes a scientific approach will depend on the degree of development of a particular field..." (p2).

In this critical respect, Eysenck's views are quite unique. By his clear and repeated statements over many years [19,21,22], science proceeds in a perfectly straight line from "hunch" to hypothesis to theory to law. An idea with little or no confirmatory evidence is a hunch; if sufficient supportive evidence can be found, it will eventually shuttle along to become a law. He explained this with a diagram on p3 of "General Features of the Model" [19], entitled "Demarcation theories of science: a unified point of view."

Unfortunately, this is pseudo-philosophy. It is surprising that the same erroneous opinion appeared in print so many years apart because, using his bizarre approach, truism will become "scientific law" before a highly improbable but accurate hypothesis. More than ten years after this peculiar exposition of his ideas, in a paper entitled "Biological Dimensions of Personality" [15], Eysenck repeated his opinions on how science ought to proceed. Psychology, he finally admitted, was a "weak theory" as opposed to physics and other "hard sciences" that are strong theories. Therefore, he believed, psychology should be developed in accordance with pre-war ideas on the logic of science.

1936 was a good year, he opined: "...in order to deduce the proposition P from our hypothesis H, and in order to be able to test P experimentally, many other assumptions, K, must be made (about surrounding circumstances, instruments used, mediating concepts, etc.). Consequently it is never H alone that is being put to the test by the experiment—it is H and K together. In a weak theory, we cannot make the assumption that K is true, and consequently failure of the experiment may be due to wrong assumptions concerning K, rather than to H's being false. In a strong theory, enough is known about K to render empirical failure more threatening for H. This argument suggests that positive outcomes of testing H are more meaningful than negative ones. The former imply that both H and K are true; the latter that either H, or K, or both are false. In other words, failure does not lead to any certain conclusion" (p 250).

In the first place, as Scriven had described, psychology is notorious for its many unstated assumptions. But Eysenck's main point is the central issue in Popper's rejection of verification as a demarcation criterion, a point which clearly eluded Eysenck. He could not see that if both the hypothesis and the other assumptions are true, then it may by due to either a unique case (chance) or, more significantly, to the fact that, while true, the entire hypothesis and its nested assumptions are boring. Eysenck's oft-repeated "methodology" will necessarily elevate banality to the level of "strong science" before an accurate but highly improbable theory. This is exactly what has happened with his utterly banal psychology.

In addition to his perilous methodology, Eysenck's theories fail on quite separate grounds. Eysenck is a psychologist, specifically, a personality theorist, meaning he has devoted his very long career to elucidating the nature of human personality. As a psychologist, he is a behaviorist, in that he uses as his field of data only observable human behavior. All talk of unseen causative mechanisms of that behavior is forbidden; hence his well-known antipathy towards psychoanalysis and other folk psychologies. His psychology tries to describe the generative mechanisms of human behavior without mentioning unobservables and without relying on evidence from outside the narrow field of behavior. A series of questions springs from this stance. Can there be a theory of personality based in evidence from one dimension only? Just what is a theory of personality that does not mention "hidden generative mechanisms," and finally, what is the mechanism by which observable behavior is generated?

The first question, can there be a behaviorally-based theory of personality, raises a number of prior questions: what is a theory in psychology, what is personality, and what behavior can be used as evidence for a theory of personality? Eysenck has said that personality is a constellation of dispositions to act; the evidence for these dispositions comes entirely from observable behavior. For him, there is no limit to behavior: if humans do it, it's behavior. So even though he talks about tough-mindedness, for example, he is not talking about mind but about behavior, specifically, the behavior of reporting statements that are classed as "tough-minded attitudes", even though everybody knows there isn't a mind and attitudes are mentalist. What the subject may believe his statements about his attitudes signify is inconsequential. His belief, say, that his attitudes control his behavior and are themselves controlled by the stars, is of no import. The Eysenckian behaviorist reports all this dispassionately, making no judgments and offering no opinions.

Immediately, it is clear that a genuinely behaviorist account of "personality" is inductive; all conclusions are temporary only, held pending further evidence and subject to revision by somebody who has asked different questions. Hence the constant bickering between psychologists as to how many personality factors there are [22]. It all depends on how you ask the questions, as Eysenck clearly explained: "By a suitable choice of additional questions we could make the correlation between E and N (Neuroticism) assume almost any value between -0.2 and +0.2; clearly there is a good deal of subjectivity involved in the whole process, and a question about the real state of affairs is meaningless ... thus the question we are dealing with really involves properties which we desire our scale to have, rather than properties which some concept existing independently of human thoughts, desires and aims may have—some immaterial *Ding an sich* which in the nature of things we could never comprehend ... *If the theory says that extraversion and neuroticism are independent, then a measuring instrument will be constructed and chosen which will give independent readings for the two concepts...*" [19, p 25, my emphasis].

We can conclude from this that even opinions concerning behaviorist concepts of personality, or behaviorism itself, are temporary. By denying the possibility of meaningful theories of mentality, thereby restricting themselves to a single dimension of data, behaviorists are forced to equate behavior and mind. While you and I can talk about our neighbor's mind, psychologists can only report his behavior, even when that includes him complaining that their questions are driving him out of his mind. It is pure description, vast, encyclopedic, true only insofar as it occurred, and incapable of supporting any more than boring, inductive conclusions.

The question of whether Eysenck equates behavior and mind is not clear. At times, he has talked about mind in the perfectly ordinary, mentalist way of a "reciprocal influence of body and mind ... psychologists will have to learn to accept a mind-body continuum" [23]. This would be unremarkable were it not for his acerbic criticism of frankly mentalist theories in psychology—even in that particular paper. I suggest, however, that Eysenck has not equated behavior and mind in the sense that whatever can be said in "mentalese" (the language of folk psychology) can immediately and with no loss of meaning be translated into the language of behavior. His approach seems different. In his work, most mentalist talk has been eliminated as meaningless, the implication being that the remainder can be brought to account by an adequate description of behavior. This is not the same as equating mind and behavior as we normally use the terms, but takes an impoverished definition of mind and argues that a behaviorist account is functionally equivalent.

In brief, a behaviorist theory of personality is not a theory of mind in that it does not give an account of intellect, memory, the experience of emotion and perception, etc.. In addition, he has discarded common terms such as wish, desire, aim, etc. replacing them with statements of dispositions to act. Thus, in an Eysenckian analysis, the fact that I experience a burning desire to finish this work is of no account. What matters is that I work long hours at it, writing and rewriting, then repeatedly submitting it to publishers despite the fact that the editorial responses are anything but reinforcing. While in this particular case, it may be true that my desire amounts to naught, pretending it does not exist does not convey to you the intent that I hope you will apprehend. The fact that I have a burning desire to go fishing but never get there because I don't have any money cannot be adequately described behaviorally.

A theory of personality based in data from the single dimension of observable behavior cannot be developed beyond the point of mere description of the types of behaviors the subject habitually reports. That is, it can never be anything but a typology of human behavior. If it cannot postulate hidden or unseen causative mechanisms of that behavior, then it will remain wholly inductive. It can never have true predictive value, in that it cannot make any interesting predictions about a person unless we already know the answer to the question from another person of a similar type.

Eysenck would strongly disagree [15, 19]. His theory, he has argued, has real predictive value, particularly in the biological sphere. He is of the opinion that it has reached a high level of development, such that it can generate interesting predictions about people. Well, how interesting? In his paper "Biological Dimensions of Personality" [15], he describes in great detail experiments involving dropping lemon juice on the tongues of different types (note that word) of people. This is physiology, and a very old and tiresome sort of physiology at that. His descriptions are tedious and pointless: they tell us next to nothing about people as creatures with minds. If the only predictions his theory can make are of the type he describes in this paper, then the theory amounts to very little.

A description of personality types does not amount to a theory of personality. A theory of personality just is an attempt at an explanation, but descriptions are never explanations. A theory of personality has to extend beyond the available (behavioral) data [24] to hypothesize about the unseen mechanisms or processes that cause the observable behavior. If the term "personality" has any meaning, it's not about what we see, it's about what we don't see. All behaviorally-based, dimensional systems of personality classification fall into this simple error. A theory of personality that pointedly does not mention "hidden generative mechanisms" is a waste of time.

Eysenck has repeatedly disparaged the many frankly mentalist theories of personality, including Freud, Adler, Erikson and Maslow, among many others: "They fail essentially because for the most part they do not generate testable deductions; because where they do so the deductions have most frequently been falsified; and because they fail to include practically all the experimental and empirical studies which have been done over the past fifty years" [23, p774]. But if all theories of a causally-effective mental apparatus fail to qualify as science, what does Eysenck himself believe causes behavior?

On this point, the normally-forthright Eysenck is remarkably coy. Of his book, *The Biological Basis of Personality* [1967], he said: "...an attempt is made to deduce extravert-introvert differences ... in terms of differences in cortical arousal, mediated by the reticular formation." This quickly becomes confusing. At times, he intimates that the difference between the two types (introvert and extravert) just is the difference between their measures on the physiological parameter; at others, he suggests they manipulate their own experiences to give themselves the level of arousal they prefer [19]. More recently, he has identified E with cortical arousal as mediated by the ascending reticular activating system, while N is "closely related to the activity of the visceral brain, which consists of the hippocampus-amygdala, cingulum, septum and hypothalamus" [15, p248]. A careful reading of this paper indicates that the psychologist sees an identity relationship between the psychological (meaning behavior) and the physiological, although it has to be said that, at times, he is vague to the point of confusion on this point.

We could go further: if he wishes to avoid mentalism (it is not at all clear whether he does but, as a good behaviorist, he ought to), then Eysenck has to postulate a direct relationship between brain states and observable behavior. Otherwise, he opens his theory to intervening variables whose nature cannot be restricted by his theory (just because it says nothing about intervening variables), i.e. the intervening variables he doesn't want to talk about may well be mental. The relationship he appears to prefer is identity, meaning that as a matter of contingent fact, psychological states just are brain states. Now the doctrine of brain-behavior identity solves a number of problems for behaviorists. Firstly, it protects them absolutely from any and all charges that they have covertly smuggled in mentalist concepts, a charge against which Eysenck is certainly not immune (for example, see his "mind-body continuum" [23]).

Secondly, it encompasses within a materialist framework everything that mentalists regard as important in humans. Thus, they can avoid being the butt of the old joke that behaviorists don't believe in beliefs, they think that nobody thinks and, in their opinion, nobody has opinions [25, p158]. Thirdly, it provides psychologists with a ready-made scientific research program, albeit one belonging to another discipline (neurophysiology), but one that would immediately provide them with scientific respectability [23]. Finally, it would allow them quietly to drop their exhausted behaviorist program [7] without anybody raising the embarrassing suggestion that psychology is an "emperor with no clothing" [9].

These are the advantages, and Eysenck is certainly aware of them. The disadvantages, of which he betrays no awareness, are based on the premise that Mind-Brain Identity Theory (MBIT) fails the critical second point above, that it must provide a materialist (reductionist) explanation for strictly mentalist concepts. Proponents of MBIT believe that it provides a rational account of such ephemera as society, culture, personal experience, etc. [26, 27], i.e. everything. Its opponents argue that when it attempts to stretch it to cover these quintessentially mental matters, MBIT collapses into incoherence [28, 29]. At this stage, the proponents are in disarray; the consensus is that MBIT will not satisfy the hopes psychologists have placed on it, and Eysenck will therefore not be able to save his theories by this means.

Despite his oft-repeated claims, Eysenck did not write the definitive human psychology and his work cannot form the basis of a general theory of human psychopathology. All he had to offer was a human typology that he attempted to relate directly to brain function. This is Mind-Brain Identity Theory, with all its attendant problems. While of some research value, his typology is superficial and cannot generate a single interesting prediction about an individual's life which, after all, is what psychology is all about. After fifty years, it has not gained a foothold in ordinary clinical practice. Eysenck might disagree, citing evidence such as the accuracy of the "predicted changes in auditory thresholds of introverts, ambiverts and extraverts with change in the intensity of ambient illumination" [19,p15]. Or he might quote results of parotid salivary flow stimulated by lemon juice applied to the tongue [22, p254]. This is physiology, not psychology, and very dull and outdated physiology at that. Neurophysiology passed by this kind of work several generations ago, picking up the methods of behaviorist psychology *en passant* but leaving behind the theories (such as they were).

It is my belief that Eysenckian psychology will never satisfy the enormous, even outrageous, claims its founder made for it. His typology has more direct value and, suitably refined, may make a longer-lasting contribution as an aid to research programs. But until it can do better than talk about such arcane trivia as electrodermal responses in ambiverts, it will amount to very little.

2-6. Conclusion

As mentioned above, some eighty years ago, a reviewer said of Watson's Behaviorism: "Perhaps this is the most important book ever written. One stands for an instant blinded with a great hope" [7]. After his very thorough examination of the rational basis of behaviorism, McKenzie concluded: "What behaviorism ... can be said to have left us ... is some portion of the tools appropriate for building a science—but not the science itself, and very little even in the way of durable preliminary structures which can be taken into the science" (p170).

One hundred and twenty five years after Wundt opened the first psychological laboratory, psychologists have reluctantly admitted that they have spent a century wandering around in a dead-end. Quietly, they have dropped behaviorism in favor of mentalism ("cognitive behaviorism") while continuing their noisy claims to be the only group properly equipped to investigate the mind.

Without behaviorism, the research discipline of psychology will shrink to being little more than part of the very broad field of neurosciences. The practice of psychology is already blurring as social workers, nurses, and anybody with a printer sets up business as a "generic counselor." Consequently, there are no grounds whatsoever for believing that behaviorism can form the basis of a general theory for psychiatry, and no grounds for psychologists to criticize psychiatry for its lack of a firm scientific foundation.

<table>
<tr><td>

3

</td><td>

Mentalism in Psychiatry: Psychoanalysis and Cognitive Psychology

</td></tr>
</table>

3-1. Introduction

There are many mentalist theories of mind; what they have in common is the idea that minds are real and causally significant. Most of them would also say that the mind is irreducible, but that's not central to the idea. By mind, I mean what everybody knows the word to mean: the private, inner experience of myself as an effective agent experiencing meaningful interactions with the real world. The concept of mind includes a range of mental matters such as memory, current perception, emotion, cognition, volition, etc. [1].

For most people throughout most of our history, the mind was and still is more or less synonymous with the spirit or soul, which has all the properties of the modern mind but is immortal as well. That is, most people have no doubt that what they are experiencing today will continue in one form or another after death, which brings us straight to the major problem with all mentalist theories: their relationship with the supernatural.

If I want to talk rationally about my mind, where do I start and what can I talk about? The easiest place to start is my immediate experience—the vast, private picture theatre in my head. In it, I have a sense of self that appears to be separate from such things as my memory, my emotions, my plans and hopes, my willpower (or lack of it), and so on. I have the clear impression that if I want something and make the effort, then whatever I want will come to pass provided it doesn't cost too much. I appreciate that this is "mentalese" but, for me, my private inner life is very real, constantly active and, through the agency of my body, acts on the real world. How any sensible person could doubt that my mind exists, I will never know. Well, there are over six billion sensible people who could doubt that my mind exists, just as I can toy with the idea that you are nothing but a clever automaton.

The reason you can doubt I have a mind is quite simple: you can't see it, touch it or measure it in any way. And if the mind is something we all accept exists but is forever beyond independent confirmation, then we can't complain if different people have different ideas of what it is and does. You may believe that the mind is just an emergent property of the intricate organization of the brain, one that therefore cannot survive the death of the brain, while your neighbor believes that something with all the properties you attribute to your emergent mind is in fact immortal. Somebody else may believe that his mind can nip out for a stroll around the garden, or that he can read other people's minds or bend spoons just by concentrating on them. Nobody can prove another person's idea of the mind wrong, especially for someone who believes that spoons won't bend in front of a skeptic. Once we open the door to mentalism, a whole range of academically undesirable ideas will scamper through as well. Nobody has ever found a way of letting rational mentalism in and keeping irrational spiritualism out.

In order to formalize this problem, we can use Popper's approach which says that there is no feature or demarcation criterion that reliably distinguishes between the concept of a rational, emergent mind and the most fanatically mystical and supernatural beliefs. Concepts of mind range from very narrow, cognitive models right through to some truly Gothic masterpieces. Where I choose to stand on this continuum is entirely a matter of taste.

The ordinary model of mind is what Dennett [2], probably following Wilhelm Wundt, calls "folk psychology." Folk psychology is what ordinary folk would expect it to be, an account of the mind as a busy, private executive station in the head where I check what is happening in the world "out there" and make my decisions. I model my understanding of your mind on my own experience and, usually, I can make fairly accurate predictions about your behavior. Folk psychology doesn't imply the immortality of the mind, although it doesn't preclude it.

While we can predict each other's behavior quite well, even in highly competitive settings (such as love and war), our *Voelkische psykology* is wholly descriptive, not explanatory, and thus has two major failings. In the first place, it's based in what I personally think or believe, so it isn't very reliable when dealing with people who think differently from me. Secondly, it doesn't say much about the extremes of life experiences, mainly because, being descriptive, folk psychology doesn't have enough experience of extremes to draw any conclusions. For example, folk psychology can't explain phobias. Ordinary people know they exist but have no explanation for them.

This particular shortcoming of commonsense psychology was well appreciated in the latter part of the nineteenth century. At the time, the French neurologist Charcot was experimenting with hypnosis and found he could duplicate many of the symptoms of hysteria. This greatly impressed a visiting Austrian neurologist, Sigmund Freud, who, on his return to Vienna, started to work with patients suffering from this affliction. His subsequent history is well-known: far from being convinced that hysteria was an hereditary degeneration of the brain, which was the standard explanation, Freud soon came to believe that it was the result of psychic trauma. Over the next fifty years or so, he and his followers elaborated a vastly complex theory that they believed not only accounted for the whole of normal and abnormal mental life, but dictated a form of treatment as well.

3-2. The Logical Status of Freudian Psychoanalytic Theory

Psychoanalysis, as it became known, was the first substantial attempt at a coherent, natural theory of mind. It exerted a powerful intellectual attraction, dominating Western ideas for the greater part of the twentieth century. Yet it is now crumbling into disuse. Was this decline predictable? I say it was because, almost from the beginning, many people had raised serious objections to the theory. If these had been pursued, then several generations of effort would have been saved. Unfortunately, very few of the psychiatrists who believed in Freudian psychoanalysis could also understand the objections. Even if they had, they would have been given short thrift from the psychoanalytic establishment, which was remarkably intolerant of anybody daring to question its ideas.

Psychoanalysis was never as dominant in Britain, Australia or New Zealand as it was in the US. In these countries, psychiatry was cast in a biological mold long before Freud's ideas gained currency. Nonetheless, psychoanalysis stands as the most highly developed of the materialist mentalist theories, and general criticisms of analytic theories also apply to non-Freudian mentalist notions.

Early critics of Freud's theories were quite blunt: the author Vladimir Nabokov is said to have called Freud a charlatan and his psychoanalysis the worst sort of quackery. By the 1920s, positivist philosophers had mounted very substantial attacks on the theory but by then it was too well-established—not the least because there simply wasn't anything that could compete. The philosopher Karl Popper reported a conversation with Alfred Adler in 1919, when he began to suspect the ease with which analytic theories were confirmed in daily clinical experience: "It was precisely this fact—that they always fitted, that they were always confirmed—which in the eyes of their admirers constituted the strongest argument in favor of these theories. It began to dawn on me that this apparent strength was in fact their weakness" [3, p 35].

From this type of work, Popper developed his notion that there is a discrepancy between the weight that must attach to instances of verification or refutation of a theory. Verification only tells us that the theory was right on that occasion; it says nothing about whether it will always be right, i.e. whether it is an interesting general truth, a truism or just randomly true. Refutation, on the other hand, tells us with absolute certainty that the theory was wrong at the time of the experiment, and therefore cannot be generally true. Refutation thus became his critical criterion, the point of demarcation between true scientific theories and metaphysics. Science, of course, is subject to empirical confirmation or denial while metaphysics never is.

Popper made no secret of his view that, since psychoanalysis could not be refuted, it was non-scientific. There was no evidence that would convince a committed analyst that his theories were wrong; therefore, the theories were no better than other ideas accepted on faith alone (i.e. religion): "But what kind of clinical responses would refute to the satisfaction of the analyst not merely a particular analytic diagnosis but psycho-analysis itself? ... The criterion of falsifiability ... says that statements or systems of statements, in order to be ranked as scientific, must be capable of conflicting with possible, or conceivable, observations" [3, p 38-9]. Popper first aired these ideas in the early 1920s but criticisms of this type did not impinge upon the analytic consciousness for many years.

Popper's work was suppressed by the Nazis in Europe and was not widely available in English until the 1960s. The quotes above were finally published in English in 1972. Thereafter, the notion that there was something seriously wrong with psychoanalysis percolated slowly through the psychiatric world. In 1973, the former editor of the British Journal of Psychiatry, Eliot Slater, published a critique of analytic theories that drew heavily on Popper's ideas [4].

More recently, there have been major critiques of Freud's work that suggest he actually falsified his results [5].

3-3. Saving Freudian Theory

Popper's criticisms are unassailable: psychoanalysis can no longer lay claim to scientific status. But having dominated the mentalist wing of psychiatry for so long, analysts are not about to give up without a fight. From time to time, mainstream psychiatric journals publish defenses by analysts against the main objections raised to their theories. In the past quarter century, Freudians have shifted their position, from maintaining that theirs is the only truly scientific theory of human psychology, to arguing that it is a system of interpretation lying outside the scope of science. One such defense was published some years ago as an editorial in the *Australian and New Zealand Journal of Psychiatry* [6]. In fact, it can be read as a defense of all elaborate mentalist theories, not just of psychoanalysis itself.

In this paper, Bracken argued that psychoanalysts should abandon their claims to scientific status. Current concepts of science are too restrictive, he claimed, and science is anyway far less rational than we've been led to believe. Unfortunately, his paper contained a number of subtle shifts of position so his case wasn't easy to follow. His main points seemed to read as follows:

1. Because of its pursuit of objective knowledge by means of empirical tests, science is often said to be radically different from other forms of human activity;

2. Some people have said that unless psychoanalysis can be fitted into this concept of science, it is doomed as a system of ideas;

3. However, science isn't quite as objective as these people would have us believe: "Progress in science depends on innovation and imagination ... New insights in science depend on intuition and often fantasy." He quoted the philosopher Thomas Kuhn in support of this view, concluding there are no "transhistorical or transcultural" criteria of validity or rationality (roughly, that all objectivity is mere intersubjectivity): "The problem of paradigm choice (in science) is in the same psychological realm as political choice or religious conversion, and the history of science becomes comparable to the history of literature, art and the other humanities." He then quoted Foucault on the cultural relativity of "objective science" (roughly, that truth is just a shared delusion).

4. Therefore, he argued, "It is untenable to defend psychoanalysis by appealing to its ultimate scientific validity ... there is no such thing as a universal model of science by which it can be judged ... psychoanalysis allows us to elaborate and create knowledge of our world but does not lead to discoveries of objective facts that are universally applicable." But, he added, nor do chemistry, biology or physics. This was his defense against Popper's criticism: "To aspire to a psychoanalytic science that is empirically testable is to aspire to an outmoded concept of science."

5. Finally, he concluded: "Psychoanalysis is a method whereby we can elaborate valuable knowledge about ourselves. Its truths, like the "truths" of all sciences, are never universally valid but can be of enormous immediate

benefit. Psychoanalysis provides a basis for emotional articulation and empathy and, as such, its value for human beings is assured."

On closer reading, flaws appear in his argument. It is not clear from his paper which of the following propositions he accepts:

P1. Modern scientific methodology is excessively rigid and restrictive, and psychoanalysis is far too valuable to discard just because some unimaginative scientists say we should, or

P2. Historically, modern science has shown itself to be highly flexible, imaginative and creative, and psychoanalysis, which is all of these things, therefore fits neatly into the realm of true science.

The reason for his dilemma lay in a major error in his argument: he conflated two quite separate areas of enquiry in the philosophy of science, namely the methodology of science, and the comparative analysis of its history, or historiography. This error led him to draw what I believe to be the wrong conclusion regarding psychoanalysis. In order to clarify this opinion, it is necessary to reconsider the purpose behind the debate over the scientific status of psychoanalysis, and then look briefly at the fields of scientific methodology and historiography.

3–4. Critique of the Apologists

The continuing disputes over the status of psychoanalysis are concerned with the single issue of whether we need to take it seriously or not. Is Freud's project in the class of, say, nuclear physics or molecular biology, or should we discard it along with phrenology and pyramidology? For the practicing psychiatrist, the interest in pursuing psychoanalysis lies not in whether it can help some people feel better some of the time (as novels and sunny days can do), but whether it can actually make most people better most of the time, like exercise or antibiotics. Governments and insurers want to know why they should pay for a hugely expensive form of treatment of questionable value.

Bracken started with the strongly partisan view that psychoanalysis is a Good Thing, then cast around for convincing philosophical reasons to justify his stance. However, that is not philosophy: philosophy is about analysis. One philosophizes (i.e. analyses in a philosophical manner) rather than "uses" philosophy to win arguments. A philosophical enquiry into psychoanalysis is necessarily concerned with the question of methodology, rather than with historiography.

An analysis of the latter type would consider psychoanalysis in its historical context, comparing it abstractly with, say, Wundtian introspectionism, with Pavlov, Watson and Skinner, etc. One cannot justify a science by an appeal to metahistorical analysis. By way of illustration, Eysenck [7] used many of the same authors as Bracken to argue that his version of behaviorism is the "correct" science of psychology. It is not possible to use the same evidence to argue two incompatible points of view; the cynic is justified in saying that neither of them needs be taken seriously.

A theory is a set of propositions that attempts to go beyond the available facts. It is a conjecture or informed guess at what might be the generative mechanism underlying the observable facts. Theories are "best guesses," and anybody who forgets that point runs the risk of slipping into religiosity.

Bracken's blunt assertion that science "...is viewed as a form of discourse that secretes universal truths about the world and ourselves ..." is just not true of any of the major philosophers of science nor, I suggest, of any enlightened scientists. Only religions "secrete" universal truths, because only religions deal in universal truths. Science is much more prosaic, so how do we distinguish between science and religiosity?

In Popper's view, the proper objective of scientific research is to formulate better and better approximations of the true state of the material universe. He explicitly and repeatedly denied that there is such a thing as "scientific certainty." Instead, he argued that the only truth in science is either truism (a proposition that could not be other than true and is therefore boring) or mathematics, which is non-empirical. Mathematics is a scientific tool but is not part of the corpus of empirical science.

A large part of Popper's prolific output concerns two questions, firstly, finding a means of separating science from metaphysics, and secondly, how to choose the better of two competing scientific theories. In his carefully argued view, science is an empirical endeavor, that is, its theories are based on observation of the material universe and are open to refutation by subsequent experience. Non-scientific theories, or metaphysics, are based on existential statements. Theories of science are empirically falsifiable while theories of metaphysics are not. This is Popper's "demarcation criterion" of falsificationism and, while disarmingly simple in its definition, it is actually very complex in its application. His emphasis on the concept of falsifiability derives from the logical impossibility of determining when a metaphysical theory is incorrect, as a metaphysical theory can be "immunized" against refutation by a variety of different ploys. However, if a theory can be shown to be wrong just once, then the researcher is in the very much stronger position of knowing that his theory is not a general truth. This is the only certainty available to a scientist. In its outcome, the falsification criterion is neither subtle nor trivial.

With regard to the choice between two competing scientific theories, Popper has elaborated Tarski's theories of language [8, Ch.2] in order to formalize the notion of each theory having a truth and falsity content. Although the notion is largely intuitive, he has rendered it in axiomatic form, and the modern psychologist is therefore in a strong position when it comes to evaluating the competing claims of, say, psychoanalysis and radical behaviorism. Freud's theories were cast in the form of science current in the mid- and late nineteenth century, a form that was soon superseded because of its deficiencies. In the history of Western science, it was long believed that knowledge of the natural world (natural philosophy) could be absolute, meaning of a form such that our understanding could not be otherwise. The model of absolute knowledge was the Aristotelian syllogism:

> All dogs have four legs;
> This animal is a dog;
> Therefore, this animal has four legs.

Given the premises, the conclusion could not be otherwise. People long believed that science matched this model of inference closely, if not precisely. Unfortunately, since the natural world could not be described in an ordered series of syllogisms, deduction was not the way to go.

The failure of the deductivist model led to Baconian induction, in which the scientist attempted to draw universal truths from a limited set of observations. In fact, this is how we run our daily lives and it serves us very well. From a collection of neutral observations, the natural philosopher hoped to derive law-like generalizations. Scientific knowledge would therefore progress smoothly and inexorably via the accumulation of bigger and better sets of observations by ever-more dispassionate researchers.

This was Freud's modus operandi. He tried to devise a general psychology that could provide an answer for all possible human behavior but, in so doing, he immunized his theory against refutation: "No description whatever of any logically possible human behavior can be given which would turn out to be incompatible with the psychoanalytic theories of Freud, or of Adler, or of Jung" [8, p 38]. The infinite theoretical plasticity of the group of psychoanalytic theories places them very firmly in the metaphysical camp, not in the scientific. In this respect, Crews noted: "(Freud) thus overlooked the most fundamental requirement of investigative prudence, mistaking the mere thematic coherence produced by his method for proof that it was the single reliable method. We begin to approximate empirical rigor only when we ask whether some rival set of assumptions might make plausible sense of the same data while levying fewer demands on our trust..." [9, p 94].

Unfortunately, Freudians are blind to this criticism. A recent example of irrefutability can be seen in a careful, academic summary of basic Freudian theory [10]. Psychoanalytic theory, the authors stated, rests upon a number of basic assumptions, including that of "psychological adaptation," which they defined as "Essentially ... the assumption that the (mental) apparatus functions (among other things) to maintain a 'steady state' ... (In) the face of constant disturbances of that notional state ... all behavior and experience can be related to the processes of psychological adaptation ... This approach to adaptation is radically different from that that emphasizes adaptation to the social environment only. From the psychoanalytic point of view, even the grossest antisocial or self-damaging behavior can be considered to be the outcome of attempts at psychological adaptation" (p 145). That is to say, all behavior is necessarily the result of attempts at adaptation, meaning there is no conceivable example of human behavior that could disprove the theory. The principle of adaptation is clearly irrefutable, and is therefore non-scientific.

A potential objection to this conclusion would be that psychoanalysis can't be proven wrong just because it is correct and represents the true, objective state of human psychology. If that were true, the theory would be able to make very accurate predictions, which it most certainly cannot do: psychoanalysis is incapable of making any predictions whatsoever. In addition, the theory could be rendered as a set of axioms, essentially making it into an algorithm, and psychoanalysis could be performed by the average home computer. This isn't the case, and the objection must therefore fail.

In its application, a considerable part of the remarkable theoretical elasticity of psychoanalysis derives from the concept of ego mechanisms of defense. Despite the fact that his theory depended absolutely on this concept, Freud didn't spend much time developing it. His daughter, Anna, herself a renowned analyst, wrote the definitive monograph on the subject [11]. Freud *Pater* explained the notion metaphorically: "Let us ... compare the system of the Unconscious to a large entrance hall, in which the mental impulses jostle one another like separate individuals. Adjoining this entrance hall there is a second, narrower room—a kind of drawing-room—in which consciousness ... (also) resides. But on the threshold between these two rooms a watchman performs his function: he examines the different mental impulses, acts as a censor, and will not admit them into the drawing-room if they displease him ... it does not make much difference if the watchman turns away a particular impulse at the threshold itself or if he pushes it back across the threshold after it has entered the drawing-room ... If they have already pushed their way forward to the threshold and have been turned back by the watchman, then they are inadmissible to consciousness: we speak of them as repressed. But even the impulses which the watchman has allowed to cross the threshold are not on that account necessarily conscious as well; they can only become so if they succeed in catching the eye of consciousness." [12].

In this quaint little metaphor, the watchman constitutes the ego mechanism of defense, laboring to protect the ego or eye of consciousness from forbidden impulses. The "occupant of the drawing room" or ego is not aware of the watchman. It is clear that the model is homuncular, a classic infinite regress and, on this point alone, is not scientific. It amounts to having little bits of "mind" scattered around making decisions that are good for the larger mind but about which it knows nothing. How do these clever little defenses know what is good for me? How is one or other of the defenses switched on when a particular impulse tries to force its way into consciousness? How can the defense convert an impulse into a derivative? These types of question cannot be answered within the body of psychoanalysis. The essence of this model is that it functions as "little men inside the larger man," as unknown and (above all) unanalyzable functional components of a larger machine. They are little black boxes within the big black box that the theory was supposed to explain in the first place.

But there was never just one watchman. Later authors described many, quite a number of which are now in common use: projection, intellectualization, rationalization and reaction formation, etc. It was by virtue of these slippery defenses that any particular conscious trace could be attributed to any id impulse, and vice versa: any id impulse could be linked to any conscious element. Thus, liking bananas is sexual and not liking bananas is also sexual. This was the basis for Popper's damning criticism that there was nothing a patient could say or do that could ever convince a committed analyst that the theory was wrong (this is actually a tautology; all analysts are intensely committed otherwise they don't get through the training).

In practice, psychoanalysis was only of value as a *post hoc* justification of what was already known, a road map that can tell you where you've been but can never say what lies over the next hill. That is, psychoanalysis could never make a single prediction on which it could be found wrong, meaning it isn't science.

3-5. Other Logical Errors in the Freudian Model

The complexity of the psychoanalytic mental apparatus is one of the most striking features of Freud's theory [11]. Yet this apparatus exists in a world of its own. On the one hand, it cannot be related in any way to the vast body of empirical knowledge now known as the neurosciences while, on the other, it is incapable of generating empirically testable hypotheses [14]. In fact, in human psychology, all hypothetical mental structures are in principle irrefutable so we have to be very careful what we say about them. But how can we say anything interesting about psychology without proposing a mental structure?

One way out of this impasse is Dennett's "Intentional Stance" [15] in which he argues, among many other things, that behavior cannot be analyzed in isolation from its underlying purpose. People do things for a reason, to achieve future goals. By means of rational mental processes, we set our own priorities and work towards them. While this says nothing about the form of our self-perception, how we determine our priorities, order them or plan our activities in line with them, we can make some valid generalizations about "priority-setting, goal-directed" beings. Firstly, intentional beings need a means of comparing their current situation in the environment with their priorities, of making choices based on the available information and of putting those decisions into action. That is, they have to function (to some extent) as information processors. Secondly, every step in the process of making choices, from perception to action, must ultimately be explicable in rational terms. We can neither invoke the supernatural nor leave any gaps or loose ends in the explanatory account. Thirdly, a rational being's priorities would be ordered and internally consistent such that there would be no conflict between them.

The Freudian mental structure doesn't satisfy any of these constraints. It actually consists of a welter of homunculi, as Freud's own analogy of the ego mechanisms of defense shows. In the quote above, the homuncular (non-explanatory) nature of his "explanation" is glaringly apparent. It is mere description of a process masquerading as a structural explanation. The point about this type of pseudo-explanation is that it perforce requires a structure. In the psychoanalytic approach, a complex behavioral process is related to a physical analogy. The analogy is then broken down into its sub-parts but no further explanation of them is given. In the case of defenses, there were door-men, guests, antechambers and salons, etc. All this constitutes the theoretical "structure" but the structure is irrefutable, not the empirical behavioral process itself.

In non-explanatory analogies, a theoretical structure or apparatus becomes unavoidable. The purpose of a mental apparatus is to explain the black box of the human head; there's no point in explaining one big black box by another big one. The mental structure must give at least the illusion of an explanation, otherwise it defeats its purpose. If one postulates that the human head is full of little human heads, as Freud did, then they must acquit their functions as an organized structure or production line or they lose their *raison d'être*. The original purpose of the analogy was to render an unseen, complex process comprehensible as a series of finite steps. To this end, invoking non-explanatory sub-entities such as the ego, the id, ego defenses, etc., necessarily leads to an irrefutable mental structure just because the sub-entities are non-explanatory.

3-6. Modern Mentalism: Cognitive Psychology

If psychoanalysis represented Victorian hydraulic and mechanistic physics applied to mental life, then its modern minimalist counterpart is seen in the loose group of cognitive psychologies. This term must be used carefully as it has a number of meanings. The first, cognitive neuropsychology, is the research program that investigates the intact brain's many cognitive functions, i.e. those functions subserving knowledge that bridge the gap between neuroanatomy and physiology and human mental life. It is closely aligned with neurophysiology, perhaps not even a separate field, and some of its most interesting work is actually done in neurophysiology laboratories. For example, Alexander Luria, a major figure among early cognitive psychologists, worked in the Burdenko Institute of Neurosurgery in Moscow where he conducted seminal research on the huge numbers of brain-damaged Soviet soldiers from the Second World War [16]. Studies of memory, perception, motor control, etc., would be incomplete without the contribution of this particular branch of psychology, which leads directly to (and from) the philosophy of mind [17].

However, this rarefied type of research is not what most people mean when they use the term "cognitive psychology." In treating a disorder, a "cognitive approach" implies a much more practical and less rigorous idea than laboratory-based research. In its various manifestations, it is widely used today but, for psychologists, it represents more or less a complete rebuttal of all they have stood for over the past century. It would not be unfair to say that, in the last thirty years, psychology has quietly abandoned behaviorism in favor of its former *bête noir*, frank mentalism. How can this be reconciled with the fact that, in epistemological terms, it represents a theoretical path which, many years ago, Skinner himself [18] declared a scientific dead-end?

In an essay entitled "Why I am not a cognitive psychologist," Skinner assailed the Enlightenment idea of humans as thinking, calculating beings who control their lives by rational thought processes. He drew a picture of cognitive psychology as the notion that the conscious mind assesses information of the outside world perceived via the senses, drawing on the memory banks and other sources of knowledge to reach a decision as to the next move. This, he argued, is not an explanation of behavior but simply shifts what needs to be explained (decision-making, say) from the whole person to a "little man" or homunculus inside the head. The reason it doesn't explain anything is because, inside the little man, there must be hidden another little man who is doing the same thing for him, i.e. it is an infinite regress, and is therefore not scientific. What he said was quite correct but there are two qualifications to remember. Firstly, while it might be non-scientific, we all do it all the time and it works. Secondly, his objection will fail if and when somebody devises a model of decision-making that doesn't invoke anything like a conscious mind or such like.

In the first place, we all rely on being able to guess what other people are thinking or feeling most of the time. We have a commonsense or folk psychology model of other people's minds which, as far as models go, does a pretty good job most of the time. The commonsense model of mind tells us how people will see things, how they will react and so on, and can even tell us how to second guess people who have something to hide. However, in strict terms, it is not a model of mind because it doesn't exist *qua* Model of Mind. We do it intuitively: children, indeed, are very good at it. At a very early age, they can "sense" when somebody is happy or angry, they respond empathically to grief or fear, they can tell when somebody isn't being fair or truthful, and so on. They are responding to an innate concept of other minds: not one of them has taken lessons but a child who didn't have this ability would be in serious trouble. Autistic children don't have this ability.

Of course, as educated adults, we have developed our ideas a little beyond playground level but, as a matter of a scientific concept, that's where it is stuck. Our "cognitive model of mind" can't define emotions, it can only give examples of them. It cannot explain decisions; it only takes account of the fact that we make them. It uses memory, but cannot explain it. Granted, we can analyze the conditions under which memory works better or we can rely on the Buddhist notion that attachments cause pain but these are commonsense concepts, not true scientific constructs. They describe, but do not explain. No practicing cognitive psychologist has a formal, explanatory model of mind that goes beyond mere description of the observable phenomena; they cannot define mind independently of the observations they must explain. Yet it still works, far better than the counter-intuitive Freudian model.

In the second place, Skinner's objection will fail the day somebody devises a rational explanation for a single mental phenomenon. In fact, that has already been done. Dennett's explanatory account of decision-making removes the clever little homunculus from the cognitive model, replacing it with swarms of dumb homunculi [15]. This is the data-processing model of decision-making that I am using to write this essay. A decision is broken down to its constituent parts, to the point where a mindless machine need only answer Yes or No to a lengthy series of elementary questions. When these are reassembled, they give the solution to the complex decision that the person had to make. It breaks the infinite regress without invoking magic or non-explanatory entities.

This is a crucially important point. It gives us the germ of an idea capable of transforming the intuitive cognitive notion of mind from a descriptive pseudo-explanation to a genuinely explanatory model of mind. In Parts II and III of this work, I will expand on this point at length but, first, it is necessary to dispose of a few lesser theories in modern psychiatry.

3–7. Conclusion

Freud's error was to attempt to write a mentalist psychology without having a means of tethering it to observable reality. He accepted the classical division of mind from body, accepted the mind as a sort of reality, and applied the then-current notions of science to it. Unfortunately, the mind doesn't obey the crude hydrodynamic notions that prevailed when he studied medicine in the 1870s. Science has moved rapidly to encompass the information-processing model, but psychoanalysis is so rigid that it can't be adapted. Before we are too far into the twenty-first century, economic pressures alone will mean it is just an historical curiosity. Unfortunately, its passing will leave a gap as nobody else has devised a system of psychology so vastly satisfying to its practitioners as psychoanalysis. Whether it satisfied its patients is another question.

As it stands today, cognitive psychology is a technology, but it lacks the explanatory capacity to account for the great bulk of mental disorder. In order to do that, it would have to be endowed with a mental structure but the simple or commonsense model would then be at risk of falling into the same trap as psychoanalysis. It needs a rational, non-question-begging model that can explain the different aspects of mind, such as memory, current perception, emotion, cognition, volition, etc., and not merely describe them. Later in this essay, I will argue that such a model is within reach.

<table>
<tr><td>

4

</td><td>

Classic Dualism:
Selves and Brains

</td></tr>
</table>

4-1. Introduction

Many of our most traditional notions of the world and of our role in it are essentially dualistic, in the sense that the whole as we perceive it results from the interaction of two profoundly different parts. Humanity is composed of males and females, and in turn forms a unity with an immortal godhead. We perceive good and bad, night and day, the objective and the subjective and, central to our existence, the mind and the body. This last pairing, an awareness of dual aspects of ourselves, is deeply engrained in many cultures, perhaps all. It forms the basis of many religions and is central to most concepts of folk psychology. From early childhood, I experience myself as a thinking, feeling mind, hidden inside a physical body which I alone control by my thoughts.

Classic mind-body dualism is now usually known as Cartesian dualism, after the French mathematician and philosopher, Rene Descartes (1596-1650) who elaborated and formalized the central ideas of dualism within a Christian context. By a process of systematic doubt, Descartes arrived at a self-evident proposition so basic as to precede even belief in the Creator. Merely by thinking, I establish the incontrovertible truth that I exist: "Let the demon deceive me as much as he may," he said, "he can never bring it about that I am nothing, so long as I think I am something … (that) I am, (that) I exist is certain, as often as it is … conceived in the mind" (Meditations). He summarized this as *Cogito, ergo sum*: I think, therefore I am.

Cartesian dualism reflects an apparently unbridgeable gap between the two, fundamental aspects of human existence, the mind as "active, unextended thinking" and the body as "passive, unthinking extension." Several questions quickly follow from this stance. Firstly, what is the nature of the mental or spiritual component? We could also ask What is the nature of matter, but this question has devolved to physicists. Secondly, how does the mind or soul arise, and thirdly, how does it interact with the body? The second question, the origin of the soul, leads to another, which has probably occupied as much human thought as any other single topic, namely, what eventually happens to it?

There are many dualist theories of mental life, the great majority being of a religious nature. Since the religious mind or soul has supernatural powers, these accounts don't have to answer the three questions listed above. For them, the soul is a purely spiritual entity that arises through divine intervention, it interacts with the body miraculously, and it is usually (but not necessarily) held to be immortal. Because a religious ontology must be accepted on faith, these views aren't open to question. They can be profoundly irrational, but if they made sense, they wouldn't involve faith and therefore wouldn't be religion.

Being largely descriptive, folk psychology doesn't attempt to answer these questions beyond saying: "Well, that's just how it is." The deficiencies of this approach were well known and, early in the twentieth century, helped propel scientific psychology into the uncompromising antidualism of behaviorism. From about the same time, Freud's rigidly materialist doctrine of psychoanalysis dominated western thinking. Notions such as the subconscious and ego defenses entered common parlance, while fields as diverse as psychiatry and criminology incorporated the Freudian model almost without question.

But as the fortunes of psychoanalysis declined, helped along by frequent, often vituperative attacks by behaviorists, so too did those of dualism. Outside departments of philosophy, the concept of a non-mystical dualism became a casualty of the rush to denounce psychoanalysis. For those unwilling to embrace the mindless sterility of behaviorism, this was a very real problem as there was nothing to take its place. Dualism as a rational, materialist doctrine seemed headed for the history books. Where could the ordinary scientist turn?

Eschewing doctrinal religiosity, unable to accept the counter-intuitive excesses of psychoanalysis yet repelled by behaviorism, many people retreated into a vapid eclecticism while they waited for something better. In due course, something arrived that, at first, seemed very much better. In 1977, a quite remarkable book was published, remarkable not just for its intellectual scope, but because of the unique collaboration of its authors. *The Self and Its Brain* [1] was the result of an extended colloquium between two distinguished scholars, Sir Karl Popper and Sir John Eccles, both of whom were then well into their seventies. The three parts of their book were intended as a substantial assault on antidualism.

4-2. Popper's Case for Dualist Interaction

In the first part of the book, Popper elaborated the case against a concept basic to all materialist theories of mind, that of the closed material universe. There is more to the world, he argued, than mere physical processes; conversely, purely physical theories (of matter and energy and their interaction) can't account for the whole universe as we perceive it. He hoped to derive a theoretical case for mental-physical interactionism: "...I wish to state clearly and unambiguously that I am convinced that selves exist ... I could say of myself 'I believe in the ghost in the machine'" [1, pp 101, 105]. By virtue of its capacity to act on the real (physical) world, the mind or self must be accepted as real, albeit a different sort of reality: "...the brain is owned by the self, rather than the other way around ... The active, psycho-physical self is the active programmer to the brain (which is the computer), it is the executant whose instrument is the brain" [p120].

However, when asked to specify just what this self-thing comprises, Popper was uncommonly agnostic: "A discussion of the self, of persons and of personalities, of consciousness and of the mind, is only too liable to lead to questions like 'What is the self?' or 'What is consciousness?' But as I have often pointed out, 'what is' questions are never fruitful, although they have been much discussed by philosophers ... (They) are liable to degenerate into verbalism—into a discussion of the meaning of words or concepts, or into a discussion of definitions... such discussions and definitions are useless" [p100]. Thus, after an uncharacteristically loose discussion ("...my somewhat scattered remarks on the self..." p100), he admitted: "I do not think that what I have said ... clears up any mystery" [p129].

Perhaps Popper should have overcome his dislike of asking 'what is' questions, accepting that the "discussion of the meaning of words and concepts" can be valuable, if only as a preliminary. That way, he may have avoided his unhappy blurring of terms such as self, mind, consciousness (p129), personality, etc., because in ordinary use and in technical language, these terms aren't the same. Their differences reflect our awareness of different aspects of mental life. Ideas exist; of that much he was certain, but how they arise, where they exist, and how they relate to the physical world, he could only indicate in the most general terms.

I suggest the reasons for his failure to clear up any mysteries lie in the way he defined his field. At the outset of his case, Popper offered criticisms of a series of monist theories: "...a consistent materialist view of the world is only possible if it is combined with a denial of the existence of consciousness" (p98). Ideas exist, he said, and monist theories of mind are excellent examples of highly-developed ideas. Yet any materialist who would espouse them is forced to deny their mentality. However, and despite his rebuttal of restricted (naive) materialism, denying a rational basis for monism is not the same thing as outlining just what dualism is (a 'What is?' question). Popper did not set himself this task. Rather, he wanted to focus on the role of his (undefined) self, on: "...what it does, or what function it performs and so to a biological approach to the self" (p108). He wanted to sketch the logical status of dualist theories in general "...just because I do not believe that men are machines or automata" (p5), but not to write the definitive theory, because he didn't believe it could be done: "But I also think that complete understanding, just like complete knowledge, is unlikely ever to be achieved" (p37). The central questions of dualism (the origin and nature of mind and mind-body interaction) he left unanswered, just as when Descartes framed them some 350 years ago.

4–3. Eccles' Outline of Dualist Interaction

In their joint work, the philosopher outlined the logical necessity of a dualist interactionist theory of mind. To the neurophysiologist, Sir John Eccles, fell the Sisyphean task of attempting an explanation of Descartes' enigma of dualist interaction, of just how a non-material mind might interact with the material body. While neither author could describe the "Self" in any detail, if the brain was not of a form that could admit extracorporeal intervention, then their theory was still-born. Eccles undertook his task with a full awareness of the limitations of the neurosciences in the mid-1970s. At the outset, he warned bluntly: "It is not claimed here that our present scientific understanding of the brain will solve any of the philosophical problems that are the theme of this book" (p226). But note that, by concentrating on the function of the Self, Popper had also declined to accept the challenge of some of those questions.

The brain, Eccles argued at length, is a "machine of almost infinite complexity and subtlety," organized in such a way that it can be influenced by non-material events. Residing in intimate relationship with this clever but mindless machine is a non-physical entity, the Self-Conscious Mind (SCM) which, essentially, comprises the human element in our animal bodies: "...the SCM is an independent entity that is actively engaged in reading out from the multitude of active centers in the modules of the liaison areas of the dominant cerebral hemisphere. (It) selects from these centers in accord with its attention and its interests and integrates its selection to give the unity of conscious experience ... It also acts back on the neural centers ... (It) exercises a superior interpretive and controlling role upon the neural events by virtue of a two-way interaction across the interface between the (physical world and the world of mental states)" (p355). In simple terms, Eccles' Self-Conscious Mind is the traditional Spirit that our grandparents said separated us from "the beasts of the field" (this does not imply that animals don't have some sort of awareness).

4–4. Metaphysics and Dualist Interaction

But what is this remarkable thing that, "...in a sense plays on the brain, as a pianist plays on a piano or as a driver plays on the controls of a car" (Popper, p495)? This is the crux of their case, the point on which the whole, elaborate theory hangs. In fact, it just *is* the theory. The rest is mere background material whose truth or falsity doesn't affect the central idea. Their central idea, that there is a non-material Self, mind or whatever, is wholly a metaphysical assertion, i.e. any empirical evidence you can bring to bear on the question can also be shown to support an alternative view. In fact, it is surprising that Popper in particular allowed himself to be drawn into conjectures of this type, as he had often declared himself to be totally opposed to existential statements, blind assertions of the form "There is..." [2, p68 *et seq*]. His reason for opposing theories of this type is that they are not falsifiable, and therefore do not fall within the ambit of science. But the whole book depended on unquestioning acceptance of the existential statement: "Selves exist." If you don't accept that point, then don't buy the book.

So, at the outset, their joint theory fails Popper's own test of what constitutes science and, despite its lather of neurophysiology, their book remains a bald exercise in metaphysics. When we search Eccles' contribution for his account of the nature of the SCM, we find only blunt assertions that it exists and that it can influence the brain. He also showed that the brain was ineffably complex; what he didn't show was that it was of a form that could be influenced by non-material events. But these, surely, are the points their theory needed to answer before any credibility could attach to it. At the crunch, all they could say was: "We believe this to be true."

Perhaps this is unfair. Eccles set himself the task of showing how a non-material entity (the SCM) might interact with the material brain, not of explaining the nature of the SCM itself. Since Eccles argued his case from the point of a neurophysiologist, while Popper took the more general case. If either author had that duty, it should have been the philosopher. In effect, Popper argued that it was in theory both necessary and possible to build a bridge across the chasm (of the Mind-Body Problem), while Eccles assembled the ramps on and off the bridge. But at the critical point, where the bridge was supposed to meet in the middle, there was a gap. Messages were passed from one side to the other (from mind to body) by a spirit, which is more or less what animists have been saying for millennia. Daniel Dennett dismisses this type of solution to the problem as tantamount to saying: "And then a miracle occurs." Granted Eccles had in mind only a very small miracle that wouldn't do much to disturb the fabric of the real universe, but we should still reject it, like the stern father whose weeping daughter pleads: "But daddy, I'm only a little bit pregnant!" Let a little miracle through the gate, and big ones will get through, too.

There are many other, substantial failings in this work, the majority of them in Eccles' part, mainly because of the difficulties of translating the theory into practice. For example, there is a very real problem with sleep. What happens when we go to sleep? Crucial parts of the brain shuts down, meaning there is nothing for the SCM to read. We therefore have no memory of these periods until, during REM sleep, the cortex is activated in a disorganized way and we dream. But why do we have no memory during deep sleep? While the brain closes down, why doesn't the SCM continue its own party? The memory banks are still alive, they're still working. General anesthesia, epilepsy and protracted coma confirm that when the vital brain centers temporarily stop functioning, there is nothing, no awareness, not even an awareness of nothing. So we can have proof of the existence of the SCM only when it has access to the intact brain's memory stores or its sensory input, etc. What does the SCM do that a materialist model of brain can't?

We have no knowledge of thinking or of other mental events taking place in the SCM independently of its interaction with the fully functional brain. But if we can't test for it, then it can't be presumed to exist, except that, in Eccles' theory, the SCM must have memory capacity of its own (it selects "according to attention and interest..." p495: there can be no coherent interest without memory). Attention, however, is purely a physiological function, so if there is no testable memory in the SCM, it is well on its way to becoming superfluous. Similarly, if we argue that the brain sleeps in order to give the SCM a rest, we have introduced an homunculus and thence an infinite regress. On the other hand, if we argue that the SCM is a mindless parasite, functioning only by accessing brain functions, we defeat the purpose of having it. Popper and Eccles' theory of the Self-Conscious Mind is supposed to be a theory of mind, not of mindlessness.

All this suggests Eccles was unwittingly arguing a case for monist materialism, not substance dualism. Teased out in this manner, Eccles' apparently convincing physiological arguments continue in endless circles. This is unavoidable, simply because the fundamental ideas are metaphysical and empirical evidence is therefore completely beside the point. In many areas, his evidence was at least equally supportive of the materialist case. *Ignoratio elenchi*: Eccles argued the wrong case. At its core, their theory was philosophical, not neurophysiological, but they didn't answer the critical philosophical questions.

While the book was interesting, particularly after so many years of rigid antidualism, it did little to advance answers to the questions posed by Cartesian dualism. Armstrong summed it up succinctly: "I don't think it is a very good book. The Eccles material doesn't do anything to prove dualism ... The great dualist counter-attack has still to be launched" [3, p 35]. Central to Armstrong's critique is the notion that anybody espousing dualism has to prove his case: only religions and politics don't require proof. Popper and Eccles didn't prove their case. It would appear that the reason for their failure was because their entire argument rested on a fundamental misconception, that they believed there cannot be a materialist form of dualism.

In Eccles' section of the book, his bias was perfectly clear. He believed in the immortality of the soul (p 555) and assembled a supportive theory that was an open affront to the laws of physics (p 355). That's quite legitimate, but there should be no doubt that one cannot hold spiritualist beliefs within a strictly materialist ontology. In fact, Eccles nowhere states that he is working within a strictly materialist ontology. He seemed to be under the impression that materialism had very clear limits and could be discarded whenever it didn't give the answers he wanted. Unfortunately, it appears that in this respect, the neurophysiologist was led astray by the philosopher, as Popper had previously mounted an extensive case against what he called materialism.

In his third chapter, entitled "Materialism Criticized," Popper argued that the central notion in materialism is that the physical world is closed and must therefore be understood entirely in terms of physical processes. While some materialist theories accept the idea of mental events, they do not assign a causally significant role to the mind. Given this definition, Popper listed four fundamental types of materialist theory:

1. Radical materialism, in the form of radical behaviorism, in which mental and/or conscious processes are deemed not to exist;

2. Panpsychism, which allows the existence of mental processes but, because it depends on the doctrine of parallelism, denies them a causative role;

3. Epiphenomenalism, which says that mental events exist but are of no causal significance; and

4. Identity theory, which says that abstract knowledge does not exist.

It should be recalled that the colloquium on which this book was based took place in 1974 but, even then, Popper's list of materialist philosophies was old-fashioned and incomplete. It implies that there cannot be a materialist form of dualist interactionism, a conclusion that would surprise many modern philosophers [4, 5]. Popper's restrictive view of materialism is flawed, for example, in his assertion that identity theory denies the existence of abstract knowledge. What identity theory says is that, as a matter of fact, all mental events just are brain events. This includes those events that comprise knowledge of abstract theories, including, of course, the theory of the identity of mind and brain. It is also not the case that panpsychism denies mental events a causative role. Panpsychism doesn't say anything about what minds can or can't do, all it says is how minds arise. I can be a panpsychist materialist, or a panpsychist spiritualist, as the fancy takes me.

Thus, Eccles launched into his account with a license to range beyond the confines of materialism. Neither he nor his co-author could ever complain, then, if somebody else took their license and drove a little further than they did: to tree-nymphs, for example. If we open the door to one sort of magical spirit, we open the door to all of them, which is what Popper's concept of a demarcation criterion is all about.

The most interesting difference between the co-authors lies in their attitudes to immortality. Eccles was emphatic: "I cannot believe that this wonderful gift of a conscious existence has no further future, no possibility of another existence under some other unimaginable conditions" (p555). Popper was equally emphatic: "I don't look forward to an eternity of survival. On the contrary, the idea of going on for ever seems to me utterly frightening" (p556). There is no a priori reason why their Self should be immortal. The only requirement for ghosts is that they be immaterial: why can't their "ghost" be as mortal as the "machine" in which it rides? This leads to the question of whether there can be a natural mentalism an idea which, until quite recently, did not have a large following.

4-5. A Note On Skinner's Anti-Dualism

As previously outlined, Skinner's radical behaviorism more or less equated mentalism with the supernatural. His theory demanded the removal of all traces of mentalism as a causally significant factor [6]. Skinner saw only two aspects of the inner world, the physical realm of the body, and a fleeting, inconsequential world of experience, etc. Despite everything he said, he dismissed the latter as of no causal significance. All that counted was biological: "A small part of the universe is contained within the skin of each of us ... eventually, we should have a complete account of it from anatomy and physiology" [7, p24].

This is quite a clear statement of reductive materialism. Introspection, he averred, could tell us nothing of note: "An organism behaves as it does because of its current structure, but most of this is out of reach of introspection." While Skinner insisted his theories did not dismiss mentalism as either unobservable or as subjective, he certainly acted as if it were both. He claimed that a proper understanding of the effects of the environment on the organism allows us to dispense with all mentalist talk. This is partly because "(s)ome can be 'translated into behavior'... (while the rest can be) discarded as unnecessary or meaningless" [5, p19].

In common usage, mentalism equates with dualism, which has long meant Cartesian 'substance dualism.' This is unfortunate as 'dualism' need not imply two substances. It merely implies two very different things that, taken or acting together, amount to a new unity. The material universe consists of the interchangeable dualism of matter and energy. The Manichaean dualism of good and evil does not imply any substances at all, yet it is nearly as old as recorded human thought. Mentalism as such is compatible with a whole range of dualist theories with no implication of immortality or other supernatural powers. But dualism doesn't need to stop with mind and brain; perhaps mind itself is a further duality of, say, perception and decision-making which are only contingently related in the brain. For a natural account of mind, this would be most convenient. Followed to its limits, this approach could help materialism because we already have very good, natural models of dumb decision-making [6].

Following his program to its limits, a goal Skinner acknowledged was beyond him, would lead to an account of behavior with no room for mentalist "intervening variables." Under his enormously powerful influence, generations of psychologists were trained in the notion that anything less than the most rigid monism was mere fantasy. This included the highly influential Freudian theories that dominated psychiatry and many other fields. The critical question for Skinner, which he never answered, was: Can there be a non-mentalist psychology? His whole work hinged on this question, which was logically prior to the questions that occupied him throughout his long career. He made no attempt to answer it. But if a non-mentalist psychology is impossible, then what form should the ensuing dualism take?

4–6. Conclusion

It has previously been argued that there cannot be a non-mentalist human psychology. Mental events cannot be reduced to mere brain events, nor can we dispense with mentalist predicates, meaning we cannot have a fully explanatory, non-mentalist theory of psychology. The lesson from Skinner is therefore twofold, that a non-mentalist psychology is necessarily incomplete, while mentalism itself does not equate with the supernatural.

Popper and Eccles work showed again that metaphysical questions cannot be answered using empirical knowledge. If we are committed to dualism, meaning we need some immaterial element to complete the causative chain, yet we wish to remain within a materialist ontology, we need to devise a natural form of mentalism *before* anybody tries to say how the ghost, spirit, self, mind, etc., will interact with the body. This is not a minor point, because, fully articulated, a naturalistic theory of mental life would not have a mind-body disjunction. A naturally-occurring mind should be able to interact with the equally natural body without violating any known physical principles: that's what natural means. If we wish to talk about a "ghost" in the human machine, we need to remember that ghosts don't have to be supernatural: insubstantial, yes, but insubstantial does not imply supernatural. If the physical body is run by a virtual machine based in or deriving from an information-processing realm, then the physical principles on which we base our understanding of the Universe will remain intact. This point will be explored in detail in Part II.

5 The Concept of An Eclectic Psychiatry

5-1. Introduction

With the clarity of hindsight, it is easy to look back critically at the main theories used in psychiatry over the last 120 years or so and wonder why they were ever accepted. While their errors are now obvious, the answer is surely because, at the time, they seemed convincing, far better than what had gone before. Thus, it has been suggested, perhaps we should avoid making any strong commitment to a particular theory in case it too turns out to be wrong.

The idea of picking bits from a range of theories or schools, thereby forming a new whole, is quite old. In the seventeenth century, artists and philosophers who followed this approach were named eclectics, from the Greek "to select." It is not clear when the term was first used in psychiatry, because it has traditionally been applied only to the humanities and not to scientific fields. Nonetheless, it has become widely used in psychiatry. An eclectic psychiatrist is one who practices a moderate type of psychiatry, using whatever seems likely to work, while deliberately avoiding the more extreme schools.

In an eclectic department of psychiatry, it is possible to hear the staff talking about one patient in behaviorist terms, about the next from a strictly biological viewpoint, and the third wholly in psychodynamic terms. Practitioners try to fit the theory to the patient, rather than vice versa, and there is a lot to be said for this pragmatic approach. Indeed, as first psychoanalysis and then behaviorism came under accurate and sustained criticism, eclectic psychiatry came to be seen as eminently sensible. Eclecticism became a mark of moderation in an intellectually unstable world. Polite psychiatrists felt no qualms in adopting the middle path while they got on with helping people get better.

In large parts of the English-speaking world, eclecticism also served to conceal the fact that, very often, its supporters knew next to nothing about the theories they were pirating. By avoiding commitments, people were able to make a virtue of the necessity forced upon them by their intellectually barren training. The fact that nobody had ever attempted an intellectual justification of eclecticism was not seen as a disadvantage; the justification of moderation is self-evident.

5-2. Eclecticism as a Virtue

One such attempt was published as part of an essay competition in 1995. Trainee psychiatrists were invited to expatiate upon a quote from an esteemed Australian psychiatrist: "Although science is an essential part of psychiatry, it is not its essence." Subsequently, the editors published one paper [1] because they regarded it as an "excellent" commentary on the subject, and therefore included it after the competition's winning entries. The author searched for the "essence of psychiatry" somewhere between the rock of "Freud's metapsychology" and the hard place of the neurobiological tradition of Santiago Ramon y Cajal. He couldn't find it: "Given the countless tributaries that flow into mainstream clinical psychiatry, it goes without saying that psychiatry is an eclectic discipline ... Psychiatry certainly makes use of a bewildering array of explanatory models."

While this approach had its value, it evoked in him a particular fear, that because psychiatry is "intellectually vulnerable" ("vulnerable" long ago replaced the word "weak" in psychiatric circles), it has the damaging, cyclical tendency to rush madly after "fundamentally incoherent" practices. This urge must be resisted: "A more avowed eclecticism in which competing paradigms are held in an uneasy equilibrium might serve as a pragmatic way to avoid being carried in by one tide and out by the next." Despite the fact that eclecticism can "...lead the clinical psychiatrist into a good deal of tightrope walking," he saw a lack of theoretical commitment as an advantage: "An eclectic psychiatry mirrors a diverse world, a world wracked with uncertainty and overloaded with information."

But, he warned, eclecticism is a double-edged sword. It allows or even encourages psychiatrists to become "intellectual jackdaws," whimsically chasing after "...rubbish, odds and ends that don't fit together in any particular way, baubles selected only because they happened to glitter brightly..." Eclecticism must be subject to a guiding principle, and he felt that empiricism is just that principle, although he warned that it "cannot be brought to bear on everything that lies within the domain of psychiatry." He concluded: "The more questions psychiatry tries to answer, the more eclectic it must become, and the more ... it has need of an empirical methodology to make sense of the world. Perhaps this is the essence of psychiatry."

5-3. Eclecticism as a Vice

It is perhaps revealing of the state of theorizing in psychiatry that the journal's editors, who lauded Knight's paper, did not detect its many errors. For example, Freud did not write a metapsychology. Metapsychology is philosophy. Freud wrote a metaphysical psychology, meaning a psychology based in premises that could not be determined empirically, i.e. straight metaphysics, in the worst sense. Also, and despite our long misuse of the term, eclecticism does not apply to matters scientific. It applies to art. One can be an eclectic sculptor, an eclectic cook, even an eclectic architect, but not an eclectic scientist. Eclecticism means borrowing freely from styles which differ only on aesthetic grounds. So when psychiatrists boast that they choose freely from such diverse fields as neurobiology, psychodynamics and behaviorism, not to mention every social fad that wafts past, they are effectively claiming that these schools can only be distinguished aesthetically, not scientifically. In making this claim, they surely can't expect to be taken seriously.

In a real science, there is a larger discipline governing what the practitioner will believe (read: accept as provisionally true). I cannot be a Lamarckian evolutionist just because the fancy takes me. I have to bend my prejudices to the prevailing scientific ethos, not vice versa. But in psychiatry, I can formulate a patient's present state in a variety of mutually irreconcilable ways and nobody can criticize me. In fact, psychiatrists see this kind of rubbery intellect as a virtue, not realizing that an eclectic science is a solecism. Furthermore, a psychiatric eclecticism cannot be modified by empiricism just because many of the fundamental questions bedeviling our field are wholly metaphysical, and by definition, cannot be decided by empirical evidence. Metaphysical means non-empirical.

But if people claim [1, 2] that psychiatry is an eclectic field, what exactly are they saying? The immediate implication is that practitioners can pick and choose, more or less as they see fit, from what is on offer within the field and, quite likely, from outside as well. If so, this would be a strange form of science [3], but eclectics may retreat from this charge, saying that psychiatry isn't a science. To some, this is not a handicap [4]; to others, it is a definite weakness [5]. In a practical field such as ours, one can be eclectic in three distinct areas: in theory, in research and in the practice of getting people better. Taking each of these areas in turn, I will show that there is no virtue in the idea of an eclectic psychiatry.

5-4. Theoretical Eclecticism

Theoretically, a psychiatrist can embrace the biological approach, any one of many psychodynamic stances (including cognitive psychology), adopt one or other school of behaviorism or be wholly sociological. An eclectic would not feel restricted to one or other of these, but would be free to pick and choose *ad lib*. In fact, this is how psychiatry is normally practiced throughout most of the world. People accept that some conditions are biologically-determined, while formulating others in behaviorist, cognitive or psychodynamic terms.

Unfortunately, the various schools are incompatible, and only one, if any, can be right. If biological psychiatry is correct, then introspective psychotherapy is a waste of time and money. Similarly, if the psychodynamic approach is correct, then using drugs to suppress symptoms of critical psychological significance would be culpable. More likely, they are all curate's eggs, good in parts and bad in others. But the rationale for the picking and choosing is historical. There is nothing in psychiatry that will allow us to look at a condition and say: "Yes, this is necessarily biologically-determined, but that one could not be other than psychological." The allocation of a disorder (if we agree it is a disorder) to one category or another is determined not by a pre-existing formula, but by argument from authority (the ICD and DSM systems), by votes (DSM III and homosexuality), by fashion (meaning where one trained), serendipity (where the patient is admitted) and by economics (if the psychotherapy is expensive, then the condition must be biological; see [6]).

So how does the budding psychiatrist choose the correct theory? Truth is, he doesn't. Trainee psychiatrists are taught what their teachers believe; they are most definitely not encouraged to question what their teachers believe. And where did the teachers learn their theory? From other, older psychiatrists who were in turn expanding on what they were taught way back in the thirties and forties. As long as everybody agrees to be eclectic in the same directions, to pick and choose roughly the same dishes from the smorgasbord, as it were, there won't be any friction. For example, homosexuality was a mental disease until we all agreed that it wasn't.

The notion that one can assemble a rational, coherent theory by pinching bits and pieces from other people's theories is not to be taken seriously. I have never heard anybody claim it can be done, but people commonly act as though it can be. Anybody who thinks it is possible is shouldering a heavy burden of proof. Pending such a proof, I assert that theoretical eclecticism is pure caprice (from the Latin for goat).

5-5. Eclectic Research

The psychiatric research program should be dictated by the accepted theoretical position [3], but that's a bit difficult when we don't have an accepted position. At present, biology rules the roost, as demonstrated by the pendular swing in the American psychiatric literature over the past twenty-five years. A generation ago, the American psychiatric literature was largely an exercise in latter-day Freudianism. Nowadays, it is mainly about neurochemistry, genes and fMRI scans, and the more abstruse, the better.

In poorer countries such as ours, we spend our research budgets counting things. Cheap computers have made everybody an epidemiologist. Who are more likely to experience orgasm with masturbation, young women with bulimia or matched controls? [7] How does the significance of this little gem change if bulimia is biological, if it is psychological, or sociological? Who smoke more, Chinese patients with schizophrenia or Western? Before answering, note that nicotine alters the firing rate of ventral tegmental dopamine cells, leading to an increase in dopamine levels in the nucleus accumbens. In rats [8]. It looks like science, but I assert that this type of "knowledge" is mere scientism, the uncritical application of scientific or quasi-scientific methods to inappropriate fields of study.

It is commonplace in science for disciplines to borrow freely from the methods or techniques developed in other fields, which may be why some people believe that science as a whole is an eclectic pursuit. For example, behaviorist methods have been used with striking success in neurophysiology, physical research into isotopic decay soon led to tracer techniques in physiology and pathology and, of course, a statistical method is no sooner developed than it is grabbed by everyone. No field has a prerogative over methods. Methods belong to the scientific community, and if they can properly be applied to another field, then it would be improper not to apply them. But methodological eclecticism is not in itself science, nor does it render the whole scientific program eclectic.

The problem in psychiatry is that no other scientific endeavor has developed a methodology suitable to the peculiarities of our field. Research into human mental life has had to adapt to the highly restricted methodology of positivist science, not the other way around. So long as we continue to borrow other people's techniques, we can comfort ourselves with the idea that our research follows the very best available procedures. That they are often not appropriate does not impinge on the collective consciousness, and we therefore feel no compulsion to develop our own.

Thomas Kuhn [4] distinguished between what he termed 'revolutionary science' and 'normal science.' Normal science is the steady, pedestrian exploration of a theory or paradigm to its limits. Normal science "...seems an attempt to force nature into the preformed and relatively inflexible box that the paradigm supplies. No part of the aim of normal science is to call forth new sorts of phenomena; indeed those that will not fit the box are often not seen at all" [p 24]. 'Normal' psychiatric research is not designed to show the existing theory's weaknesses, as the examples given above clearly demonstrate. Its function is to reinforce the status quo, although how most published research manages that is not entirely clear.

The research program in biological psychiatry was set nearly 150 years ago when the British alienist Henry Maudsley announced: "Mental disease is brain disease." Bolstered as it was by the early discovery of the cause of GPI, there has never been a proper examination of this hypothesis [5]. Since then, the program aimed at forcing psychiatry into a biological box has soldiered on, oblivious to the total lack of proof of the underlying thesis. This doesn't deter anybody; as Kuhn observed forty years ago, normal science isn't designed to shake the foundations of the ruling paradigm. Indeed, psychiatry's research program would suggest that pointless results are often preferable to shocking results. The world of "normal" psychiatric research just is not about changing the dominant paradigm.

5-6. An Eclectic Psychiatry in Practice

Practice, of course, should be guided by theory and controlled by research, but in psychiatry, practice is a matter of grabbing whatever seems to work. Sometimes this approach works (e.g. the sedative properties of some drugs discovered by antihistamine researchers in the early fifties) and sometimes it doesn't (frontal leucotomy, insulin therapy and deep sleep therapy, to name but a few). Lacking a guiding theory to determine in advance which therapies are acceptable and which aren't, we are forced to make this crucial decision by consensus, usually after the event.

The periodic catastrophes in psychiatric practice are not mere aberrations against which we have no protection, but are rendered highly likely because of the nature of our field. We lack a coherent theoretical basis to our practice but practitioners are desperate to do something for their patients. Encouraging people to pinch bits from other fields as they push further and further into the unknown inevitably puts us at risk. Because we operate by consensus, and because nobody knows enough theory to say unequivocally whether something is loopy, and because the profession is locked into self-justification, not self-criticism [9], nobody can stop the adventurers until it is too late. Somewhere out there, an exuberant soul is cooking up our next scandal—and nobody can tell him not to.

5-7. Conclusion

The problem of 'eclecticism' has the insidious effect of licensing those who don't like the party line to try whatever takes their respective fancies. At the same time as they are quietly and ominously exercising their creativity on the fringes, the social trends in science outlined by Kuhn are working within the mainstream to suppress innovation. Despite opinions to the contrary [4], there is no historical or logical reason to suppose that truly innovative changes will arise within the orthodox heartland of the profession. Classically, new ideas are contributed by recent recruits to the field or by the intellectually dissatisfied. Also classically, their ideas are resisted very strongly by the "recognized authorities." Kuhn quoted the glum conclusion of the nuclear physicist, Max Planck: "...a new scientific truth does not triumph by convincing its opponents and making them see the light, but rather because its opponents eventually die" [p 151].

Psychiatry is not like nuclear physics. Not only can the professors not say why the unorthodox psychiatrist shouldn't be doing what he is doing, but we won't in fact know what he is doing until after the damage is done. This is because people who don't accept standard views are rapidly marginalized. There is no place in a university department of psychiatry for heretics. As is true of orthodoxy in any system of human ideas the world over, orthodox psychiatry doesn't like being questioned. Trainees are rewarded not for original thought, but for creative regurgitation of the party line, as in the essay competition mentioned above. As Kuhn noted, those who challenge that line are quickly pushed away from the intellectual center. But, and herein lies the problem for psychiatry, unorthodox trainees will have been well-trained in the habit of raiding other disciplines for ideas before they are finally shown the door. The intellectually restive young psychiatrist will then be left to his (sometimes her) own devices, politely ignored by the mainstream and free to do more or less as he pleases—until the police come knocking on the door.

Eclecticism in psychiatry is a dangerous myth. It allows us to avoid the unpleasant realization that we are the only medical specialty without a sound theoretical basis to our practice. It helps to provide orthodox psychiatry with a sense of immunity against accusations of theoretical inadequacy. It fosters the notion that techniques are more important than theories, and permits a smug self-satisfaction in the face of our failure to develop methodologies appropriate to our field's requirements. Above all, it encourages psychiatrists who feel alienated from the mainstream to experiment without being subject to normal processes of accountability.

I can't see any point in encouraging budding psychiatrists in the type of emollient displacement activity represented by the essay competition. We should urge them to follow Popper's injunction and submit our theories to severe criticism. Meanwhile, trying to justify the unjustifiable, such as "empirical eclecticism", serves only to shield us from admitting that, in the main, we haven't a clue what we are doing. Despite arguments to the contrary, an eclectic psychiatry is pure humbug (n. 1. a person or thing that tricks or deceives, 2. nonsense, rubbish).

6

The Biopsychosocial Model in Psychiatry

6-1. Introduction

For several decades, many psychiatrists throughout the world saw eclecticism as a more reasonable stance than any of the mainstream theories, but eclecticism was never a body of knowledge and doesn't dictate practice. Being an eclectic was really more of a moral position, a moderate and moderating ontology that says only: "Forget the theory, use what works." But what works for one person may not work for the next, so it could never tell, say, a junior psychiatrist how to treat a particular case. It could only justify a low-key approach more or less in keeping with what the neophyte was going to do anyway, which was in turn more or less what his teachers would have done themselves.

Eclecticism was never a body of knowledge. There were no authorities on the topic, no journals of eclectic psychiatry, no conferences or seminars. While there were plenty of departments that would proudly have said they were of an eclectic orientation, not one of them had the word on a door or a letterhead. There were eclectic professors, but no Professors of Eclectic Psychiatry. In truth, being an eclectic psychiatrist was a claim so broad and so general as to be meaningless, a courtesy but never a challenge. Occasionally, somebody might comment that being an eclectic was a euphemism being too frightened to make a commitment, but psychiatrists saw their moderation as a virtue.

6-2. The Need for a Moderate Approach

In its daily application, eclecticism had to be rephrased or recast in a form that was both moderate and recognizably scientific. The vacuum between theory and practice was eventually filled by a working and very practical psychiatrist, George Engel. In a series of papers starting in 1960 [1-5], Engel outlined what he saw as deficiencies in the dominant "Biomedical Model" as it applied to medicine in general and to psychiatry in particular. He characterized the Biomedical Model as reductionist ("...the language of chemistry and physics will ultimately suffice to explain biological phenomena" [2, p 130]) and dualist, i.e. it separated the intangible mind from the physical body. Despite the undoubted success of the Biomedical Model (in the 1960s, it seemed very successful), Engel saw its drive to discount mental life as a major fault. Humans are not just biological preparations, he argued, but exist as sentient beings in a causally significant psychological and sociological matrix, of which the Biomedical Model gives no account. A true science of human affairs would be able to incorporate these settings.

He acknowledged that his complaints against the dominant ethos were not new, that "psychosomatic medicine" had been offered as the bridge between the "two parallel but independent ideologies of medicine, the biological and the psychosocial." That particular bridge had failed, he believed, because it was forced to conform to "scientific methodologies basically mechanistic and reductionist in conception and inappropriate for many of the problems under study," i.e. psychoanalysis [2, p 134]. In his view, the psychosomatic model failed because it was based in Freudian and Meyerian concepts, and he implicitly acknowledged that there was no way these could be formalized into a system compatible with the Biomedical Model. In the first place, the methodology of modern science could not analyze constructs based in these theories and secondly, empirical research failed to validate crucial elements such as the disease-specificity model. Therefore, in order to advance where psychosomatic medicine had become mired in irrelevancies, he offered a new approach, the Biopsychosocial Model. This, he claimed, was a scientific model where the psychosomatic had not been. In place of the unproductive Freudian concepts, he suggested that a new approach, Von Bertalanffy's General Systems Theory (GST) [6], provided a suitable orientation. Its particular strength lay in its purported capacity to permit scientific investigation across the different levels of a hierarchy without attempting to reduce higher levels to lower, or even dispensing with them, as the reductionist Biomedical Model did.

After a final tilt at the prevailing "impersonal and mechanical" teaching in US medical schools in the mid-seventies, Engel concluded: "The proposed biopsychosocial model provides a blueprint for research, a framework for teaching, and a design for action in the real world of health care. Whether it will be useful or not remains to be seen" [2, p 135]. This chapter will argue that any value that may have derived from Engel's Biopsychosocial Model has been entirely fortuitous, because it is not a model at all. Furthermore, even if there could be a genuinely biopsychosocial model, George Engel never wrote it.

6–3. The Role of Models in Science

Models are absolutely fundamental to the progress of science. All the more surprising, then, when we realize just how little of the philosophical work on defining what a model is or does [7] has percolated through to the scientific literature. My dictionary gives nine definitions of the noun 'model,' mostly about toys or young women in expensive clothes. The ninth definition states: "A simplified representation or description of a system or complex entity, esp. one designed to facilitate calculations and predictions." This is the technical sense in which we use the word in psychiatry, but as with so many of our technical terms, the word has lost much of its specificity over the years. While we may believe we have models, the following brief review of the literature will show that, in fact, we don't.

In ordinary usage in the non-medical literature, two meanings of the word 'model' are readily apparent. These need to be considered in some detail, in order to show how far we have strayed from the theoretical mainstream. Lacey's dictionary of philosophy states: "A scientific model is normally a theory intended to explain a given realm of phenomena, or a sort of picture intended to explain a theory by replacing its terms with more perspicuous ones" [8]. This is not entirely perspicuous itself: is a model a theory or is it the realization of a theory?

To Beer [9], the matter is less opaque: a model is "a representation of something else, designed for a special purpose ... All models have one characteristic in common ... the *mapping* of elements in the system modeled onto the model" (p 394-5, his emphasis). He distinguished isomorphic models, in which every element of the larger system is mapped, and homomorphic, in which complexity is deliberately sacrificed. He also saw a difference between physical models (as in the model aircraft used in wind tunnel experiments) and systems of mathematical equations that "model the behavior" of the particular theoretical system.

In *The Nature of Explanation*, Achinstein [10] did not explain the difference between a theory of explanation and a model of explanation, although it is clear from his usage that theories and models are conceptually quite different. A theory is a broad, general statement while the model of the theory is the actualization of the theory, the (truncated) theory at work, as it were. In the field of semantics, Leech [11] emphasized this important difference between theories and their models: "Whereas theories claim to tell us what reality is like, models claim to tell us what reality can and could be like—given certain speculative assumptions."

The work of the philosopher Karl Popper was entirely devoted to theories: how to distinguish scientific theories from non-scientific, why we should prefer one theory to another, how science progresses via its successive theories, etc. To Popper, theories were ideas of the highest and most abstract kind. He used the term "model" sparingly, and almost always in a real and mechanical sense [12, e.g. pp 172, 358-9]. In Popper's evolutionary view, the value of theories is that we can let them die in our places, but we will also construct a long series of models before suspecting the theory itself. The theory of heavier-than-air flight survived many crashed models.

One of the most influential modern philosophers of mind, Daniel Dennett, has, at times, tended to use the terms "theory" and "model" interchangeably while, at others, he has distinguished clearly between the theory and the model that simulates the theory in action [13]. Theories are ideas, he says, and as such, they can have only logical consequences. By contrast, the whole point of models is that they are "experience generators," acting rapidly to generate an approximation of the material consequences that flow from the application of the theory. He emphasizes that models must be distinguishable from the real things they model. Nobody can get wet from a computer model of a hurricane (p 191) derived from a larger theory of weather.

At this stage, the two meanings of the noun "model" are quite clear. A minority of authors use theory and model more or less interchangeably to represent any abstract idea or notion. The majority use the terms quite separately, reserving theory to nominate large, unembodied concepts or abstract notions, and model for the class of smaller real things, usually simplified diminutives of the unseen objects and processes outlined in the theories.

In the somewhat less disciplined social sciences, things are never quite so clear. Ryan [14] accepted the Popperian notion of submitting theories to severe or critical tests: "Given a (theoretical) generalization, we want to see if it holds under unusual conditions ... successful causal laws are those which apply under the most improbable conditions" (p 64). He saw it as important to "unravel the distinction between theories and such close relations as models, maps, metaphors and analogies" (p 76). Theories, he suggested, make existential claims about the world, i.e. they say that this is how things are. Models, on the other hand, do not. They simply say it is *as if* this is how things are: "Those who produce models do not make existential claims about the world; but those who produce theories generally do..." (p 95).

The common element in these accounts of models (physical, diagrammatic and mathematical), lies in their function: models model. What do they model? They model theories or theoretical constructs, meaning they embody, actualize or realize an idea, notion or concept. The original idea consists of a series of propositions (a belief system) regarding the nature of reality. Such propositions are almost always metaphysical, and therefore lie outside the purview of science as we now define it. Nonetheless, there is no escaping them: our science is suspended in a web of metaphysical assumptions. But to be science, the propositions must be cast in a form that permits empirical testing, which is where the model comes into its own.

Simply stated, the purpose behind a model is to see if, at a first approximation, the theory works, to actualize its logical consequences and thereby subject it to the kinds of "severe tests" that Popper saw as essential to scientific progress. In this sense, models are real and their material consequences can be measured. Theories are ideas and, while their logical consequences can be predicted, they can no more be measured than daydreams. Model-building separates the theories with a future from those that will always remain dreams. What is the relationship between a theory and its models?

Beer [9] listed five steps in building a theoretical (mathematical) model:

"1. The variables to be used in characterizing and understanding the process must be specified;

2. The forms of the relationships connecting these variables must be specified;

3. Ignorance and the need for simplicity will ensure that all relationships other than identities are subject to error and so, for purposes of efficient statistical estimation, these error terms must be specified;

4. The parameters of the model must be estimated and the extent of its identification ascertained; if this is inadequate, the model must be reformulated;

5. Finally, the model must be kept up to date and used, so that an impression can be formed of its robustness and reliability" (p 394).

While these steps are idealized, they indicate the rigor that must accompany model-building in its broader sense. A model must be a formal and recognizable embodiment of its theory. Models derive directly from their theories; without a theory, there can be no model even though there are plenty of theories that can't yet be modeled. Finally, regardless of the validity of the theory, if the model is wrong, investigating it is non-science.

6-4. The Biopsychosocial Model

It is wrong to criticize an earlier theory because it was not formulated according to modern standards but, knowing that standards change, it is legitimate (in fact, necessary) to reassess older theories to see if they still meet acceptable standards. So where does Engel's biopsychosocial model stand?

The first thing we have to decide is whether it is a theory or a model. Engel was quite explicit: it is a model. However, since his construct does not satisfy any sense of a model as a formal, working representation of an idea, this cannot be accepted. At most, it could be a very general theory, but even as theory, it is seriously flawed. Engel relied on von Bertalanffy's General Systems Theory (GST) to validate his assertion that the (positivist) scientific method could be used to investigate different levels of human activity. However, there is nothing in any of that author's writings to justify that opinion. Engel tacitly acknowledged this: "For medicine, systems theory provides a conceptual approach" for studying the biopsychosocial concept. At no stage did he indicate it was any more than conceptual.

Von Bertalanffy's writings provided the conceptual approach Engel needed, but turning that approach into a methodology required another step. For that step, Engel turned to other writers, primarily Karl Menninger [15]. All other authors citing GST do so, too. But there is no methodology in that book, either. All Menninger said was that he thought GST was an interesting idea, one which might be able to render psychosocial issues amenable to scientific analysis by the extant (1950s) methodology. That has never happened, and, in my opinion, never will because, extended outside its narrow physical and mathematical basis, GST became utterly banal. It could only line up rough analogies and try to extract broad, inductive generalizations about them. It could never constitute a general methodology of human affairs, not the least because nobody has ever shown that the critical matter-energy transfer functions are applicable to the mind-body problem.

It is not possible to build a model of mind based in a theory of systems: it is the wrong sort of theory. Models of mind have to be based in theories of mind (although we may organize the theory of mind according to the principles of a general theory of systems). In essence, a vital element of Engel's program was missing, but this objection pales when we realize that Engel never actually wrote his Biopsychosocial Model.

A strange thing happened in his seminal paper [2]. He set the scene by arguing at some length that the dominant model (he meant theory) in medicine, the Biomedical Model, was producing generations of doctors as technicians who cost a fortune and weren't very nice to patients. He showed where this model had arisen, subsequently sketching an outline of what he thought a new model would need to do in order to overcome the Biomedical Model's failings (p 131). He then argued generally that "a biopsychosocial model" (and note the indefinite article) would satisfy those requirements if it could incorporate scientifically the "impact of nonbiological circumstances upon biologic processes" (p 134). He continued to use this general term without specifying what form such a model would take: "The development of a biopsychosocial medical model is posed as a challenge for both medicine and psychiatry".

Next, he argued that GST could provide the basis for a biopsychosocial model, followed by another critique of "dogmatic biomedicine," after which he suddenly announced the birth of his model: "The proposed biopsychosocial model provides a blueprint for research, a framework for teaching, and a design for action in the real world of health care." Note the change from the future conditional tense to the present, and from the indefinite article to the definite. But of the model itself, there is nothing to be seen. Engel simply demonstrated a need for a particular approach, described what it might do then announced that he had found it. He had not. All he offered was an emotive case for more humanity and less technology in medicine. It was hardly a theory, and it was certainly not a model.

In a subsequent paper [5], Engel described the clinical application of his putative model. "(The) biopsychosocial model," he argued, "enables the physician to extend application of the scientific method to aspects of everyday practice and patient care heretofore not deemed accessible to a scientific approach ... The biomedical model can make provision neither for the person as a whole nor for data of a psychological or social nature..." He then outlined his "model" but once again, it was not a model in any practical sense of the term. It was an earnest plea for a model, a description of where such a model would fit in medical thinking, but not the model itself. The rest of the paper was devoted to a detailed discussion of a case where psychological factors complicated a man's myocardial infarction (heart attack). His discussion was interesting, but nothing revolutionary.

6-5. The Concept of a Model

It is worth recapitulating some basic elements in the epistemic status of psychiatry. Our ontological position is materialist, i.e. we operate within a system that asserts there is nothing in the Universe beyond matter and energy interacting in a time/space matrix. But being curious creatures, we like to investigate the Universe, and there are lots of ways of doing this: armchair theorizing, listening to prophets, reading chickens' entrails, or by a rule-governed, empirical project aimed at elucidating the nature of the Universe independently of all but our most basic prejudices. This last method we call science, and because the fundamental elements of our materialist Universe are restricted, so too is the scope of our science.

But the Universe itself is so large: what is the intellectual starting point for our investigations? For a starting point, we have theories, which often aren't much more than somewhat better-articulated guesses of how things must be behind the scenes. Theories must proceed logically from our ontology, with no sudden discontinuities. Since materialist science can't investigate concepts that are in principle unobservable, we rule them out of court, i.e. a scientific theory cannot invoke non-empirical concepts. To this extent, the rules governing the proper subject matter of science and how it is to be studied help determine the form of those theories. At the end of this logical chain sits the model as a working demonstration of "...what reality can and could be like..." [11], something built to test the theory in action.

It is all very restrictive—and circular. Ontology determines the content of theories and the rules of investigating them; the rules themselves help restrict the form of the theory and a model must exemplify the theory in such a way as to permit its investigation within the common ontological stance. There is a clear line from the most general statements of what we believe the Universe to be, right down to, say, a working model of a better mousetrap. Mousetraps can't defy any of the more general rules or principles on which their function depends, and there is only one test of a good mousetrap.

It is immediately clear that this restrictive view of science excludes a great deal of what we regard as quintessentially human. If what we think and feel matters, then we must either find a way of handling these slippery notions within the field of science, or else change our rules of science. Unfortunately, changing the rules of science is not so easy, not the least because they derive directly from our ontological stance. Since psychiatry hasn't yet been able to enlarge the arena of science to include things that are in principle unobservable (because they also include the supernatural), we are caught, as Eisenberg noted [16], between the Scylla of mindlessness and the Charybdis of brainlessness. Traditionally, psychiatry has fudged this critically important issue, formerly by tolerating a number of incompatible theoretical schools, but more recently by espousing a vapid "eclecticism."

Engel's 'biopsychosocial model' was an attempt to steer a course through this unhappy impasse. He wanted to retain all that was best in the western scientific ethos, yet find a way of rendering our unobservable mental life amenable to rational analysis. His attempt foundered on a number of points, meaning that, theoretically, we are back to where we were forty years ago, when all the main theoretical schools in modern psychiatry weren't far off their centenaries.

6-6. The End of the Biopsychosocial Model

Even if we allow that his model had its imperfections, could it be saved by showing the model at work? This won't happen, for two reasons. Firstly, a description of a model at work is not the same as a definition of the model itself. The act of nominating a model by demonstrating its output cannot simultaneously serve to define it separately from all other models that may have a similar output ('What is this?' is necessarily different from 'What does this do?' as other things might be able to do it by totally different means). Engel did not define his biopsychosocial model; instead, he hoped its definition would emerge by example, through a description of how it might function, with the emphasis on 'might'. His model can therefore never reach scientific status: a description of what something does can never be an explanation of why or how it does it, and science is about explanation.

In the second place, it might be argued that an approach that considers biological, psychological and social factors necessarily amounts to a biopsychosocial model but, for several reasons, this is not the case. To begin with, we must clearly distinguish theories with real predictive value (i.e. they can predict something we didn't know or that was counter-intuitive) from those that can only rationalize what we already know. The former are science, but the latter are just self-reinforcing prejudice. Only highly improbable predictions can test a theory's basic assumptions. Furthermore, researchers who gather data from a variety of theoretically unrelated fields will not be able to test the basic assumptions that led them to collect just those data and not others. They may be able to detect associations but, critically, not errors in their own basic assumptions. Only a model with true predictive value can do that, and then not always.

Unless there is an integrating theory already in place, gathering biological, psychological and sociological data about people will only yield scattered lumps of information that don't relate to each other in any coherent sense. Without an over-arching theory to integrate the fields from which the data derive, associations between differing classes of information are meaningless. For these reasons, Engel's description of his model at work must fail as an attempt to define the model itself.

A critical reading of his paper [5] does not reveal anything that would not be known to any reasonably sensitive practitioner. But what he argued powerfully is that too many modern physicians are not reasonably sensitive, for which he blamed modern medical training: "The reductionist scientific culture of the day is largely responsible for the public view of science and humanism as antithetical ... The triumphs of the biomedical model all have been in the areas for which the model has provided a suitable framework for scientific study." That is, biomedical science was very successful as long as it didn't stray too far from the same theoretical position as veterinary science.

In practice, if we want to know whether Engel's biopsychosocial model is truly a model, or just a case of wishful thinking, then a simple test will decide the issue. Try making, say, a prediction about a man's psychological state from his biological data, or vice versa. Or perhaps try to predict wholly from sociological data which girls will develop post-partum mental disorders as young women or psychoses in their old age. Since nothing like this can be done, Engel's "model" is not a model in any interesting sense of the term.

Can his approach be saved? As a model, it cannot. To be a model, it must be based in a well-formulated theory. Regrettably, one thing psychiatry doesn't have is well-formulated theories. Biological psychiatry has been shown to be restricted in its scope. Psychoanalysis is in retreat; behaviorism is reeling under philosophical attack and naive cognitive psychology falls into the trap of the infinite regress, meaning it can never be scientific. Without the theories, there can be no models.

The biopsychosocial approach is widely accepted, especially for teaching purposes. What everybody wants it to do is to drag mentalist psychology and sociology into the scientific arena so these ephemera can be lassoed by the ropes of the current (positivist) scientific methodology. Throughout the history of modern western science, this has proven impossible. Eventually, and in despair, people have tried the alternative, which was to declare human mental life non-scientific, expelling it from the field. As early as 1913, the psychologist JB Watson declared: "The time seems to have come when psychology must discard all reference to consciousness, when it need no longer delude itself into thinking that it is making mental states the object of observation" [17]. He announced that he wanted his students to know as much about the mind-body problem as students of physics and chemistry, namely, nothing at all. MacKenzie [18, p 17] characterized Watson's program as "mechanistic, elementaristic, associationistic, peripheralistic, environmentalistic—and correspondingly anti-teleological, anti-purposive, anti-nativist, and anti-emergent." And it failed. It was in just this intellectual setting that Engel proclaimed his humanist revolution. Unfortunately, it is one thing to announce the need for a revolution, something else again to write its manifesto. He never did.

6-7. Conclusion

Engel's attempt at a new model should be seen in its historical context, as a reaction against the woolly excesses of psychoanalysis and the sterility of behaviorism. That his theory didn't work first time is not altogether surprising, but he did a service to orthodox psychiatry in that he legitimized the concept of talking to people as people. His 'model' promised to fill a sorely-felt need, that of uniting the disparate elements of human life in such a way as to legitimize an holistic approach. Arguably, that need remains as strong today as it was forty years ago.

Nobody would argue that reductionist science has not served us well but, as Engel noted, only in the areas in which it could work. The inescapable conclusion is that in human psychology (which, for this purpose, includes psychiatry), our concept of science has failed its subject matter, not vice versa. What we need is a new methodology, new ropes for catching these wraith-like constructs, as the old ropes are too inflexible [19]. But a new scientific methodology will only work in a new scientific arena: if we wish to move beyond crude biologism garnished with well-meaning humanism, we need a new concept of science [20].

This is not to suggest that we should abandon materialism just as we start to get to the really interesting bits. Materialism involves more than just matter and energy. Today, we accept that information, its transfer and manipulation, rest firmly within a materialist ontology. Information is very much a material matter. Thus, if mind consists of the manipulation of brain-based information, then we have a materialist theory of mind, i.e. interactive substance dualism that does not breach any natural laws. This type of approach would be entirely consonant with the emerging field of cognitive neurosciences. But for the present, psychiatry is and will remain the only branch of medicine lacking a well-formulated theoretical basis and logically-derived models with true predictive power.

7
The Categorical System of Diagnosis: Personality Disorder

7-1. Introduction

Central to the entire modern system of thinking in psychiatry is the notion that the different disorders recognized by psychiatrists represent fundamentally different classes of disturbance of mental life. There are some caveats to this broad assertion, in that they are all seen as disorders of brain chemistry but, within that limit, they are regarded as quite as distinct as, say, coronary artery disease and rheumatic carditis. It is held that the clinical manifestations accurately chart unseen "biochemical imbalances" with different etiologies, which necessarily mandate different forms of treatment. A very large part of the psychiatric research budget is spent on epidemiological studies aimed at isolating pure examples of the separate conditions as a prelude to discovering the genes responsible for their underlying disturbances. This is not questioned at any level. If, for example, the psychiatric syndromes were to be found to be just subtle variations on a single theme, say, sociologically-determined responses to a single axis of distress, then biological psychiatry would lose a large part of its *raison d'etre*.

I believe we can dispense with that idea fairly quickly. Human mental function is far too complex for anything to be represented on a single axis. However, the concept of distinct mental disorders raises another crucial question, namely, can there be separate categories of mental disorder? This is very important, not the least because of its role in biological psychiatry, but also in management and prevention.

The current system of diagnosis in psychiatry depends not only on the notion that there are separate categories of mental disorder, but also on the more basic concept that mental illness is as different from normality as, say, pneumonia is from normal health. I doubt that this is true, and want to explore the basis of the categorical system using the example of personality disorder. I appreciate that personality diagnosis is by far the weakest link in the categorical chain, but what better place to start to unravel it?

The categorical system of personality diagnosis used in psychiatry since at least the 1920s has long been recognized as having its shortcomings [1-5]. The editors of DSM-IV [6] acknowledged this in a brief note on the alternative approach to the subject. Their view, that "Personality Disorders represent qualitatively distinct clinical syndromes" (i.e. categories, p 633), is opposed by the dimensional model in which personality is conceived as a multidimensional construct. This states that "...personality traits merge imperceptibly into normality and into one another." While noting that the matter remains under "active investigation," they mentioned that the DSM-IV clusters of personality disorder "...may also be viewed as dimensions representing spectra of personality dysfunction on a continuum with Axis I mental disorders" (p634).

This is not entirely lucid. The question of whether categories of personality disorder are in fact qualitatively different is empirical, and is of a form readily answered using existing techniques. If the clusters themselves are on a continuum with formal mental disorder, then the question becomes metaphysical, namely, what is the nature of mental illness and how does it stand in relation to character? A satisfactory answer to the question of the nature of mental disorder will depend on an answer to the question of the nature of mental order, i.e. normal mental function. As it stands today, there cannot be a continuum of mental disorder-personality disorder, as they are understood to be different concepts, and different concepts cannot be measured on the same axis. The suggestion in DSM-IV that mental illness and personality disorder were continuous was necessary for empirical reasons (p 632) but weakened their assertion that categories of illness and of personality disorder are qualitatively different. If they are continuous, they are not qualitatively different, but if they are qualitatively different (distinct categories), then they are not dimensionally distributed.

In a detailed study of 110 outpatients with "minor psychiatric diagnoses", Nurnberg et al [7] scored each patient on all the 112 DSM-III-R criteria used to diagnose personality disorder. 68 patients met criteria for a total of 155 diagnoses, including 37 patients averaging 2.3 diagnoses each. The remaining 42 patients in the survey "...met a substantial number of criteria for personality disorders." The clear presumption was that not one of the 110 subjects could be considered a normal personality. The authors noted: "Insufficient attention has been paid to the fact that every study of Borderline Personality Disorder (BPD) finds substantial and variable overlap with other psychiatric diagnoses ... Patients who meet DSM-III-R criteria for BPD constitute a very heterogeneous group with unclear boundaries whose overlap with neighboring personality disorder categories is extensive." They concluded that it was necessary to move away from the categorical system of personality diagnosis toward a dimensional model.

In a similar study, Dolan, Evans and Norton [8] found that 35% of 274 undergraduates met criteria for one or more personality disorders, with an average of 3.4 diagnoses each (the point of using students is that they are deemed a normal population). They considered the number of diagnoses per subject gave a rough indication of the extent of disturbance rather than a definitive statement as to the type. Forty-five of their subjects (16%) scored diagnoses in all three clusters of personality disorder, while at least one case managed nine separate diagnoses.

Results such as these are not viewed by all as mere "blips" to be overlooked in the manner Nurnberg et al suggested is the norm. In an incisive essay, Ellard [9] criticized the categorical approach to the classification of personality disorder. He argued his case from three points of view:

1. Since we do not have an adequate conceptualization of personality, "...is it possible to make any useful statements about the different sorts of personalities?" He concluded that it is not.

2. Apart from the most banal applications, the very concept of categories is so vague and so open to bias that it cannot meaningfully be applied to human conduct: "Assigning a thing to a category does not necessarily tell us anything definite about it."

3. Given these overwhelming difficulties, no synthesis can succeed: "...the pursuit of specific categorical personalities is the pursuit of a dream, the sculpturing of smoke."

In summary, he stated: "...if one uses dubious criteria to categorize an indefinable entity, the results may be confused and conflicting to the point of absurdity." And, he warned, we pursue the dream at our peril.

The greater part of Ellard's paper was rather gentle *reductio ad absurdum*: if the consequences of a proposition are absurd, then the proposition itself cannot be taken seriously. However, his case against the categorization of personality was brief, an analogy to show that in the absence of a sound conceptualization of personality, attempts at classification become little more than "...an exercise in the politics of committees." In the first part of this chapter, I wish to examine the notions behind categories in order to test the validity of the current categorical classification of personality. In the second part, the dimensional system will be considered.

7-2. The Psychiatric Concept of Categories

In the sense in which we use it in psychiatry, the term "category" has more in common with the mathematical notion of sets than with the classic, Aristotelian sense [10]. In addition, we do not follow the usage outlined by Ryle [11] in his concept of "category errors." Classically, categories are classes of ideas or thoughts, essentially predicates attaching to perceptions of real things. Aristotle recognized about nine categories that can attach to or qualify substances or real things, including quantity, quality, relation, possession, action, etc.: "(Categories) represent the specific ways in which whatever exists does exist or is realized... Aristotle did not consider these categories or these classifications as artificial creations of the mind. He thought that they were actually in existence outside the mind and in things" [12, p 84-5]. Since classic times, other philosophers have developed the notion further without, it must be said, attaining a large measure of agreement.

Ours, however, is the commonsense and non-metaphysical notion that, based on their observable properties, things can reliably and meaningfully be placed in valid categories, classes or sets of similar objects. These features— reliable, valid, meaningful—were fundamental to Ellard's somewhat allegorical critique of our current approach to personality disorder.

Everything except raw perceptions can be named and described, usually according to a number of parameters such as size, structure, purpose, provenance, etc. We can readily nominate categories by means of descriptive parameters of the things in question, making the groups thus formed as big or as small as we want. The category of insects is huge, whereas that of my cars is small (one member). The category of insects is defined by the usual means: six legs, head, thorax and abdomen, reproduction by egg, larval and pupal stages, etc. These are not just positively defining parameters, but they also exclude other possibilities, such as two, four, eight and more legs. So one criterion for the category of insects says: "Six (and not two, four, eight, etc.) legs..."

The notion that categories are defined both by inclusion and by exclusion is important because, without it, there will be such a degree of overlap as to render the exercise meaningless. Normally, the exclusive criteria are understood, not stated, but they come into their own when there is a dispute about where an object is to be categorized. After an encounter with a small boy, a beetle limps off with just five legs. We save the case by saying: "All things being equal, six legs...' This particular concept of categories is quite precise but, in practice, the definition of unambiguous individual categories depends on allowing them to multiply to their limit, such that each member of the field will fit in one and one only. The limit to the number of elemental categories in any field is the number of objects in the field.

It is important to remember that categories are often not directly comparable. Ellard asked: "A sofa is furniture; is the cushion on the sofa also furniture?" This is another type of category error, comparing elements of a collective category with the collective itself. In a hierarchical categorical system, like can only be compared with like. Overlooking this rule leads people to believe that the concept of categories itself is at fault.

To be of any value, categories are defined according to the principle that items within each category are more like each other than they are like members of other categories. In order to make the categories internally consistent, we devise inclusive or positively-defining features. In order to separate or distance the category thus formed from all others, we use exclusive or negative definitions. The purpose is to prevent overlap. A categorical system that cannot reliably separate its field of elements into their ultimate categories is a waste of time. This feature is most important in considering categories of personality disorder.

This leads to the last point, the purpose or meaning of forming categories. Members of the category must have more in common than their defining feature, otherwise they will be so different from each other that forming the category is pointless. One of the critical features of a useful category is its internal consistency, such that what is true of its existing members will also be true of new members. To be of any purpose, categorizing something must imply or predict a lot more than it says. What do members of the category of blue objects have in common? Only their blueness. We can't predict anything more about them. This requirement is especially important in science, where predictions are central to the progress of knowledge. Thus, the inclusive and exclusive defining criteria of categories determine the validity, the reliability and the meaning of the categories as they are formed.

In practice, however, we cannot simply go through life defining categories as the fancy takes us. When I think of all the categories of things in even so restricted a field as my home, there are many hundreds of them. After letting them multiply to their limit, as suggested above, we need to be able to sort them into a system that quickly defines them according to a larger purpose, otherwise we may be comparing categories of different levels of complexity – and completely bewildered. This implies hierarchies of categories, or sub- and sub-sub-categories. This is practically second nature to us. Almost without thinking, we sort the objects of the world into broad classes, then we split each of these in turn and keep on splitting until we decide enough is enough.

The best example of a cascading or hierarchical categorical system is the Linnaean binomial system of nomenclature that forms the basis of modern biology: Kingdom, phylum, order, family, genus, species—a place for everything and everything in its place. Linnaean taxonomy is valid (the species exists as the ultimate separate category), reliable (a living thing will always be correctly categorized in its species) and meaningful (knowing something about a member of a species allows predictions about its co-members, and defines their relationships to all other living organisms). It is also simple, parsimonious and empirically objective. Can psychiatry boast anything like it?

7–3. Categories of Personality Disorder

Using the concept of categories outlined above, it is immediately obvious that the system of categories of personality disorder described in DSM-IV has grave deficiencies. In the first place, it is not part of a larger system, the categories float independently in an undefined space with no clear indication of how they should relate to each other or to the larger taxonomy [13]. Axis II (personality disorder and mental retardation) is deemed to be independent of Axis I (clinical disorders *qua* mental illness). How personality disorder and intellect relate to each other is not explained in the Manual, nor is there any explanation as to why personality, which necessarily precedes mental illness, should come second. They are not axes in any formal sense of the term, just unrelated domains.

The separation of these domains is problematic. The editors note that their use of different axes for personality disorder and for illness does not imply different etiologies (p 26) and concede (p 632): "It may be particularly difficult (and not particularly useful) to distinguish personality disorders from those Axis I disorders ... that have an early onset and a chronic, relatively stable course." For example: "Many individuals with Generalized Anxiety Disorder report that they have felt anxious and nervous all their lives ... over half ... report onset in childhood or adolescence..." (p 434). Yet there is no category of anxious personality; anxiety is deemed an illness unless it leads to avoidant behavior, in which case the behavior becomes a personality disorder and any underlying "Social Phobia, Generalized" retains its separate status as an illness (p 413). A more parsimonious account would be to say that lifelong anxiety represents an anxious personality manifest as avoidant behavior, with the social phobia therefore being a subcategory of the anxious personality.

However, assuming for the minute that there are suitable, operationalized demarcation criteria between personality and illness familiar to all psychiatrists, we see substantial problems within the category of personality disorder. In the first place, the three (super-) categories or clusters of personality disorder are defined only by inclusion criteria. They are (p 629-30):

Cluster A (paranoid, schizoid and schizotypal): Odd or eccentric people;

Cluster B (antisocial, borderline, histrionic and narcissistic): Dramatic, emotional or erratic people;

Cluster C (avoidant, dependent and obsessive-compulsive): Anxious or fearful people.

Are we to assume that paranoid people are not erratic, that avoidant individuals are not also odd, or that eccentric people are never anxious? As they stand, the clusters are largely meaningless because the different groups within them have so little in common as to deny any value in clustering them together. Schizotypal people are harmless, which would not generally be said of paranoid individuals. The "obsessive-compulsive" personality keeps the country running while some dependent people may think the country runs for their benefit.

Putting this objection aside, the clusters are not reliable. People are allocated to them according to unrelated criteria, when everything we know of categories says that like must be grouped with like. The DSM-IV system is akin to devising, say, three clusters of transport systems according to whether they are marine, noisy or yellow. These are not comparable. It is not possible to have different clusters at the same level of a hierarchy determined according to totally unrelated parameters. To be of any value, the DSM-IV clusters would need to be devised according to significant differences on one parameter, such as behavior or emotional state. If, however, the clusters were determined according to the individual's score on any one of three unrelated factors, then there would be twenty-seven of them, not just three. We can have clusters of big dogs, medium dogs and small dogs, or of white, black and brown dogs, etc., but not just three clusters in which all dogs must fit, one of big dogs, another of white dogs and the third of expensive dogs. Where would the small, brown mutt fit?

Because there are no exclusion criteria in personality diagnosis, people can be categorized by whatever strikes the interviewer as most obvious. Anxious psychiatrists may well over-rate aggression, particularly in big men who don't speak much English; conspiratorially-minded interviewers will not condemn someone who sees a plot at every turn, while grandiose psychiatrists are hardly likely to damn their adoring clientele as "dependent." There is nothing to stop this happening. The lack of exclusion criteria affords too much potential for the circumstances of the patient's presentation and the interviewer's bias to prejudice the diagnostic process. On any objective basis, avoidant personalities are as odd or eccentric as schizoid, and anybody who gains the confidence of a schizoid individual will quickly realize how anxious they are. It's just that, normally, they don't talk about it.

Moving beyond the clusters, the separate categories are most definitely not reliable. Too often, inclusion criteria of one category are duplicated in another, albeit in slightly different language [3]. This fault is actually conceded: "Other personality disorders may be confused with BPD because they have certain features in common" (p 653). Of course, if the authors had specified exclusion criteria, this wouldn't happen. Other examples of duplication are readily apparent, although the wording of the lists of criteria tends to indicate differences that are less real than apparent. For example, the borderline personality makes "frantic efforts to avoid real or imagined abandonment..." whereas the dependent personality "urgently seeks another relationship ... when (one) ends". The avoidant personality "...views self as socially inept ... unappealing ... inferior to others" while the dependent personality has only a "...lack of self-confidence in judgment or abilities...," feels helpless and unrealistically fears having to manage alone. There are numerous pairs of criteria written as though they were different when, in practice, they are different only to the eye of faith.

Other features actually occur in different categories but are simply omitted because their inclusion would render the categories less distinct. For example, paranoid ideas or illusions occur in paranoid personalities, of course, but also in borderline and schizotypal personalities (p 653). However, narcissistic (NPD, p 653) and avoidant personalities (p 665) merely over-react to perceived criticism. Of NPD, we read that "...criticism may haunt these individuals and may leave them feeling humiliated, degraded, hollow and empty (sic: presumably metaphor). They may react with disdain, rage, or defiant counterattack" (p 659), not unlike, one presumes, most paranoid people. In addition, prickly sensitivity is not uncommon in the obsessive-compulsive personality (p 671), while suspicion and uncontrollable jealousy are frequently seen in antisocial personalities (p 642). Thus, clear-cut paranoid traits are a common element in no less than seven separate categories of abnormal personality. Quite clearly, it would be impossible to use paranoid ideas in any exclusive sense, meaning the core concept of categories starts to break down.

The validity of the categories of personality disorder within the larger clusters suffers from the same failings as the clusters themselves, but is intensified by the strong tendency of the lists of criteria to be swollen by dubious rewriting of attributes. For example, we learn that schizoid people do not want or enjoy close relationships and almost always choose solitary activities; hardly surprising, then, that they should have "...little, if any, interest in ... sex with other people (p 641)." Onanism follows naturally from the first two criteria. Not only do these people not desire or enjoy close relationships (criterion A1, p 641) but they lack close friends or confidants (A5). By even the most restrictive interpretation, (A5) follows logically from (A1); it is not an independent criterion. These people are also indifferent to the praise or criticism of others (A6) as well as showing emotional coldness, detachment or flatness (A7), which is clearly just another way of saying the same thing.

These are not isolated examples. In the criteria for Avoidant PD, criteria A2/A3/A5, and A4/A6 are merely variations on themes. Individuals with Antisocial Personality Disorder show impulsivity (A3), lack of remorse (A7), and "irritability and aggressiveness, as indicated by repeated physical fights or assaults" (A4). They also display a "reckless disregard for the safety of self or others" (A5), which clearly flows from the first three features.

The question of whether any meaning can be attached to the separate categories of personality disorder is best answered by considering results such as those of Dolan, Evans and Norton [8]. In their series, many individuals scored diagnoses in all three clusters, while some subjects even managed to score all eleven separate personality diagnoses. The mix of diagnoses was largely random; given such clear empirical evidence, the idea that we can say anything meaningful about a person by choosing, without a prior system of rules, just one aspect of his personality seems not just unfair but also unscientific.

7–4. Discussion of Categories of Personality Disorder

However broadly we define behavior, if we take any behavioral parameter, certainly any one of the 79 listed in the personality disorder section of DSM-IV, and score each person in the population, then the parameter will distribute dimensionally, not categorically. That is, there will be a smooth gradation from the unfortunate with the highest score to the person with the least. Therefore, there can be no factual basis to the notion that we can define a cut-off point on any dimension, such that all individuals below are normal while those above it are abnormal. Unfortunately, the notion of cut-off points is a *sine qua non* of any categorical system. Psychometricians avoid this problem simply by nominating the individual's statistical distance from the norm. They recognize that, by definition, traits, including abnormal traits, are never all-or-none phenomena.

A graded distribution is true of such mundane traits as obsessionality or self-adornment, but also of the more striking such as paranoid attitudes, which the editors of DSM-IV concede may even be normal in certain circumstances (p637). By their frequent use of such terms as excessive, markedly, persistently, etc., the editors implicitly acknowledge this point. For example, they cannot define normal suspicion: their apparently tight operational criteria turn out to be remarkably elastic in practice [8]. Clinicians are free to apply the criteria as broadly or as narrowly as they please, which often leads psychiatrists into disputes in court.

The evidence for a dimensional distribution of all human behavior is overwhelming. Therefore, a system of classification of personality that depends on the concept that there are "qualitatively distinct clinical syndromes" rests on spurious foundations. The most that could be said is that the categorical system of personality assessment is a procrustean bed for a dimensional construct.

This point notwithstanding, psychiatry's categorical system of personality diagnosis rests on a profound misapprehension of the nature of categories. This is the idea that reliable categories can be formulated by inclusion criteria alone, without reference to exclusion criteria. By omitting negative criteria, we lull ourselves into believing that there are diagnostic features that occur only in particular personality disorder categories. But the editors of DSM-IV freely admit the characteristic features of any diagnosis are not distinctive, that there is considerable overlap. It is definitely not the case that the inclusion criteria for one category are present in that group only and absent in all others; only by a convenient fiction do we ignore them in all but the particular one in which we wish to place the subject.

When an assiduous researcher asks every criterion of all subjects [8,13], multiple diagnoses are common. That is, people do not fit the categories psychiatrists have constructed for them, but blur across the boundaries with no regard for the effort that went into drawing them: "Insufficient attention has been paid to the fact that every study of borderline personality disorder finds substantial and variable overlap with other psychiatric diagnoses" [7, p 1374]. In any categorical system, if the elements don't sort into discrete groups, then the clear implication is either that its architects have used the wrong system of categories (e.g. pre-Linnaean biology, pre-atomic chemistry), or that there weren't any categories at all (e.g. phrenology).

The notion that anybody can have more than one personality disorder is certainly not intuitive, and psychiatrists now use the term "comorbidity" to encompass it [14]. This appears to be based upon the notion that Smith can at once be classed as a husband, father, brother and son, or that he can simultaneously be suffering alopecia, halitosis and piles. Once again, this represents a serious misconception of the nature of categories. Smith is indeed a son, brother, etc., but not to the same person. It is true that he can be placed in a number of different categories at once, but only if they are not mutually contradictory. This can be known only if the categories are defined by both inclusion and exclusion criteria. He can be both a friend and an enemy but, because these are contradictory categories, not to the same person at the same time. Without exclusion criteria, we slip into "category errors" [11].

The alopecia-halitosis-piles argument collapses when we recall that poor Smith has all these ailments, but not in the same organ. The body is composed of discrete subsystems that can be separately disordered. Joint pathology in these systems is contingent, i.e. neither necessary nor impossible. Using the same argument as for the physical body, anybody who wishes to say that the personality can be "multiply-disordered" must first show that the normal personality is composed of discrete and more or less independent subsystems. Use of the term "comorbidity" begs at least part of the question that the concept of personality disorder is designed to answer.

The notion of functionally independent subsystems of personality is not so outlandish as at first it sounds. Just as Dennett [15] "decomposed" intelligence, or Luria [16] showed movement to be the outcome of orchestrated action in many subsystems, so my need for attention may be quite independent of my desire for order. But once again, scores in the separate subsystems will distribute dimensionally throughout the population, not categorically. Thus, if we use categories, we will be compelled empirically to accept "comorbidity," but if we explore the notion of multiple pathology to its limit, we arrive at a dimensional system which, of course, doesn't require "comorbidity."

The fact that one person can meet criteria for all ten or so personality disorders reduces the notion of separate diagnoses to an exercise in pseudoscience [5, p 467]. More pertinently, it negates the basis of the categorical argument by showing empirically that all parameters are distributed throughout the population, i.e., epidemiology supports a dimensional, but not a categorical system. It also raises another question. By definition, everybody has a personality. Since any definition of personality will necessarily start with the sum total of the individual's behavior, regardless of how bizarre it may be, it follows that nobody can have more than one personality, even if his behavior is of the type some people call "multiple personality." If everybody has but one personality, how can anybody have several abnormal personalities? Whatever his behavior, that just is his personality.

The notion of "personality disorder comorbidity" or "multiply-disordered personality" is specious, and arises through a tautology. Smith, poor fellow, has nephritis. We do not say he has "nephritis disease" because nephritis just is a disease state. We can say he has Bright's disease as Bright is not a disease. Sadly, Smith is also a nasty fellow. He has an antisocial personality. But he does not have an "Antisocial Personality Disorder," because an antisocial personality just is a disordered personality. Descriptively, we could say that Smith has an abnormal personality characterized by aggressive, paranoid, anxious and rigid traits (a dimensional approach, of course). This would allow us to stop tying ourselves in knots each time we say that, even though he has only one personality, Smith has half a dozen Personality Disorders.

As they exist, the clusters of personality disorder are totally unnecessary. They do not add to our knowledge of the individuals placed in them, allow no meaningful predictions and so on. Our knowledge of personality disorder would not be diminished if they had never been devised. They give the appearance of a larger system but, on closer examination, that system does not exist. Furthermore, the lists of criteria for the differing categories of personality disorder appear different only by virtue of creative writing and the selective omission of common signs and symptoms. Science is not supposed to be deceptive.

Finally, in the last note in the chapter ("301.9: personality disorder-NOS" p 673), the validity of the DSM-IV categories of personality is shown to be illusory. The editors recommended that if a person doesn't fit any of the categories on offer, then the clinician should feel free to devise a more appropriate one. There are no constraints on this freedom which, if it were exercised to its limit, would give us one category for every living human being: *Reductio ad absurdum.*

7-5. Alternatives to Categories: The Dimensional Approach

Nurnberg et al stated: "A better understanding of personality disorder awaits a paradigmatic shift away from discrete nosologic categories..." [7, p 1376]. This is, of course, a polite call for the rejection of our current concepts of personality disorder. As mentioned, the editors of DSM-IV accepted that there were arguments for and against the opposing models, the categorical system and the dimensional approach. Dimensional models of personality are essentially the province of psychology, having long been the subject of considerable research effort. However, one of the most influential living psychologists, HJ Eysenck, has gloomily concluded that personality research lacks a proper paradigm: "It has become almost a joke to see the proliferation of concepts and tests in the personality field..." [19, p 3]. Further, he stated: "There is no agreement on definitions, models, methods, results or indeed anything whatever; all is confusion, with no effort used to sort the chaff from the grain. The result ... is simply a Dutch auction ... No wonder that 'hard' scientists do not take psychology seriously as a science...." [17, pp 773-74].

If, as has been argued, the categorical system is inadequate to the task set it, and a personality theorist of Eysenck's stature concedes his own field is hardly worth serious consideration, where does this leave psychiatry? In the rest of this chapter, I wish to consider the dimensional approach to personality to decide whether it can satisfy our needs.

Within psychology, there are many approaches to personality, the majority of them formulated in such a way as to render them non-scientific [17]. These include the theories of Freud, Jung, Adler, the neo-Freudians, Maslow and many others. Non-metaphysical theories of personality are essentially behaviorist in nature, i.e. eschewing the unobservable, they take measurable behavior as their sole source of data. By subjecting it to statistical analysis, they derive a small number of general behavioral parameters. These, it is held, allow every person to be classified empirically in a schema of individual differences that can "...deal with the definition, origin, and interrelation of traits of human personality" [17, p 775]. This, in behaviorist terms, just is a theory of human personality, and it was this approach that the editors of DSM-IV offered as an alternative to their categorical notion of personality disorder. Since Eysenck's tri-dimensional model is the most highly developed, and has the widest acceptance in psychology, it is appropriate to use it as an exemplar of dimensional systems.

Over the past fifty years or more, Eysenck has developed his concepts of personality using questionnaire data which, after sophisticated analysis, yield three fundamental groupings of human behavior. These are named extraversion/introversion (E), neuroticism (N) and psychoticism (P). He distinguishes between transient behavioral states and enduring traits; his dimensions are conceptualized as "the most far-reaching, aggregating behaviors characteristic of a given person over many years" [17, p 776]. These dispositional dimensions are held to have a genetic basis and, through their interaction, determine the individual's behavior to a very large extent. Approximately 80% of personality variance is said to be governed by these factors. While arguments rage as to the number of dimensions, it would be fair to say that Eysenck is convinced his three correctly represent the scientific truth of human personality.

There are, however, very real problems with dimensional approaches in general and, before rushing to embrace one or other of these models, psychiatrists should be familiar with their shortcomings. Firstly, as previously detailed, his own account of the nature of the scientific endeavor indicates that truism is likely to be accepted as a "general scientific law" before a highly improbable but correct theory. I suggest that this is what has happened with Eysenck's half century of statistics. His three behavioral parameters are excessively reductive, leading him to assemble a model which, while true, is not enlightening. The differences, which are really what we want to know about, are swamped by the similarities. Using his three dimensions, every human must fit into one of just eight groups. By contrast, DSM-IV offers ten groups (down from eleven in DSM-III) and, since multiple diagnoses are common [7], the potential number of clinically-recognizable groups is very large. In this sense, Eysenck's model is regressive.

Secondly, and despite his frequent claims, Eysenck's concepts do not represent a theory of personality so much as a typology of behavior. This is unavoidable: his work is based in behavior (which he takes to include verbal behavior and cognitions [20]) and therefore cannot extend beyond its data base without invoking unobservables—anathema to a behaviorist. But a theory has to go beyond its data; it has to move to another realm or dimension, otherwise it is limited to restating the obvious, albeit in different terms. A theory of personality has to say more than just that Smith acts thus and thus. To be of any interest and, more significantly, of any predictive value, it has to say why and how he acts so.

I am not aware that Eysenck has ever actually said how he believes behavior arises, but it is clear from his writings that biology plays an extremely important part. At one stage, he defines his personality factors as dispositions to behave; at another, he talks about the "biological substratum of behaviorally defined dimensions of personality" [20, p 244]: "Genetic factors play a predominant part in the causation of individual differences in personality ... Genetic factors cannot directly influence behavior or cognitions, of course, and the intervening variables must inevitably be physiological, neurological, biochemical, or hormonal in nature" (p247). That is, cultural, educational and environmental factors (presumably including the psychological) are expressly considered to be of very much lesser importance than the biological.

On the other hand, there is a considerable tension between his biologism, and his awareness that social influences are significant. In the beginning of one paper, he condemns mentalist theories of personality as non-scientific but, at the end, concludes: "...psychologists will have to learn to accept a mind-body continuum" [17, p 785]. Is there a mind or is there not? If so, what is its nature, and is it causally significant? And what is meant by a "mind-body continuum"?

Behaviorists are severely restricted in the theories of mind they can embrace, mainly because they deny the existence of causally-effective minds. For Eysenck, the only escape from behaviorism's self-imposed trap is via Mind-Brain Identity Theory (MBIT) which says that, as a matter of contingent fact, mind and brain are identical. While this would immediately relieve the tension in his work, as everything significant about humans becomes biological, I have previously argued that MBIT cannot provide a complete account of human behavior. There are always significant aspects of human conduct that cannot be reduced to the biological. Unless he formally invokes the notion of a non-reductive mind, Eysenck's approach to personality will necessarily be incomplete, meaning it should be viewed as part of a larger (psychobiological) theory of human conduct, but it is not the whole theory itself.

This point leads to a third criticism, that because Eysenck's work is just a descriptive typology of behavior based on a restricted field of data, it cannot be expanded to provide an explanatory account of behavior. It must be understood very clearly that a description of something is not the same as its explanation, i.e. mere description can never constitute a model or theory (see Chapter 7). Eysenck's description of clusters of human behavior is, while perhaps a little pedestrian, nonetheless as accurate as modern sampling and cluster analysis techniques permit. But his parameters are dispositions to act, mere statements that because Smith has always acted this way in the past, he is likely to continue to do it in the future, and that because most people of his type also act in a particular way, then it is statistically likely that he will do so, too. But statements "that something happens" are never statements "why something happens." In order to have a theory of personality, as distinct from a description of types, Eysenck would need to expand his explanatory field to another, unobservable realm."

Now Eysenck would certainly argue that he has done this, pointing to his long-standing biological research program. In his 1990 paper, "Biological Dimensions of Personality" [20], he summarized evidence relating to causative elements in the biological substrate of behavior. He specifically mentioned genetic and environmental factors, but did not say which type of environment he meant. This paper is worthy of close study because, although Eysenck has written prolifically on the biological basis of personality over many years, it is one of his most recent statements in a field that rapidly goes out of date.

The paper begins with a brief outline of the differences between taxonomic (descriptive) and causal theories, then quickly launches into a prodigiously-detailed resume of some seventy-five years of research in the area of human biology and personality. The encyclopedic level of detail is typical of this author. The problem with it, apart from the fact that it is so indigestible, is that there is no basic hypothesis. All we know at the end is that he is convinced there is some very close link between behaviorally-defined personality and the individual's genetic endowment. Now this is hardly novel, the ancient Greeks were also convinced of this. But he needs to prove it and, on such a critical issue, the only standard of proof is that it could not be otherwise. Until then, all the suggestive evidence in the world is beside the point. Until we have a clear definition of personality, there is nothing to be gained from talking about genes and personality; in the absence of a uniting theory, lemon juice dropped on the tongue tells us nothing beyond the fact that different people may react differently to the same biological stimulus, which is not a novel finding.

In conclusion, he states: "All in all, considering the youth of the subject and comparatively small amount of effort that has gone into its investigation until quite recently, results are not too disappointing" (p 270). His optimism is not contagious. In this paper alone, he quotes hundreds of studies, and reviews dozens of books and papers, which together cite thousands more. The biological program in personality research has been active for over eighty years but the results have not had any significant effect on the daily practice of normal or abnormal psychology. The simple truth is that this essential part of his program lacks an adequate philosophical basis, is conceptually outdated and, in terms of its objective, the vast corpus of work amounts to remarkably little. And until the notion of personality is properly articulated, this gloomy conclusion is not going to change.

7–6. The Limits of Dimensional Models

To summarize this very brief review of a major part of twentieth century theorizing in human affairs, Eysenck's program is based in behaviorism, a theory that has been shown to be incapable of fulfilling the expectations placed upon it [23, 24]. It is supplemented by Mind-Body Identity Theory, which has also been found to be unable to support a general theory of human conduct. Anybody who follows the program or form of science outlined by Eysenck runs a serious risk of endorsing mere truism as science.

His biological research program lacks essential first steps, namely a clear definition of personality that extends beyond the base data of 'mere behavior.' He needs to explain how the physical realm can influence the behavioral which, in his definition, includes speech, attitudes, beliefs, etc., attributes that most of us lump together as 'mind.' Eysenck does so, too [17, p 785] but, by his self-imposed convention, everybody ignores the amount of work the concept of mind has to do in his ostensibly behaviorist theory. Until the metaphysical question is answered, all he can do is assemble encyclopedic lists of unexciting correlations between biology and behavior, without any convincing explanation of how these actually come about.

Historically, psychologists wanted to bypass the apparently empty speculations of generations of philosophers, deriving an empirical theory of mind where metaphysics had so signally failed [25]. But since everyone knows that an empirical theory of mind is a solecism, they had to give it a new name. They called it personality, but their new creation's job was indistinguishable from that performed by the old-fashioned Mind. Since psychology dealt only with observable behavior, early theorists necessarily had to equate behavior and mind (Eysenck's rubbery "mind-body continuum," for example), hoping they could thereby throw an empirical harness over the slippery metaphysical horse. They couldn't do it.

All they gave us was a drab and ultimately sterile typology of behavior. Since a description of the output of a machine is not an explanation of how the machine effects that output, behavior is not equivalent to mind. In his aphorism, "All human behavior is over-determined," Freud understood this perfectly well. In psychology, and hence psychiatry, an empirical typology of behavior is not the same as an account of the generative mechanisms of that behavior, mechanisms otherwise known as mind. In order to derive a general theory of mental abnormality, of which personality disorder will be an essential part, psychiatry needs an adequate theory of mind.

7-7. Conclusion

Deficiencies in the categorical system of personality classification have long been recognized. I believe they are now overwhelming, and the system should be abandoned. At present, it isn't possible to derive a general account of personality disorder from a system of dimensional constructs based solely in behavior. Behavioral descriptions can't explain how the hidden mechanisms generate observable behavior. By discarding the categorical account in favor of a dimensional approach, the editors of DSM-IV would simply swap a square wheel for one that keeps falling off.

Categories of mental disorder fail to satisfy any reasonable concept of the word "category." In the first place, the need for categories is based in a misdirected biologism and, secondly, the categories that have been devised to satisfy this need are themselves dependent upon a false understanding of what categories do. The present use of the notion of separate mental disorders leads us to think in terms of "comorbidity," which is just another epicycle trying to keep the non-scientific biological model of psychiatry up in the air.

8 When Does Self–Deception Become Culpable?

8-1. Introduction and Review

So far, I have reviewed the main theories used in modern psychiatry. Chapter 1 looked at Biological Psychiatry, arguing that its reliance on reductionism and on Mind-Brain Identity Theory (MBIT) is totally misplaced. Chapter 2 examined Behaviorism in several incarnations, finding that each of them is fatally flawed. In Chapter 3, Mentalism, as psychoanalytic theory and as naive cognitive psychology, was shown to be beyond repair. Chapter 4 looked at a classic form of substance dualism, concluding that everything ever said against it was true. Chapter 5 moved away from "applied philosophies of mind," towards the actual theoretical basis of psychiatry as it is practiced. Eclectic psychiatry was shown to be a pseudoscientific myth. In Chapter 6, the Biopsychosocial Model was shown to be hollow. Finally, Chapter 7 looked at a fundamental aspect of modern psychiatry as a branch of medicine, the categorical approach to mental disorder, and concluded that it rests upon spurious grounds.

It is a striking feature of modern psychology that the most influential theorists have been verbose in the extreme, and utterly incapable of accepting that their ideas may have been wrong. Psychology has reached the point where few seem prepared to challenge the "greats" simply because, having written so much, they must have secreted the truth in there somewhere. However, I believe that Eysenck's vast output of perhaps five million published words is a lesser contribution to human psychology than MacKenzies' elegantly terse essay [1], but time will tell.

Freud and his followers assembled an unprecedented intellectual edifice, but the conduct of the analytic movement was more typical of a fanatical religious sect than of a sober scientific body. Many of its adherents became notorious for their scandalous ideas and behavior [2]. Yet, in my training in psychiatry, there was absolutely no mention whatsoever of any criticisms of Freudian ideas. The calm air of certainty among our lecturers made me wonder whether I had was correct in believing I had detected errors or whether I was simply deluding myself. In those early years, some mention that all was not well in the world of psychoanalysis would have been very helpful.

This was also the case for the little bit of behaviorism to which psychiatric trainees were exposed in the 1970s. Despite the fact that in 1977, when his book was published, MacKenzie was a lecturer at the University of Tasmania, there was no mention of it nor, more significantly, anything like it in the series of lectures given our small group of trainees in Western Australia. We heard no hint of a suggestion that the foundations of behaviorism were creaking badly, and that behaviorists themselves would soon be deserting their "science" in droves. In fact, all we heard from psychologists was how dreadful psychiatrists are.

Self-criticism was not and still is not part of academic psychiatry. Psychiatrists are not trained in the ancient art of criticism, and papers critical of the mainstream are rare indeed. In the ten years 1996-2005, the *Australian and New Zealand Journal of Psychiatry* published 1082 full-length articles and reviews, as well as 94 brief reports or commentaries. Of the 1176 contributed papers, only ten were critical, and of those, seven were mild, mostly arguing that their authors' special interests (e.g. religion) deserved more attention. Only three papers (0.25%, or about one in four hundred) challenged the mainstream view in any substantial way. Of these, two were by overseas authors and one was mine.

Practically all the remaining 99.75% of publications sympathetic to the standard view will vanish without a trace, forgotten even before the dust has started to settle on the bookshelves. In biological psychiatry, vast sums of money have been poured into research programs without a proper *a priori* analysis of the likelihood of the program being successful. The search for the elusive schizococcus (now the schizosubviral genetic inclusion body) roars ahead, with absolutely nothing in the way of realistic results to support its continued funding. Quite probably, no theoretical field in science has seen so much investment with so little return, yet money is always available for yet another analysis of season of birth of schizophrenics or PET studies of ADHD data processing. The idea that we should examine the basis of the entire biological research program is not popular among the funding committees, probably because most of the members got their seats via biological psychiatry. I doubt that any person has ever served on those committees just because he was a critic.

8-2. Caveats

To my knowledge, this monograph is the first of its kind in the history of psychiatry. I am not aware that there has ever been an attempt to marshal the different types of theories we use and subject each of them to critical analysis. It has become the norm in psychiatry that theories are written and accepted, generations of psychiatrists are trained in them and then, years later, somebody comes along and argues that they are no good. This happens with treatments, too. Insulin coma therapy was in wide use for years before a young registrar in a London hospital showed that it was useless [3]. Psychosurgery came from nowhere in the late 1940s, exploded across the world then faded into richly-deserved oblivion, all in less than twenty years [4]. The reason is just because psychiatrists were too frightened to say: "*Sondern traegt der Kaiser nichts*"—But the emperor is wearing no clothes! So much for the theoretical basis of late twentieth century psychiatry.

This is not to say that mentally-disordered people are no better off today than their great-grandparents were in 1900, because they are. To suffer a psychotic condition in those days was more or less the end of one's life. Until just recently, the certificate of admission to a mental hospital in Western Australia had written on the back: "Late Residence," just as appears on death certificates. But such changes as have occurred have largely been fortuitous.

Theories have not helped mentally-disordered people in the way they have the physically-ill. And this is psychiatry's loss.

But a hundred years in the intellectual wilderness teaches certain lessons. In the first place, it should now be obvious that there cannot be a non-mentalist psychology. In view of the wealth of material on this topic, it is no longer acceptable for people to claim they can write a non-mentalist psychology.

Secondly, a reductionist account of human behavior will always be incomplete. The wild claims made by biological psychiatrists are unjustified—and unjustifiable. There are huge swathes of human conduct that will always remain beyond the reach of reductionist materialism. That is, there are concepts with no direct or indirect parallels in the world of physics just because they are formulated in symbols, and symbols are necessarily removed from the things they represent. The disjunction between symbols and the physical realm cannot be bridged by fiat just because it is their nature to be different. It is like the old argument that induction can be as reliable as deduction. Yes, it can, but it won't be induction any longer. It is the very essence of symbols that they are non-physical in nature: attempting to reduce them to "mere physics" denies the reality of their existence as non-physical entities.

Thirdly, a substance dualism of the natural realm and the supernatural can only complicate matters. Short of miracles, any means by which a supernatural soul could interact with the body is also available to a natural "spirit" or whatever. The only value supernatural dualism represents over the natural form is in conferring powers of immortality and reincarnation, telepathy, telekinesis, etc. It must be admitted that these ideas exert a strange pull over people, but wanting them is not the same as showing that these properties exist. Anyway, adopting them would be to abandon materialism just when it is getting to the really difficult questions of mind, matter and the nature of reality.

Fourthly, we want no infinite regresses in our theorizing. These delay the day of reckoning, but never for very long. At the same time, there is no place in a theory of human affairs for elements that are unobservable in principle. This is a little difficult, as the light cast by neurophysiology does not extend very far into the cranium, and, of necessity, we need to invoke unobservables to provide any sort of explanatory theory. But there is a profound difference between Freud's Byzantine theorizing, and other ideas simply awaiting further biological developments, such as Gregor Mendel's spartan outline of genetics.

Several times, I have referred to the reluctance of psychiatrists to see criticism as the engine that powers scientific progress. I have said that, in its response to criticism, my profession acts more like a closed religious order than a section of the scientific community. Can I justify this claim? Yes, I believe I can. The response of the RANZCP to my critique of Engel's biopsychosocial model is a case in point.

8-3. The Place of Criticism in Psychiatry

In his seminal historiographic work on the progress of science, Thomas Kuhn [5] distinguished clearly between what he termed normal science and its rare antithesis, revolutionary science. Normal science is what the vast majority of scientists do throughout their careers, i.e. explicating the model or paradigm of science within which they trained by steadily filling the gaps of our knowledge. Their job is to complete the model, but never to threaten it. Revolutionary science, on the other hand, results from a sudden change in the world view, the abrupt transition from one way of looking at things to another, totally different apprehension of the same phenomena. There can be no revolutions before there is criticism of the status quo. As an example, Kuhn used the Copernican revolution, in which the Ptolemaic or geocentric model of the universe reluctantly yielded to the heliocentric notion of the earth as a minor satellite of a gigantic sun. Other historic scientific revolutions include the replacement of the static, creationist concept by the dynamic Darwinian model, the change from Newtonian physics to the relativistic view and the transition from the notion of supernatural causes of illness to the germ theory. Scientific progress does not follow a straight line.

Kuhn left no doubt that, collectively, scientists are conservative and resistant to change. People who spend their lives developing a particular concept of the world are not going to abandon it in favor of every new idea that comes along. He quoted Darwin in his later years: "Although I am fully convinced of the truth of the views given in this volume (*On the Origin of Species*) ... I by no means expect to convince experienced naturalists whose minds are stocked with a multitude of facts all viewed, during a long course of years, from a point of view directly opposite to mine." Similarly, he approved Planck's pessimistic realization in his *Scientific Autobiography*: "....a new scientific truth does not triumph by convincing its opponents and making them see the light, but rather because its opponents eventually die, and a new generation grows up that is familiar with it" (p151). Criticism drives scientific progress.

8-4. The Biopsychosocial Model in Contemporary Psychiatry

Within modern psychiatry, the prevailing ethos derives from the notion that, while our field may be somewhat lacking in certainty, psychiatrists "....need to be highly skilled in multiple paradigms: biological paradigms, the psychological paradigms, the whole spectrum of social sciences, economics, ethics and political science ... the spiritual dimension of human beings and how this differs enormously between cultures" [6]. Responding to these intellectual demands, the RANZCP has endorsed what is called the biopsychosocial model. In defining what a psychiatrist is and does, the College's Position Statement reads: "By virtue of their specialist training, (psychiatrists) bring a comprehensive and integrated biopsychosocial approach to the diagnosis, assessment, treatment and prevention of psychiatric disorder and mental health problems ... An integrated understanding of the biological, psychological and social aspects of mental health problems enables psychiatrists to recognize and treat both the physical and emotional effects of psychiatric disorder" [7; see caveat].

This view is sufficiently widespread to be held as mainstream, as not requiring further justification. In a fervent case against unrestrained biologism in psychiatry, Lachter [8] did not question the reality of the biopsychosocial model. Harari [9] took a more sanguine view, arguing that "a more sophisticated formulation... such as the biopsychosocial model, enables psychiatry to study clinically relevant phenomena at various levels of conceptual integration from the synaptic to the social order" (p 729).

In one of the very few psychiatric texts published in this country, *Foundations of Clinical Psychiatry*, edited by Bloch and Singh [10], several contributing authors mentioned the biopsychosocial approach as a basis for clinical practice: "The biopsychosocial approach provides one helpful framework by postulating that clinical problems result from the continuous interplay of biological, social and psychological factors" (p 45). The authors of another chapter stated: "…there is no reason to see psychiatric disorders as different from the rest of medicine in the context of the medical model of disease. On the other hand, psychosocial factors tend to play a greater role in psychiatry than in other areas of medicine… the biopsychosocial approach … takes into account not only symptoms and signs but also environmental factors and the overall social context" (p 68).

In their critique of the descriptive or categorical approach to psychiatric diagnosis, Frances and Egger [11] warned that psychiatrists training in the "DSM era" were learning a narrow, blinkered way of thinking about patients that prevents them "….understanding the patient and his or her presentation within a biopsychosocial context" (p 164). Indeed, they were even unhappy with the very term mental disorder as it implies "…a mind-body dichotomy that is proving to be illusory." Nonetheless, they were optimistic that further progress in neurosciences would allow us to "….move from a descriptive model to an integrative model that reflects the interplay of biological, psychological, environmental and social variables affecting the expression and treatment of psychiatric disorders," i.e. the same biopsychosocial model cast in slightly different terms.

Recently, this steady flow of support was greatly supplemented by a series of commissioned articles on the contribution of the American psychiatrist, George Engel, to medicine and psychiatry. The first paper, by his son and daughter-in-law [12], was a personal account of his life's work and how this could be related to the disaster in New York in September, 2001. The second [13] was an historical outline of the influence of psychoanalysis in the development of Engel's ideas while the fourth [14] was merely "personal reminiscence." At the outset of the third paper, Smith and Strain [15] pronounced: "Medicine in Australia became biopsychosocial without knowing it … A generation of Australian medical students and psychiatry trainees have been taught (the biopsychosocial method)" (p 458). This follows from their view that "Engel's biopsychosocial model … stands as one of the most influential ideas in Medicine in the 20th Century." His model, they believed, was wholly scientific, in contrast with "counter dogmas" such as holistic or humanistic medicine. The latter "…qualify as dogmas to the extent that they eschew the scientific method and lean instead on faith and belief systems handed down from remote and obscure or charismatic authority figures." They also saw deficiencies in static, descriptive models, such as the DSM-IV system: "The integration of biology, psychology, social issues and behavior, and the interaction among them, is the hallmark of the biopsychosocial model of disease…"

Reading these papers, one might conclude that the biopsychosocial model has been fully articulated, although some authors have expressed reservations. In passing, Smith and Strain quoted several critiques of the biopsychosocial model, but they did not see any of these criticisms as compelling: "Most authors who have offered criticism call for further work on (Engel's) model rather than its dismissal."

I believe it is fair to say that Australasian psychiatrists accept the biopsychosocial model as the central intellectual element in their field, if not defining the discipline itself. Historically, the model derives from a series of Engel's papers starting in 1960 [16-20]. Dismayed by what he saw as deficiencies in the dominant "biomedical model" of medicine and psychiatry in North America in the 1960s and '70s, Engel outlined the case for a new approach directed at countering the unashamedly mechanistic-reductionist concepts of biomedicine. He believed a biopsychosocial model would bring psychiatry back to its roots as a human-centered discipline. The recent appreciation of Engel's work leaves no doubt that, at least in Australia and New Zealand, orthodox psychiatry accepts that he succeeded in his ambition.

8-5. Critique of the Place of Biopsychosocialism in Psychiatry

It is a matter of public fact that, while George Engel outlined a place for a new model and even devised a name for it, he never wrote it [21]. That is to say, it is false to state that there exists a model, theory, approach, intellectual context or frame, etc., which could meaningfully be called biopsychosocial. Despite claims [15, p 458], his 1977 paper is not an "exposition of the biopsychosocial model" because there is nothing in that paper beyond a few homilies and non-threatening pleas for a model to integrate science and humanism.

Furthermore, it is false to claim, as Smith and Strain did, that I saw Engel's "model" as merely "flawed" and supported its further development. I stated explicitly: "In its present form, (it) is so seriously flawed that its continued use in psychiatry is not justified ... (I)t is not a model at all ... not a theory ... not revolutionary ... not a model in any interesting sense of the word ... just a case of wishful thinking." Apparently, this language was not strong enough so I will therefore call for its "dismissal." In a word, the officially-endorsed biopsychosocial model is pure humbug, i.e. "(some)thing that tricks or deceives; nonsense, rubbish." I say this just because it does not exist.

This leaves Antipodean psychiatry somewhat exposed. Throughout our training, we are told Engel wrote a model, the College and its journals constantly tell us he did, most psychiatrists here seem to believe it, and our representatives tell governments and other funding bodies that we alone have it and are thereby specialists. Even Engel himself seemed to be in no doubt that he had done it but, when we look for the details, they are nowhere to be seen. There is nothing in Engel's papers that in any way qualifies as a scientific model, theory, plan, exposition or anything of the sort. If he wrote it elsewhere, I have never found it and no Australian psychiatrist has ever referred to it, nor has his son. All he did was pen a heartfelt plea for such a model, which may explain why, forty years later, Frances and Egger were still conscious of the same deficiencies in the profession – and felt driven to make the same, heartfelt plea.

This means that the work the College accepts as the theoretical basis for our existence as a separate specialty is illusory. If our *raison d'être* is only that we bring a "comprehensive and integrated biopsychosocial approach to the diagnosis, assessment, treatment and prevention of psychiatric disorder and mental health problems" [3], then we have no justification in calling ourselves specialists. This is not to say that there could not be a rationale for psychiatry, only that Engel's work does not provide it.

This conclusion is not popular with mainstream psychiatry. In commissioned commentaries on my paper, Muir [22] and Mullen [23] offered defenses of the biopsychosocial model. Muir was of the view that my efforts were misdirected because, when used in connection with Engel's work, nobody really meant model, they meant 'model,' i.e. it was merely metaphor, interchangeable with 'frame' or, as the College prefers, 'approach.' That is, nobody can criticize biopsychosocialism as a failed scientific model because it was never meant to be science in the first place, and it is only "semantics" to claim otherwise.

There are several flaws in his response. Firstly, he has simply attempted to shield the biopsychosocial model from scientific criticism by shifting it out of the realm of science. This attempt must fail as, far from defending the model, he has confirmed my case that Engel did not write a scientific theory or model. Muir's move seems unlikely to attract wide support in the profession because if the College's "biopsychosocial approach" is not science, then it carries no more weight than, say, the "mystical approach," the "homeopathic framework" or the "chiropractic context." I feel confident in stating that psychiatrists should never accept that our daily practice is guided by mere metaphor. At the very least, if 'models,' frames, contexts or approaches aren't science, they shouldn't be paid as such.

Secondly, and more to the point, it doesn't matter how psychiatrists use the word model, whether in the firm sense of the physical sciences as I defined it or in Muir's allegorical sense, the crucial point surely is that Engel didn't write one. A model must consist of more than a name: it is not possible to nominate an entity and to define it in the same illocutionary act.

In the same vein, Mullen suggested that the term "biopsychosocial model" was no more than an obvious truth, a "useful and familiar friend." Prior to Engel, we had all understood intuitively that biological, psychological and social factors influence mental disorder but Engel's phrase "...provided an articulation of these previously ill-expressed and partially inchoate assumptions. The power of an apposite word should never be underestimated." Nonetheless, he continued, nobody should take it seriously as it is simply a "rhetorical flourish and comforting commonsense" that "expresses something about the world which appeals to a significant number of people." Perhaps, he implied, it may be no more than an "erroneous and frankly silly belief" but, by virtue of its studied vagueness, it offends none and may even help some feel a little better. "Give me every time," he pleaded, "a vague, ill-defined, well-meaning froth of a notion, like the biopsychosocial model, over [reductionist biologism]." In these difficult times, he concluded, assailed by the pharmaceutical industry's dehumanizing biotechnology, we psychiatrists "need every protection we can find, even if it is a chimera."

While neither commentator attempted to argue that Engel's work was in any way scientific, it is clear from their contributions that they saw psychiatry as locked in a Manichaean battle between, on the one hand, Engel's gently humanist notion and, on the other, "reductionist materialism" (Muir) or "mean-spirited rationalizations which ignore culture and humanity, in attempting to reduce human experience to genes and neurotransmitters" (Mullen). By default, they presumed, those who don't support Engel's approach are necessarily of the "dehumanized technology" camp. I have previously argued that biological psychiatry cannot provide a general theory for psychiatry, that it is no more than scientism (i.e. the inappropriate application of scientific methods or concepts to non-empirical questions) but I see no reason to accept that the way to deal with rampant reductionist materialism is to retreat into "erroneous and frankly silly" non-science.

Engel, as one of his students revealed, was "driven by a narcissistic belief in his own 'specialness'" and saw himself as a "medical Darwin" [14]. Throughout his long career, he reiterated a major problem for reductionist psychiatry, that humans are more than just lumps of meat. What he failed to do was provide a solution to the impetus of "dehumanizing biotechnology." His disciples, however, are in no doubt: "What no one can deny is that he [left] a towering edifice...." [14, p 471]. Yes, I deny it. I say his legacy is mere homily or a mnemonic and cannot form a basis for a general theory of psychiatry. He indicated where the towering edifice should be built and told us what the view from the top might be like, but he didn't even sketch a plan for it, let alone test its feasibility.

8-6. Conclusion

The establishment's defense of their whimsical 'model' is self-contradictory. It is not clear why the editorial board of a scientific journal that claims to be both ethical [24] and of an international standard [25] should publish the frank view that the conduct of psychiatry is based in non-science. Never having met Dr Muir, Professors Smith or Mullen or any of the other invited authors, I am sure they are all charming, well-read and well-meaning men. If, however, they were to say to the Minister of Health: "Sir, we psychiatrists are the keepers of chimeras and purveyors of rhetorical flourishes. We offer comforting commonsense and vague, ill-defined, well-meaning frothy notions, if not erroneous and frankly silly beliefs, yet we expect to be paid handsomely for our services," then I suspect the honorable person might show them to the door.

"Gentlemen," I hear him say, "pixies may express something about the world that appeals to a significant number of people, but we don't pay those who profess to conjure them up. Good day to you." And well he might because, in their misdirected defense, the editor's champions have exposed truism where the intellectual heart of our profession should be.

In an editorial, Bloch [26] opined: "...it is salutary to note in the article on the level of interest in psychiatry among medical students ... that an unattractive feature of our profession is its 'perceived absence of a scientific foundation.' This is clearly not an accurate portrayal..." Bloch is wrong; the students correctly recognized that scientific truth is not established by dint of repetition of a falsehood. By endorsement of the establishment, of which former editor Bloch is a pivotal member, modern psychiatry is a prescientific hodge-podge of random observations, serendipity, tradition and "rhetorical flourishes" held together by the gossamer of wishful thinking. Of our intellectual leaders, Max Planck, a committed revolutionary to the end, would simply laugh and say: "Wait until they die, and their chimera will die with them!"

Orthodox psychiatry is attempting to convince the general public, the funding bodies and, most significantly, the younger generations of students and psychiatrists, that it has articulated a rational model which grants it special and unique knowledge of the etiological processes and phenomena of mental disturbance. However, by admitting that it knows full well there is no such model, psychiatry exposes itself to charges of the very grossest intellectual neglect. Worse still, if anybody wished to accuse us of perpetrating a scientific fraud, practically anything we could say in our defense would simply look dishonest.

If psychiatry as a discrete profession is eventually broken apart and the bits left to general practitioners, psychologists, social workers and all the others who fancy they can do our job better, then, by their lack of intellectual leadership, our own establishment will bear full responsibility. Had Thomas Kuhn known of our failure to develop an adequate scientific model, he would surely have said we deserve our historical fate. I believe that if we can't do better than "vague, ill-defined, well-meaning froth" masquerading as "one of the most influential ideas in Medicine in the 20th Century," then we should get out.

In the next two parts, I will look at two theories of mental life that might form the basis of a general theory for psychiatry, then derive some general principles for an integrative theory of mental disorder.

Part II: The Working Mind

Any scientific theory of the mind has to treat it as an automaton.
—Phillip Johnson-Laird, 1983

9 | Functionalism and the Nature of Control in Human Behavior

9-1. Introduction

So far, our search for a general theory for psychiatry has foundered for want of a general theory of human mental life. What sort of mental state could control human behavior? This is a critically important question, but one which, for most of this century, has usually been answered with one word: "None." Both biologism and behaviorism denied the efficacy of mental states and sought to build a non-mentalist psychology and psychiatry. I have argued that there cannot be a non-mentalist theory of human psychology so, in this chapter, I want to look more closely at what sort of mentalist psychology could do the job. This might seem a little unnecessary: mentalist means mentalist, so what's the concern with type? As with all other classes of theories, there is a range of types of mentalist psychologies. Philosophy is not constrained by reality, meaning the number of available theories expands to fill the conceptual space.

In 1978, Daniel Dennett [1] briefly summarized the available theories. He noted that since 1949, when Ryle's *Concept of Mind* signaled a new era in philosophy of mind, behaviorism and many other -isms had slipped quietly from the scene. What remained were Mind-Brain Identity Theory (MBIT) and functionalism. In the thirty years since, even MBIT has gone to the dusty bookshelves of philosophical history. At the beginning of the twenty-first century, all that remains of his particular list is the group of theories known as functionalism.

Dennett suggested that the central feature of these theories is that they define mental states as functional states, meaning "states individuated by their functional role within the whole system" (p 254). Later, he argued that reproduction in any form of the "functional structure" of the human cognitive system will "thereby reproduce all the mental properties as well," including everything that we would normally call subjective experience [2]. "If all the control functions of a human wine taster's brain can be reproduced in silicon chips, the enjoyment will *ipso facto* be reproduced as well" (p 31).

This is not an intuitive notion; even Dennett agreed "...it surely seems outrageous at first blush." In the half-century since Ryle, acceptance of the subjectivity of conscious experience has not been popular. Partly, this was related to the slippery nature of the concepts, but partly also to an intellectual aversion to grasping the nettle of mentality, especially after so many great thinkers had spent so much time labeling it as a nettle. Whatever the reason, in 1991, Dennett firmly embraced functionalism in his boldly-titled book, *Consciousness Explained*. This is a little unexpected as, in its ordinary, experiential sense, consciousness is not central to functionalism and some might argue the theory doesn't need to account for it. Dennett implied a wine taster's consciousness is emergent, and thereby didn't need explaining. Perhaps he recognized this, because his 1996 book on much the same topic, *Kinds of Minds*, was merely subtitled *Towards an understanding of consciousness,* i.e. what was explained in 1991 had become unclear again by 1996 [3]. Despite his earlier optimism, the idea of consciousness was as persistent and mysterious as ever.

In 1996, support for dualism resurfaced [4], perhaps even Armstrong's long-awaited "Great Dualist Counter-attack." This time, the case for naturalistic dualism was tightly argued, even "fiendishly clever," to quote one of its reviewers. David Chalmers' attempt at a fundamental theory of subjective conscious experience left no doubt that the essential mentality of mind could no longer be dismissed. At the outset, he insisted that it is necessary to take consciousness seriously: "The easiest way to develop a 'theory' of consciousness is to deny its existence," he said. Then, with a nudge and a wink, the theorist can deflect his audience's attention from the critical issue of why, in being a conscious human being, "...there is something it is like to be that being..." (p 4). Normally, functionalism shifts interest from subjective experience to the cognitive and other informational processes that are intimately related to but entirely different from those experiences. However, with his precisely-argued case, Chalmers thrust conscious experience back to center-stage: "To analyze consciousness in terms of some functional notion is either to change the subject or to define away the problem. One might as well define 'world peace' as 'a ham sandwich.' Achieving world peace becomes much easier, but it is a hollow achievement" (p 105).

Thus, at the dawn of the new century, we are faced with the choice between those who would argue that, at most, consciousness is causally irrelevant, and those who see it as central to human existence. Therefore, in considering the nature of the controlling element in human affairs, we need to look more closely at these competing models, at Dennett's functionalism and at Chalmers' naturalistic dualism.

9-2. Functionalism

In 1978, while reviewing starters in the race to be The General Theory of Mind, Dennett named functionalism as the "prevailing favorite," even though in 1976, Lacey hadn't included it in his Dictionary of Philosophy. By 1995, Audi [5] was a little more generous, affording the idea a heading of its own. His contributor defined functionalism as "the view that mental states are defined by their causes and effects" (p 288): "If two people, on seeing a ripe banana, are in states with the same causes and effects, then, by functionalist definition, they are in the same mental state—say, having a sensation of yellow." But, the authors warned: "The status of these arguments remains controversial."

Dennett's version of functionalism places somewhat less emphasis on its logical status than on its realization. For him, the challenge is one of sketching a workable basis for a natural, non-question-begging theory of mind. Consciousness must flow from the functional organization of the brain. Accordingly, in *Consciousness Explained* [2], he expended considerable effort in attempting to exorcise the "Cartesian Theater," his term for the error implicit in all theories of mind relying on a hidden observer. Observers, he believed, are non-scientific because they imply dualism. In turn, he disparaged dualism as a forlorn and disreputable siren song which necessarily violates the most fundamental principles of the physical universe: "This confrontation between quite standard physics and dualism (is its) inescapable and fatal flaw..." [2, p 35]. He repeatedly declared his opposition to dualism: "if dualism is the best we can do, then we can't understand human consciousness" (p 39) or "adopting dualism is really just accepting defeat without admitting it" (p 41).

Strong words, but absolutely necessary for somebody who believes that, ontologically, there is no room for two sorts of stuff in the head: "Somehow, the brain must be the mind but unless we can come to see in some detail how this is possible, our materialism will not explain consciousness, but only promise to explain it, some sweet day. That promise cannot be kept ... until we ... abandon more of Descartes' legacy" (p 41-2).

A persistent theme in Dennett's work over many years is the idea that any new model of consciousness will most likely be counter-intuitive, simply because we have already tried all the intuitive ones: "I assume that whatever the true theory of mind turns out to be, it will overturn some of our prior convictions, so I am not cowed by having the counterintuitive implications of my view pointed out. Any theory which makes progress is bound to be initially counterintuitive" [6, p 6]. "I don't view it as ominous that my theory seems at first to be strongly at odds with common wisdom ... If there were (an immediately obvious) theory to be had, we would surely have hit upon it by now" [2, p27].

9-3. Problems of Functionalism

Despite the brave title, at the end of *Consciousness Explained*, Dennett admitted: "My explanation of consciousness is far from complete ... but it is a beginning, because it breaks the spell of the enchanted circle of ideas that made explaining consciousness seem impossible" (p455). For me, this was a very welcome admission as several close readings of the book had failed to reveal just where he had explained consciousness. Dennett's work displays a deep-seated tension riving an otherwise "masterful tapestry of deep insights," to quote one of his reviewers. I suggest Dennett's functionalism is fundamentally flawed, to the extent that neither it nor any other non-dualist account of mind can provide a proper basis for an explanation of mental disorder. This point will be discussed in more detail in a later section but, for Dennett's model, a series of errors has led him to argue the wrong point.

Firstly, his implacable opposition to any hint of dualism appears to be a reaction to all the bad stuff that has gone before. Despite his opinion, dualism does not imply an acceptance of the supernatural. A non-material entity able to interfere with the physical realm does not have to be a poltergeist or a cheap magician's trick. His own "virtual machine" [e.g. 2, pp 216-221] is a perfectly acceptable example of how an immaterial entity can influence the material realm provided it has the right connections. Anything can be joined to something else as long as we have the right connections. He himself gives the clue: "How can mind stuff both elude all physical measurement and control the body? A ghost in the machine is of no help in our theories unless it is a ghost that can move things around ... but anything that can move a physical thing is itself a physical thing (although perhaps a strange and heretofore unstudied kind of physical thing)" [2, p 35]. With this throwaway comment, he has just conceded his case: that a causally-effective immaterial entity just is a "strange kind of thing" coupled with the right transducers. The efficacy of a causally-effective entity lies not in its nature but in whether it has the right three-pin plug, because that's how the virtual machine becomes effective.

Secondly, Dennett bluntly dismisses all dualist ideas as substance dualism, an unwise move as it forces him to disregard any *process* that might be doing the job without being a thing in itself. Processes can get things done, without there being any *thing* to do the doing. Processes just are "doings." By overlooking the point that processes do not imply substances, he has fallen into the trap of believing that all his opponents are necessarily guilty of reification. Processes are necessarily immaterial in the sense that one can't pick them up (that's why they are called processes and not things), and processes certainly can intervene in the material realm. That's how we know that a process has occurred: we detect a measurable change in the material realm. But, if we don't know how processes are connected, they seem magical. Through this simple error, Dennett assumes the burden of giving a non-dualist account of consciousness in all its facets, a burden he finally has to admit his theory can't carry: "I haven't replaced a metaphorical theory, the Cartesian Theater, with a nonmetaphorical ('literal, scientific') theory. All I have done, really, is replace one family of metaphors and images with another" (p 455).

A third reason he failed to live up to his grand title is because there are two quite distinct aspects to the term "consciousness," the informational and the experiential, each requiring separate explanations. Conflating them only makes the job impossible. For example, he acknowledges the place of conscious experience in human affairs, then largely ignores it, repeatedly implying that an adequate account of consciousness *qua* computation of digital data flow will also explain the experience of thinking, of loving someone, of tasting wine, of acting morally or of imagining a purple cow (p 33). At no point, however, does he argue that these dual aspects of mental life are sufficiently alike for them to be amenable to a single explanatory analysis. If he wants to *explain* consciousness, a good starting point would be to decompose it into its constituent processes.

Because he failed to argue a convincing integration of conscious experience, he developed a model which is not so much counter-intuitive as plain disorganized. Of the available evidence, he used just two types, the empirical neurosciences ("I declare my starting point to be the objective, materialistic, third-person world of the physical sciences" [6, p 5]), and the brain's computational capacity vis-à-vis its informational flow (see [2], Ch. 3, and his summary (pp 253-54), in which he considers only the computational elements of consciousness). For this omission, he offered no apologies, brazenly declaring: "This theory has enough novelty to make it hard to grasp at first" [2, p254].

At one point, he warns that people shouldn't mistake a "failure of imagination for an insight into necessity" (p 48), but it would also be fair to say that philosophers shouldn't always blame a reader's failure to grasp a model on his (the reader's) supposed inability to stretch his intuition. Plenty of people found MBIT and logical behaviorism counter-intuitive, and they were right. If the reader can't grasp what is on offer, it might be that what is on offer is fundamentally incoherent. I suggest that Dennett has failed to distinguish adequately between three quite separate elements: the function of the hidden observer in the Cartesian Theater, its reification, and its consciousness (in some of that word's many meanings), which is the *sine qua non* of the observer being able to acquit the role tradition has given it.

The real problem with the hidden observer in the Cartesian Theater is not that it is necessarily made of an ectoplasm that violates fundamental physical laws: I don't believe dualism implies this and nor, apparently, does Dennett. Rather, the fault with hidden observers is that they start an infinite regress and are therefore non-scientific *regardless* of their substance. All theories of mind that rely on concepts such as a stream, river, field, stage, theater or whatever of consciousness necessarily invoke an infinite regress. This is also true whenever mental contents of any sort are invested with a quality, however defined, of consciousness, or travel to a particular part of the brain to enter consciousness, because once invested or moved, something has to inspect them. That something can only be a homunculus acting as the first step on the road to infinity. This is the real problem with the Cartesian Theater, not the possibility that the homunculus might be supernatural. We are concerned not with the nature of the "little man inside the man," but with its very its existence. "Accepting dualism is giving up," Dennett thundered—yes, but only if one side of the dualism is left as an explanatory dead-end, a fully-functional brute of a fact, as it were.

Finally, I suggest Dennett's emphasis in his functionalist theory of mind is misplaced. He attacked dualism but I believe he should have focused his efforts on the sense of self. This is the destructive element in the Cartesian non-explanation, this is the persistent hidden observer against which he cast his jeremiad. Consciousness, on which the "self-construct" is utterly dependent, is not a thing, and therefore cannot form part of a (substance) dualism in the sense of Dennett's use of the term. His particular analytic approach is eminently suited to explaining complex, reified entities based on unseen, fundamental processes or facts, but he has given no indication anywhere that it can generate an account of those processes or facts themselves. He should have applied it to the idea of self, "...the thinking thing, the I in 'I think, therefore I am'" (p 33). That was his proper target, rather than the basic facts of his model of consciousness which, insofar as they can be explained, are largely neurophysiological anyway.

9–4. Getting Around the Problems

Dennett has foreseen part of this objection. He devoted Chapter 13 of *Consciousness Explained* to "The Reality of Selves," but it is certainly not the clearest paper he has ever written. He starts with a series of biological constructions, including the immune system's 'sense of self/not self,' of spiders weaving webs, beavers building dams, and so on. Then he makes a series of small steps, using devices which, if not challenged, lure the reader to some remarkable conclusions. As it happens, some of his conclusions are correct but, in any event, he argues the wrong case.

His first device is that his basic premise doesn't appear until the very end of the chapter, where he asserts that one either believes in consciousness as a rigidly biological "extrusion of the brain," or one necessarily embraces a "brain-pearl," the "hopelessly contradiction-riddled myth of the distinct, separate soul" (p 430). This is a straw man. I can believe in a naturalistic duality of mind and brain by the simple expedient of the "virtual machine" that he himself mentions on the very next page. Also, he needs to explain the difference between an unacceptable "soul" and his acceptable self. Functionally (and I use the term advisedly), there is very little to separate them.

Secondly, his own "intuition pump" (p 400) is working overtime: "This fundamental biological principle of distinguishing self from world, inside from outside, produces some remarkable echoes in the highest vaults of our psychology" (p 414). True, but echoes aren't proofs. "Each normal individual of (*Homo sapiens*) makes a self. Out of its brain, it spins a web of words and deeds, and, like other creatures, it doesn't have to know what it's doing; it just does it ... This 'web of discourses' ... is as much a biological product as any of the other constructions to be found in the animal world. Stripped of it, an individual human being is as incomplete as a bird without its feathers, a turtle without its shell" (p 416).

This point depends entirely on his definition of 'biological.' Does he mean all words and deeds are biological, or just some? Do words derive directly from the brain, in any significant sense, or are they wholly part of the mind? Is a novel therefore biological? For that matter, is *Consciousness Explained* biological? Who can say, as Dennett doesn't answer these questions. If he is saying: "Each human is biological and each human develops a self, therefore the self is biological," then he is guilty either of banality or of begging the question. Here, he has made the same error as Skinner in *Beyond Freedom and Dignity*: he mistook a description (of the development of self) for an explanation. Indeed, this chapter reads remarkably like Skinner's polemic in which, by a series of slightly questionable steps, the reader is lead to embrace an outrageous conclusion. As a final point, Dennett's parallel between the human self, birds' feathers and turtles' shells is a very unsubtle attempt to beg the question of the nature of mental illness: is it genuinely biological or is it psychological? This type of move will not settle the debate [8].

There are other weaknesses in his story but, as mentioned, I believe his conclusions are right. The "self-construct" is important. When it breaks down in practice (and Multiple Personality Disorder is not an example of that), then the human is in many ways worse off than a naked bird or turtle because, whatever their distress, animals don't feel the need to commit suicide. The idea of a Self constructed from one's developmental experiences is not unique to Daniel Dennett. Sigmund Freud was quite at home with it. In fact, all Dennett has done in this chapter is translate some of the airier psychoanalytic notions into 'biocognitive-speak' because, unless one is going to embrace frankly religious notions, there really isn't much alternative to a "self-constructed self." However, this notion is so general as to be uninformative. Quite clearly, children do develop a sense of individual self without formal tuition, but that doesn't prove it is biological in any convincing sense of the word.

We might use Chomsky's notion of the development of language as a rough parallel. Every healthy child's genetic endowment gives it the neurological capacity to speak, but the language it uses and what it says in that language have no basis in biology. Genes, to labor a point, code for proteins, not for ideas. Similarly, each child has the genetic endowment to develop a mental life but the genome says nothing about the mental contents. As Dennett uses the term, the "self" is very much a part of the larger mind, a piece of mental furniture, as it were, but it is most definitely not written into the architect's plans for the mental stage where the furniture will sit.

If we see the sense of self as self-constructed and self-constructing, a constantly-evolving virtual machine for which we have no points of contact other than language, then we can account for the phenomenon of self without the regressive trap of the Cartesian Theater. At that, the greater part of Dennett's argument against dualism collapses, thereby weakening his functionalist claims. However, it is critically important to understand that any move towards reification of the "self" will automatically produce another homunculus. Dennett didn't seem to understand this: he cannot rail against homunculi watching theaters in the head, then invoke a fully-functional homunculus called the Self, define it as biological and think that it settles the matter.

9-5. Experience and Functionalism

At this point, I want to leave the computational side of Dennett's model to look instead at the experiential side of human mental life. He neglected this in favor of the computational and I suggest at least part of his reason for doing so was because his ideas of phenomenal experience were, well, badly computed. In his list of "conscious phenomena" [2, Ch.3: "A visit to the phenomenological garden"] he classified experiences into three types. Firstly, he said, there are "experiences of the 'external' world," ordinary sensory experiences as everybody understands the term. Secondly, he listed "experiences of the purely 'internal' world," memories, fantasies, daydreams, bright ideas and sudden hunches. Finally, he described "experiences of emotion or 'affect'," but clouded the picture by including pains, hunger and thirst in a list of more normal emotions, such as anxiety, anger, joy, humor, etc.

If this is Dennett's phenomenological garden, then it is a "blooming, buzzing confusion," hardly a proper starting point for a "scientific, materialistic" theory (p 25). His descriptions of each aspect of these three categories are heavily biased towards the data-gathering and processing side of conscious experience. Nobody would dispute that this is very important. If our proto-human ancestors couldn't distinguish food from poison or work out how fast the proto-lion was running toward them, then we wouldn't be here today. But data-gathering and processing are not the difficult parts of a theory of human consciousness because all other animals can do the same sorts of things as we can, and we are interested in the difference between humans and animals, not the similarities. In any event, Dennett had already given a masterly, non-homuncular account of intellect [7]; what is missing in his present theory is the experiential element. By clever use of an "intuition pump," he de-emphasizes experience to the point where the reader could be excused for believing that consciousness is about information. Certainly it is – among other things, and it is the experiential things that have always caused us so much trouble.

9-6. Conclusions: Functionalism Fails

I suggest Dennett failed in his ambition of explaining consciousness within a functionalist framework because he shouldn't have tried in the first place. He had the wrong method and the wrong subject matter. His method wasn't suited to explaining his mixture of neurophysiology, higher cognitive functions, current experience and brute facts. As his lengthy list of conscious phenomena clearly indicates, he saw consciousness as pre-eminently a cognitive process, a discriminating, analyzing and calculating system aimed at garnering the maximum information (note that) from the environment as an essential part of survival of the species. His approach was, however, eminently suited to decomposing a composite reification of those processes, which is what the "thinking thing" is. Having done that, he announced that he had solved all the problems of consciousness, quite overlooking the fact that phenomenal experience, the really hard part of a theory of consciousness, was buried in the mess of material he preferred not to see.

Unfortunately, a quick reading of his work doesn't reveal these types of problems. Despite his breezy style, Dennett is a clever and sophisticated writer. He packs a great deal into what, at first glance, seems to be some fairly light-weight, popularized philosophy. It is therefore worth summarizing his case in *Consciousness Explained*, just to see where the errors lie. I read his case as follows:

9-6 (i). "...YES, my theory is a theory of consciousness" [2, p 281];

9-6 (ii). It is a materialist theory: "The prevailing wisdom ... is materialism: there is only one sort of stuff, namely matter—the physical stuff of physics, chemistry, and physiology—and the mind is somehow nothing but a physical phenomenon ... We can (in principle!) account for every mental phenomenon using the same physical principles, laws and raw materials that suffice to explain radioactivity, continental drift, photosynthesis..." [2, p 33]. "Somehow, the brain must be the mind" (p 41). See also his *Intentional Stance*: "I declare my starting point to be the objective, materialistic, third-person world of the physical sciences [6, p 5];

9-6 (iii). Consciousness is all sorts of things, but mostly it is about computation and information [2, pp 43-65];

9-6 (iv). When consciousness is not about computation, the extra bits can be explained away: "...we will try to remove the motivation for believing in these (special, subjective) properties (of our internal discriminative states) ... by finding alternative explanations for the phenomena that seem to demand them" [2, p 373];

9-6 (v). Dualism always means substance dualism, which violates the laws of physics; therefore dualism is bad: "There is the lurking suspicion that the most attractive feature of mind stuff is its promise of being so mysterious that it keeps science at bay forever. This fundamentally antiscientific stance of dualism is, to my mind, its most disqualifying feature, and is the reason why in this book I adopt the apparently dogmatic rule that dualism is to be avoided at all costs ... given the way dualism wallows in mystery, accepting dualism is giving up (as in 'then a miracle occurs')" [2, pp 33-38];

9-6 (vi). Descartes' model, the Cartesian Theater, is bad, because wherever there is a Cartesian Theater, there is a hidden observer, and wherever there is a hidden observer, there is dualism, and dualism means ectoplasm and ectoplasm is antiscientific;

9-6 (vii). Selves are good because they are abstractions that can be explained in terms of the same processes that result in snails' shells, beavers' dams and bowerbirds' bowers [2, p 368]. While these natural features are interesting, "...the strangest and most wonderful constructions in the whole animal world are the amazing, intricate..." selves spun out of the brain of the primate, Homo sapiens. In constructing a self, a child no more knows what it is doing than do snails making their shells [2, p416]; therefore, the two processes are biological;

9-6 (viii). Selves, however, do not imply a Cartesian Theater: "This idea of 'mechanical' interpretation in the brain is the central insight of any materialistic theory of the mind, but (it denies the idea that) there has to be someone in there ... to witness the events ... Witnesses need raw materials on which to base their judgments. These 'sense data' or ... 'phenomenal properties of experience,' are props without which a Witness makes no sense" [2, p322]. Hidden observers need phenomenal properties, therefore getting rid of the phenomenal properties gets rid of the hidden observer. Selves do not rely on phenomenal properties because, despite appearances, consciousness isn't really about phenomenal properties anyway;

9-6 (ix). Materialism gets rid of phenomenal properties; therefore materialism gets rid of hidden observers; therefore materialism dispenses with Cartesian dualism because it is "hopelessly wrong" (p 106); therefore a materialist Self can do no wrong, even if it is immortal [2, pp 368, 430];

9-6 (x). Dennett's materialist theory explains consciousness without doing anything naughty because it explains computation without leaving any loose bits called phenomenal experiences, which nobody would want to include in a sensible theory of consciousness anyway because they're far too difficult.

It might be argued that this is not an entirely fair summary of Dennett's life's work, and one would have to concede that compressing a 455 page book to one page is not always going to do justice to its subtleties. Nonetheless, I see major errors in Dennett's analysis of consciousness. He has not established that his approach (or anything like it) can give a proper account of the nature of the controlling element in human affairs. I am including the experiential element in human affairs here: the committed functionalist could argue that the "controlling element" (my term) need only be a computational capacity; experience does not control human affairs. I disagree: art, for example, has no computational value or, to take an extreme case, depression is all about experience taking control of the computer. It is certainly true that there is no convincing evidence in any of Dennett's later publications that he can account for the experiential element in human affairs, nor that we are wrong in our perception that conscious experience is important. Because of these objections, there is no reason to believe Dennett's functionalism could form the basis for a general theory for psychiatry.

<table>
<tr>
<td>

10

</td>
<td>

Dualism

</td>
</tr>
</table>

10-1: Introduction: Dualism Re-emergent

There is nothing new under the sun and, as the new century gets off to a tough-minded, materialist start, the oldest concept of mind has just been resurrected. Popper and Eccles tried to breathe life into it, but neither of them claimed to be a philosopher of mind; perhaps unsurprisingly, their theory of mind foundered. More recently, a startling reappraisal of this most ancient of ideas has commanded attention. David Chalmers' "search for a fundamental theory of the conscious mind" firmly subscribes to a dualist model. Dennett and other functionalists may politely hide their smirks of disdain, but Chalmers' approach is not the dualism they have long disparaged.

The concept of substance dualism is now so outmoded that it is little more than facile to criticize dualism on the basis that it necessarily implies magical substances. Three hundred years ago, Spinoza outlined the notion of property dualism. Chalmers' modern version again argues the case for property dualism on the grounds that it "gives us a coherent, naturalistic, unmysterious view of consciousness and its place in the natural order" [1, p 165].

While this is a bold claim, his case for dualism is tightly and precisely argued. There is no pretence in his work that it will be easy going. While Dennett makes light of his task, using puns, cartoons and clever wordplay to slide across some rather sticky patches, Chalmers leaves nothing to chance. Every claim is examined minutely, every consequence explored to its limit, with the result that a quick reading leaves one wondering why so many words resulted in so little progress. But, as his subtitle states, this work is but a search for a (not 'the') fundamental theory of consciousness.

10-2. Property Dualism

Once again, a brief summary of a major work cannot do it justice but his main case is as follows:

10-2 (i). It is necessary to take consciousness seriously: "The easiest way to develop a 'theory' of consciousness is to deny its existence or to redefine the phenomenon in need of explanation as something it is not" [4, p xii]. There is a problem, he concedes, as he "cannot prove that consciousness exists" but one's immediate experience cannot be gainsaid. It is also his intention to take science seriously, implicitly bearing in mind Bunge's warning: "...when scientists underrate philosophical issues, they risk falling victims to unscientific philosophies likely to slow down or even derail the train of their research" [2, p 62]. Chalmers fully intended to spend a little less time in the "logically-possible worlds" beloved of philosophers and more in the here and now.

10-2 (ii). Consciousness is "a natural phenomenon, falling under the sway of natural laws," with the consequence that "there should be some correct scientific theory of consciousness." Quite what science is, we are not told, but everybody is presumed to know and he doesn't intend any unusual demands: "Consciousness lies uneasily at the border of science and philosophy ... But it is not open to investigation by the usual scientific methods" [1, pp xii-xiv]. Quite appropriately, he did not restrict himself by attempting to define the form of the new, natural laws.

10-2 (iii). He believed a formal, reductive explanation of consciousness is impossible. Neurobiological explanations, which rely on behavioral or physiological criteria for consciousness, are covert attempts to sidestep the critical issue, namely, an explanation of the link between the physical event and conscious experience. This is of particular significance for psychiatrists. The argument also applies to efforts to account for consciousness in strictly physical terms (such as, for example, quantum variations), as "...the real problem with consciousness is to explain the principles in virtue of which consciousness arises from physical systems" (p 121). Physical theories will never tell us anything interesting about experience. Eliminative materialism is simply an attempt "...to evade the problem by denying the phenomenon" (p 164).

10-2 (iv). Consciousness exists but, since it cannot be reductively explained, Chalmers is led to embrace a form of dualism. Strictly applied, materialism denies dualism, but he opts for a naturalistic form of property dualism, arguing that, as we presently understand it, materialism is false: "...the property dualism that I advocate involves fundamentally new features of the world" (p 125). While naturalism denies supernatural properties, it is not to be taken as synonymous with materialism: "All that has happened is that our picture of nature has expanded ... (T)o embrace dualism is not necessarily to embrace mystery" (p 128).

10-2 (v). He proposes that conscious experience supervenes naturally upon the physical realm. A series of psychophysical laws defines the relationship without necessarily explaining the nature of experience itself. The existence of these laws will transform a dualist theory from metaphysical mess to a comprehensible account of one of the most difficult concepts in nature: "Given the physical facts about a system, such laws will enable us to infer what sort of conscious experience will be associated with the system, if any" (p 213). The laws, however, won't necessarily be capable of further explanation themselves: they are laws of nature, not of logic.

10-2 (vi). Consciousness divides readily into two aspects, the realm of phenomenal experience and the psychological or cognitive realm. The former is the inner, subjective world, the compelling but ineffable sense of "what it feels like to be something." He restricts the term "psychological consciousness" to the knowing, informational and reportable sense of self that I can convey to you. Cautiously, he elects not to follow the modern trend of referring to the psychological realm as "computational consciousness" as this may beg the question of its nature.

10-2 (vii). Unlike functionalism, which tries to explain consciousness away, dualism was never meant to be easy. With two sorts of consciousness, we get two sorts of mind-body problems and one mind-mind problem. There is the problem of contact between the body and the psychological self, between the body and the phenomenal realm, and between the psychological and the phenomenal realms.

10-2 (viii). The mode of interaction between the psychological realm and the body is easy to grasp. There is nothing conceptually novel or difficult about transferring information between these spheres. The real trouble for dualism arises with the explanation of the nature of phenomenal experiences. Chalmers leaves these as brute facts. Just as all laws of physics rely upon notions of time, mass, charge, etc., without explaining them, a theory of consciousness must also rest on at least some brute facts. Conscious experience is not yet (if ever) capable of further explanation.

10-2 (ix). Despite their differences, the two realms of mind are closely related: "These relations between (phenomenal) consciousness and cognition are not arbitrary and capricious, but systematic ... the nature of cognition is not irrelevant to consciousness, but central to its explanation" (p 172-73). Every time there is a conscious experience, there is also a related psychological assessment or phenomenal judgment about that experience: "...information is the key to the link between physical processes and conscious experience" (p 287) and thence phenomenal judgments. There are "deep and fundamental ties between consciousness and cognition" (p 172), with the transformation from unconscious information processing to conscious experience being effected by a particular functional organization of the brain. This gives rise to a substantial problem for his theory, the paradox of phenomenal judgments: "A physical or functional explanation of behavior ... can be given in terms that do not even imply the existence of conscious experience" (p 179). Thus, claims and judgments about conscious experience "...can be explained in terms quite independent of consciousness" (p 177). He found this paradox both "delightful and disturbing" but suggested that, with a little effort, we can "learn to live" with such a counter-intuitive conclusion.

10-2 (x). Finally, in a more speculative mood, he suggested a role for information in his naturalistic dualist model: "A conscious experience is a realization of an information state; a phenomenal judgment is explained by another realization of the same information state" (p 292). But information is ubiquitous; is experience therefore all around us? Somewhat mischievously, he defends the case for a type of panpsychism, concluding: "Consciousness does not come in sudden, jagged spikes, with isolated complex systems arbitrarily producing rich conscious experiences. Rather, it is a more uniform property of the universe, with very simple systems having very simple phenomenology, and complex systems having complex phenomenology. This makes consciousness less 'special' in some ways, and so more reasonable" (p298). For some people, the idea of conscious thermostats (or primates) is absurd but, he suggested, they owe us an explanation of why it is absurd (see note).

Chalmers leaves very little to chance. His case for naturalistic dualism is everything his reviewers said: startling, fascinating and fiendishly clever. We non-fiends can do little more than abide by Lewis' conclusion: "The materialist opposition cannot go on about how he has overlooked this and misunderstood that—because he hasn't. All we can do is disagree about which way the balance of considerations tilts."

For psychiatrists, Chalmers' dualist model is a welcome relief after so many years of ducking anti-mentalist propaganda from the behaviorist camp. Whatever their public personae, psychiatrists are at least closet dualists. We deal in mental illness. We believe in illnesses of the mind, which means that, whether we boast about it or not, we believe in minds. Quintessentially psychiatric concepts, such as hallucinations and delusions, are irreducibly mental in nature. It is not possible to practice orthodox psychiatry without in some respect paying homage to the ideas implicit in the Platonic model of mind. Thus, Chalmers should soon replace Dennett as the clever psychiatrist's source of confounding quotes. On second thoughts, he probably won't because he makes no pretence of writing philosophy for claret drinkers. A psychiatric member of his audience once complained: "Professor David Chalmers expanded his property dualist theory which for all its intricate advocacy and current fashion sounds very implausible!" [3]

There are several points at which psychiatry may diverge from Chalmers' philosophy. Firstly, we can question his use of the term science. Narrowly-defined materialist science appears to have run its course. Secondly, and regardless of how we approach it, the very notion of consciousness seems to drag problems in its wake. I will argue that consciousness is a classic category error. Thirdly, Chalmers' acceptance of a central paradox (of phenomenal judgment) in his account of mental life is worrying. While philosophers can eat out on their paradoxes, science doesn't like them. I will outline a change to his use of the concept of reductivism in the psychological realm that may resolve the paradox, thereby strengthening the case for property dualism.

10-3: Expanding Materialist Science

It is no longer sufficient simply to assume that everybody knows what the all-important notion of materialist science means. Materialism, in Chalmers' view, is an ontological statement that there is nothing in the Universe beyond matter and energy: "(T)he physical facts about the world exhaust all the facts, in that every positive fact is entailed by the physical facts" (p 124). It is difficult to be sure just what this means in practice. Does it mean that, armed with the Grand United Theory of Everything Physical (GUTEP) and the instantaneous vectors of every particle in the universe, I could predict next week's stock market figures, devise unsuspected theorems or work out what Anthony said to Cleopatra? If so, then I say materialism is meaningless, mere magic dressed in scientific clothing. It is important to remember that a physical theory, even one with high predictive power, will never tell us what is going to happen tomorrow. By setting limits on events, all it can say is what may not happen. A physical theory can never predict, say, the actual course of evolution but it can tell us a lot about what cannot evolve. Even with the vastly powerful GUTEP, we can never know enough about the universe to be able to make very precise predictions. Fortunately, however, for a lot of the things that interest us, the job is simplified by their capacity for self-determination. Given the precise position of every atom in a seed, GUTEP could perhaps tell us what color flowers it will have, although working it out would be unimaginably tedious. An easier way of doing it would be to look at its parents, or simply to plant the seed. However, as I have previously argued, a physical theory can never work on human codes. As pure information, ontologically divorced from their substrate, they are a closed book to anything but a decoder operating in the same, non-physical realm.

For us living organisms, the future is not unlimited; we can do only certain things. Much as I have always wanted to, I can never soar unaided across the sky. The limits for every living thing are there for anybody to read, coded in its genome. In a broad sense, the information in DNA is just chemical 'lock and key' stuff, but there is more to it than just that. Take the example of an alien who knows GUTEP back to front, but who has no knowledge whatsoever of the existence of human beings. If we gave the alien the precise chemical makeup of the DNA of, say, Napoleon, what would he be able to say about the dictator? I suggest he would have nothing to say, because he wouldn't have a clue what the information meant. He should be able to work out that DNA is a self-replicating molecule, but might assume that it was a life-form in its own right.

Trees are an integral part of the natural world, and tree DNA is therefore an integral part of the natural world. Yet it is not strictly material in the sense that, say, a piece of dead bark is material. DNA transcends the material realm in that, given the right conditions, it can subvert the ordinary "push and pull" causality of the material world (rain, lightning, salts dissolving in water, etc.) to its own ends. It has a function that is more than simple chemical reactions. While it cannot breach the laws of thermodynamics, etc., it can temporarily (and expensively) divert their normal direction of action to produce outcomes which would otherwise be vanishingly unlikely. By subverting the thermodynamic balance, coded information shifts the natural economy toward the infinitely improbable. Despite philosophical objections to miracles, DNA achieves minor ones every day without breaking a single physical law (think of the microorganisms living in sulfurous heat vents in the abyssal depths).

But GUTEP cannot tell us anything interesting about DNA's potential because, as a physical theory, it has nothing to say about codes. Nonetheless, codes are as much part of the material world as their end products. So we have to expand the ordinary concept of the material universe and thence of materialism to include the concept of information. However, information does not stand alone: for every code, there is a decoder, since codes alone are useless. A compact disc means nothing until put into a CD player. An alien who found such a disc would soon realize it contained coded data, but wouldn't know it was meant to be changed into sound (and, if he didn't have ears, it would mean even less).

Similarly, DNA means nothing without RNA and the rest of the cell mechanisms to realize its information. The material realm is vastly more complex than mere chemistry and physics; it is bustling and bursting with information that functions to perpetuate itself by any means possible. What is essential here is that our present notions of materialism *implicitly* rely upon a natural basis of information; given that, layers upon layers of improbability develop, stretching the limits of action close to infinity, far beyond anything that would ever happen by chance. There is therefore no wholly physical theory that can predict the limitless possibilities introduced to the material realm by coding mechanisms. The physical theory only tells us what can't happen, but never what is going to happen. Physics does not tell us what gravity is, but it says there cannot be an anti-gravity machine. Nothing in the laws of physics could ever predict, say, teeth, but teeth do not break any physical laws.

Thus, in arguing that there is necessarily more to materialism than chemicals bumping in the dark, Chalmers is on fairly safe ground. Chemicals don't bump into each other in cells, they are led to each other by coded information handed on from one generation to the next. The codes have a physical substrate but the information is not itself physical: it is, in every sense of the word, immaterial, but still part of the natural world. On this view, materialism transcends itself; the converse (and decidedly less mystical) view is that there is no such thing as simple, unadorned materialism (call it naive). At least, there hasn't been since DNA and its decoding mechanisms first appeared. Nobody knows when that was, probably around 800,000,000 years ago, which is a very long time for nature to be giving the lie to naive materialism. The rather frightening corollary is that if functionally similar codes haven't emerged in other solar systems, there is no other life in the universe.

Therefore, materialism becomes the notion that there is nothing in the universe beyond matter, energy and the informational states controlling their dispositions. Granted, this puts a heavy burden on the concept of information, especially as things like the laws of physics are not informational states since they do not control anything. They are merely inductive predictions as to how material interactions will proceed. If we adopt this broader view, then a lot of objections to materialism fade away. But one thing doesn't go away, namely, an unswerving opposition to the supernatural. What is the supernatural? It is any causative mechanism or agency that cannot be explained in principle within the natural realm just because it consistently breaks the rules of the natural realm. For theorists, life would be simpler if we could use the supernatural because excluding it causes lots of problems in deciding what to do with our mental lives.

The question of what constitutes science now falls rather more easily into place. Science is the rational, empirical endeavor aimed at accounting for matter-energy dispositions throughout the universe, and the informational states that control them. It is an endeavor in the sense it is a very broad but unorganized attempt to achieve something. Science itself isn't a project, but consists of many differing and even contradictory projects. They can be contradictory because scientists often don't know where they are going until they get there. Science is rational because it proceeds according to predetermined rules. There are certain things a scientist can do to get results and plenty he can't. Some of the rules are procedural and some are ethical; mostly, they are internally consistent but sometimes they aren't. The worst thing that can happen to the rules is when they are formulated in such a way as to produce the results people want to see. Analyzing the systems of rules of science is one of the jobs philosophers do, mainly because people trained in scientific methods are rarely trained to be critical of them. This is especially true of medicine. Finally, science is empirical, meaning all conclusions are accepted conditionally, the condition being that further evidence may overturn the original conclusions. There is no such thing as absolute truth in science, only "well-founded opinions."

10-4. Consciousness as a Category Error

Can science, as defined above, give an account of consciousness? Chalmers was optimistic: "...there should be some correct scientific theory of consciousness." Let's look at this a little more closely.

Step One: define consciousness, but this he declined to do. After asking: "Why does (consciousness) exist? What does it do? How could it possibly arise from lumpy grey matter?" he defined his twin notions of mental life ostensively. He justified this move with a nihilistic quote from the International Dictionary of Psychology: "...it is impossible to specify what (consciousness) is, what it does, or why it evolved. Nothing worth reading has been written about it" (p 3).

Unabashed, he pressed on, but we can object to his optimism at two points. Firstly, there is no such thing as a "correct scientific theory" of anything. There is only today's generally-accepted theory. If knowledge is demonstrably correct, it isn't a theory; if it is inevitably correct, it is truism and truism isn't science. That's a minor objection; more significantly, he appears to have slipped into a category error by asking: "What does it do? Why does it exist?"

In my view, there is no It of consciousness. Since consciousness is not a thing in any sense of the word, consciousness is therefore not a thing of which one could properly ask: "What does it do?" There is a "doing" of conscious matters, but no Thing doing them. I suggest that the very word Consciousness is an error, a solecism, crude essentialism of the most misleading sort. So in this view, there cannot be a science of consciousness, nor a scientific theory nor books about it, nothing. We are all conscious but there is no such *thing* as Consciousness. Being conscious is a function, the integrated outcome of many separate processes, but consciousness is a facile reification. The whole idea of a thing called Consciousness is a monstrously misleading error.

If we look at biology, we can talk about blood circulating through the body. Without breaking too many rules, we can say that Harvey discovered the circulation of the blood. But we cannot say that Harvey discovered circulation (or, worse still, Circulation) because there is no such thing. Blood circulates, but there is no thing separate from, above or beyond the fact of blood moving around the body that we can call The Circulation. There is no point in the body where circulation resides, no humor in our veins called circulation without which the blood squelches to a sticky halt, nor is there a thing or object or form or anything to which the noun 'circulation' could properly be applied. If you were to say: "His circulation is quite good today," I would be correct in asking: "Yes, but how's his blood flowing?" You might then object on the grounds that the statement that his circulation is good directly implies that his blood is flowing well. Indeed, but, used that way, the word circulation is just a shorthand for a cluster of functions, and there is neither room nor need for another thing called Circulation. Take away his heart contractions, his arterial blood flow, his venous return, etc., and there isn't an abstract entity called "pure circulation" left. Blood doesn't flow in the functional space provided by circulation, nor move under its impetus. There is a process of blood circulating but no thing called circulation.

In the half century since Ryle [4], none of this is new but, when we come to mental function, people persist in asking empty questions, like: "What does consciousness do, and why did it evolve?" To see the folly in these questions, try asking instead: "What does circulation do, and why did it evolve?" The category error is immediately apparent. Circulation isn't an entity in any sense of the word, it is an event, a concatenation of circumstances, a 'doing,' a composite of instantaneous states or functions, but not a thing. The word circulation is shorthand for a variety of hematological events and functions, some normal, some abnormal, but it is most definitely not a thing.

Nobody would have any problems with this example but, because certain events take place in the head, they bring out the worst in people:

"What's wrong with Johnny?"

"Oh, he's got concussion."

"Really, where did he get it? In the head? Oh, no, how awful for him, that's the worst place to get it!"

People don't 'have concussion', they are concussed. Just as appendicitis is a cluster of functions that occur contingently in the abdomen, and circulation is another collection of functions, so too consciousness is a contingent cluster of intracranial and other bodily functions. I say intracranial in the sense that what is happening in my computer now is intra-computer, as any further attempts at localization would ask the wrong questions [4].

On this view, there cannot be a scientific theory of consciousness, although there are scientific (i.e. natural, rational and empirical) theories of seeing, of knowing, of speaking, recalling, calculating, feeling, dreading, wanting, and so on. If, for personal convenience, somebody wanted to group these theories and talk about them as though they amounted to a theory of consciousness, I wouldn't mind, as long as nobody accuses me of believing that it is a theory about a *thing*, that it commits me to believing such a *thing* exists. The same goes for a theory of mind: since there is no such thing as a mind, there can't be a theory about it. There are, however, theories of thinking, hoping, knowing, believing, planning and so on which, when lumped with all the above, and solely for the convenience of typists and TV reporters, some might call a theory of mind.

But there is no Mind, not even a mind. There are lots of mental functions, but no mind having them and, taken together, they don't amount to a Mind. There are lots of bodily functions but it is only a contingent fact that they all occur in my skin. Indeed, as a matter of physiological fact, digestion takes place almost entirely outside me, so I can't talk about 'My digestion.' Only the end-products of the breakdown of my food are absorbed. From the same point of view, babies are technically exoparasites of their mothers so it is pointless to talk about "her pregnancy."

Talking about a thing called consciousness is akin to talking about a thing called Australia. There is no thing called Australia. There are various bits of land that happen to be governed by the same abstract legal entity (including some in the shadow of New Guinea and the Antarctic Territories) even though the people in government change regularly (not regularly enough, some feel). There are lots of different people living in those lands who speak a range of languages (about 200 Aboriginal languages, for a start), who do different jobs, who believe different religions, pursue different political aims, play different sports, and so on. Lots of them, indeed, don't even like each other. There are Australian animals with no passports or citizenship, birds that migrate to Asia each year (dual citizenship? or perhaps they are Asian birds that holiday in Australia), minerals, Australian breezes that pass over South America *en passant*, Australian fish causing international problems by swimming to New Zealand, Australian seas mixing with New Guinea waters, even Australian oil which causes trouble by being found too close to Indonesia. But where is the thing called Australia? Take away Tasmania and is it still Australia? Take away the mainland and is it still Australia? When the Provinces rebelled and Rome fell, was the Exarchy at Ravenna still the Roman Empire? Only as a legal fiction.

Talking of Consciousness, of the mind, the Self, the I, or any of the other reifications used to signify this disparate group of head-based functions is of the same nature as this type of loose talk about the odd thing called Australia. While it suits sports commentators and politicians to talk about Australia as though it were a single, united thing or entity, its myriad subunits and functions conjoined by a handy metaphysical glue, it is not. While it suits all sorts of people to talk about myriad mental sub-functions as though they were single entity called Mind, they are not. Nor is there a metaphysical glue in my head holding my consciousness together (or perhaps the glue or even the field where the sticky thing sits is itself consciousness. People who use these terms luxuriate in the warm fuzziness they generate, confident that they can never be called to task for their sloppy talk) but no matter. I am fully conscious of not having a thing called Consciousness in my head.

10-5. The Paradox of Phenomenal Judgment

This recycled analysis has a dual significance for Chalmers' dualism. Firstly, his paradox of phenomenal judgments depends directly on there being some thing like consciousness. If there is no such thing as consciousness, then the problem of claims about consciousness ("Consciousness is baffling" or "Sensations are mysterious" [1, p 176]) collapses. If consciousness is a reified myth, then claims about consciousness are of the same order as claims about fairies, Sherlock Holmes, Art, alien abduction, Good and Evil and international conspiracies. It is only baffling to Those Who Believe Consciousness Exists. For the rest of us non-believers, it's a pushover, even though the separate mental functions may still be beyond us.

Secondly, if phenomenal judgments arise independently of conscious experience, we still have to explain the remarkable parallels that exist between the two for the duration of my life. There is no reason to believe that the experience is a *sine qua non* of the judgment; the judgment may come first or they may both be the effective end-points of the same prior event. In fact, there are good reasons to believe that something like this may be the case.

If I peel a banana, I simultaneously gain a peeled banana and an empty banana skin. Neither comes first and neither is the cause of the other in anything other than the most circular sense. Yet they are intimately related in such a way that, after peeling one million bananas, peeling the million-and-first is guaranteed to yield a naked banana and a skin, both of which will spring into existence at the same time. Similarly, the TV news and the newspaper may carry stories about the same incident; both drew their material from the same wire service so that while their items are intimately related, they are not causally related. By a similar mechanism, if I see a red circle in front of me and correctly classify it as such, then both events have had their origin in the preceding flow of retinal data. Again, the events (of experiencing and of naming) are intimately but not necessarily causally related.

The alternative view is that the judgment precedes the experience, as in: "I need to know that something is happening before I can experience it." There is something to be said for this view, as the attention/orientation mechanism functions to allow the organism to attend to disturbances around it even before it knows their nature. I can't know what is happening over there until I look, but I can't look until I experience a signal that amounts to: "Look over there, something's happening." What emerges is a three-or-more-step process of crude judgment at the retinal level causing orientation (a brainstem function) and simultaneously leading to a further, refined judgment and an experience, both of which are cortical functions. Remember that children and dogs can perceive things long before they can make judgments like "My, what an interesting whistle," or "Consciousness is baffling," so we shouldn't make too much of all this.

The issue is not quite as clear-cut as Chalmers suggests. As an empirical fact, a considerable part of the process of phenomenal judgment takes place outside the brain. Starting at the level of the retina in the visual system, there are color detectors, edge detectors, movement detectors (actually on/off detectors) angle detectors, and so on. For humans as biological entities, visual decision-making is largely automated, such that we only get to know the results of the decision rather than the data on which it is based. This biological fact is highly convenient, partly because automated decisions are much faster than the alternatives and partly because all other animals make decisions (often faster than we can) without any capacity for sophisticated recursive language. So while it may be perfectly true that phenomenal judgments are made independently of conscious experience, there is nothing paradoxical about the process as they are based on the same data but are made in different parts of the brain. This point is of significance in the application of his theory to mental disorder.

There is another, oft-neglected aspect to the phenomena of mental life that may show them in a somewhat less paradoxical light. I will admit to some difficulty with Chalmers' concept of the paradox of phenomenal judgment but he makes his general position quite clear, as follows: For all behavioral acts, "...if the physical domain is causally closed, then there will be some reductive explanation (of the acts) in physical or functional terms". Anything I say, no matter how abstruse, is a behavioral act for which "There is some story about firing patterns in neurons that will explain why these acts occurred...." (pp 177-78).

If I experience "some particularly intense purple qualia," then the experience is a brute fact that defies further explanation, but if I comment on the experience, then that is a behavioral act for which an explanation in terms of neuronal firing patterns is, in principle, sufficient: "...our claims and judgments about consciousness can be explained in terms quite independent of consciousness ... (even) ... in terms that do not even imply the existence of conscious experience" (p177-79). If this seems counterintuitive, then it is something we can learn to live with (p 288).

I have previously argued that the physical realm is not "causally closed" in the old-fashioned sense, but is open to intervention by the informational realm, however it may be instantiated. I have also argued that the psychological realm cannot be reduced to mere matters of neuronal firing patterns [6] since, in humans, it involves symbolic systems and, by their very nature, symbols cannot be reduced to their substrate. Furthermore, any explanation in terms of firing patterns in neurons will necessarily involve firing patterns in other neurons, *ad infinitum*. There is no point at which these patterns can be grounded. Finally, I believe there are strong empirical grounds to view the psychological and the phenomenal realms as end-points of the same data input, albeit very different end-points.

In S.10-4, I outlined the view that there is no such thing as consciousness, that it is merely a reification of a disparate group of (often unrelated) mental and intracranial functions. If we wish to use the term, we could save ourselves a lot of trouble by using only the verb, 'to be conscious.' But, possibly uniquely in the English language, this verb has three quite separate grammatical functions. Firstly, there is the intransitive verb whose synonyms are to be alert, to be awake, to be in an apt state to respond appropriately to environmental stimulation, etc.. The antonym is to be unconscious, asleep, insensible, incapable of responding, etc.. Within this specific meaning of the verb, there is a gradation of arousal from fully alert and responsive, down to drowsy, to stuporose (responding only to direct stimulation), to deeply stuporose (responding only to painful stimulation) to comatose, where the subject is unresponsive and therefore not far from death. Used this way, 'to be conscious' is strictly a neurophysiological term, one which measures the state of arousal and therefore gauges, not the contents of the mental state, but the physiological readiness or capacity of the organism to have a mental state in the first place. Philosophically, this verb is boring; what is of empirical interest is that, even while we are asleep and have no conscious experience, we can still make decisions (a sleeping mother 'decides' to wake for her baby but not for the cat or her husband).

Secondly, there is 'to be conscious' as a transitive verb which, unlike the first use, demands an object: "I am conscious of..." This equates with Chalmers' "conscious experience," the phenomenal or experiential realm in which I am conscious of or experience sensations, phenomena, qualia, etc.. It includes, of course, unimodal memory of those experiences. In our present knowledge, the experiences are brute facts incapable of further analysis. These days, nobody would bother arguing that the peripheral sensory input has nothing to do with our experiences, but how this is achieved is the crucial question.

Thirdly, there is the reflexive verb, 'to be conscious of oneself' or self-conscious. This amounts to Chalmers' psychological consciousness or realm of awareness, in the sense of knowing something about myself or my experiences: I have knowledge of all the matters that constitute my instantaneous state and, significantly, can report on them, although this is not a criterion of self-consciousness. People who experience those awful anesthetic accidents in which they are paralyzed but remain awake during the operation are perfectly self-conscious.

We can quickly dispense with "intransitive consciousness" *qua* arousal: the neurophysiology of cat brainstems tells us most of what we need to know about ourselves in this respect. However, the other two verbs are germane to a discussion of Chalmers' paradox of phenomenal judgment. In attempting to explain both the transitive (experiential) and reflexive (self-aware) uses of the verb 'to be conscious,' we will have major difficulties avoiding both an infinite regress and brain-mind identity. We can avoid this particular risk by proposing that, instead of being realized in the physical brain ("the firing patterns of neurons"), both these mental realms are instantiated in a higher-order brain function, a virtual machine [2].

In any physical system, infinite regresses are impossible purely on economic grounds, whereas in a virtual system, such regresses can be set up and dissolved as quickly as, say, standing between two mirrors. A recursive system allows the information subserving experience and knowledge to act back upon itself in such a way as to provide a basis for self-awareness and also the impression of experience "out there." Of course, a true infinite regress would cause a virtual machine to seize just as quickly as a physical but, in heavily-damped form, they could provide the experience of the first few steps on the road to infinity. Having said this, I must add that I don't like the idea of infinite regresses, but the needs of a self-reflective system over-rule personal prejudice. This is just one way a self-reflective system can be set up; I'm not saying it's true of humans.

In this schema, phenomenal judgment and the phenomena themselves are closely allied, to the extent that there would be no paradox in their realization. They are simply different aspects of the same data flow, although it is perfectly feasible that they are generated, not by one virtual machine, but by two—or many. Empirically, this seems likely, as language, which is intimately implicated in the genesis of self-awareness, is a very much later development than the classic senses. Of course, if anything like these "virtual machines" is true of cerebral function, then we may never know the brain languages or the "programs" by which they arise. However, it does mean that, on a functional basis alone, we will eventually be able to devise machines that feel pain. We will never know for certain whether they do or not, but then I don't know that of you, anyway.

The concept of virtual machines as Popper's "ghosts in the machine" [7] has, I believe, one other real value, which is to negate the risk that rocks and trees may have conscious experiences. If conscious experiences only arise in virtual machines, and these can only be generated when the requisite informational processing capacity exists, then rocks, which, regardless of their level of organization, have no processing capacity, can never generate the informational space in which conscious experience can develop. The essence of the idea of conscious experience arising in a virtual machine is that the informational machine controls the brain, not the other way around.

I suggest these considerations may lead us around the paradox of phenomenal judgment. I don't like paradoxes; they imply I've overlooked something important. In this case, I believe the error is looking at consciousness as a thing *sui generis* when, in fact, "it" is a motley group of processes and mental doings. Of all the red herrings in science, I think Consciousness is the worst.

10-6: Future Directions

At the end of the main section, Chalmers asks a series of questions which his (or a similar) theory needs to answer. In this part, he tends to lapse into evolutionary speculations, not the least because his questions are of a form that demands an evolutionary answer and, at this stage of our knowledge of human affairs, the only evolutionary answers we have are speculations. For example, he suggests that "...we need to ... understand why judgments about consciousness are produced" (p 289). Does he mean how they arise, or what we would be like without them, or what functional role they fill? We can't answer these types of questions yet but, rather than admit such limits, many people happily offer some sort of evolutionary speculation, one which sounds terribly impressive and doesn't run the risk of being refuted in their lifetimes. The short answer to why we produce judgments about consciousness is that we, along with all living things, are judgment-producing organisms (or machines). If our brains "secrete" anything, it is decisions. And if we decide there is a thing called 'consciousness,' it won't be long before we start to produce judgments about it. The long answer would best be deferred until we have a better grip on the processes of consciousness.

"When an information space is phenomenally realized," he asks, "why is it realized one way rather than another?" (p 308) Again, is he asking why colors are colorful (because they aren't pains: if they were, we couldn't tell red from a toothache), or is he asking what evolutionary advantage is conferred by seeing in color versus black and white, or why vision is so precise while smell is so unlocalized? It depends on what pertinent information can be extracted from the environment with what effort and risk, whether biological systems can transduce the energy form, how information is processed, and so on.

He continues: "How ... can one account for the unity of consciousness?" (p 309). There are many considerations here: because all my conscious experiences have happened to me; because we always overlook the many bits, such as greed, overwhelming suspicion, hypnagogic states, depersonalization, *deja vu,* hallucinations, etc., which don't reinforce the standard model of the unity of consciousness: because all languages regard the first person personal pronoun as singular; because our ethics demand it ("I wasn't in my right mind, your Honor"); because, like immortality, the alternative is conceptually so difficult and so scary that we prefer to ignore it, etc.

There is no such thing as the unity of self. It is a Tower of Babel.

For myself, I never bother with evolutionary speculations in human affairs. Evolutionary speculations are camp followers, always two steps behind the latest scientific theory but never in front. All they can do is justify what is, and then only within the context of a banal set of premises. When somebody offers an evolutionary speculation to account for crosswords, punk music, haute cuisine and evolutionary speculations, then I will take notice. Not everything we do has evolutionary significance. Perhaps, like swimming, music, poetry and athletics, they are non-lethal side-effects of other, more important matters. Even these may long ago have faded, leaving their side-effects as misunderstood epitaphs in an evolutionary graveyard. And I am fully aware that these comments will deter nobody from the endlessly fascinating game of devising ever-more clever evolutionary speculations.

10-7. Conclusion

What is the nature of the controlling element in human affairs? The central theme of Part II is that if we are going to advocate mental control, we need a viable mentalist theory. Anything short of frank mentalism isn't going to satisfy the requirements.

From the point of view of psychiatry, functionalism is an unsatisfying doctrine for the very simple reason that the essence of mental disorder (that some mental states are intensely painful and interfere with normal function) is brushed aside. Suicide is not just putting a gun to your temple. The gun is absolutely irrelevant to the infinite pain that forces a rational person to the decision that further existence is intolerable. Also, functionalism offers no explanation of the phenomena of mental disorder. For example, what does it say about the inner state that causes a person to say: "I feel thoughts being inserted into my head"? Only that it is a state that typically causes people to say: "I feel thoughts being inserted into my head." The state of profound fear that constitutes panic cannot be related to sensory or cognitive input (panic just means irrational), yet it is very real and it is the experience itself that devastates people, as effective treatment with beta-blockers shows. At first glance, panic appears to have no causes, it serves no purpose and, in itself, has no possible evolutionary significance. To say that it is a disease state and therefore doesn't need or justify a functionalist account is simply to avoid the issue by giving functionalist accounts of the easy bits of mental life and sidestepping the difficult bits.

Chalmers' naturalistic dualism, on the other hand, appears to have many of the features needed for a full account of mental disorder. It is a mentalist theory in which the dual aspects of mental life, the phenomenal and the psychological, have a reality within a materialist ontology. While the phenomenal realm remains unexplained, there is no attempt to hide it in the "too hard" basket. It shares primacy in human life; without the fuss and bother of phenomenal mental life, our inner states would be as silent as the grave. *Mea culpa*: there would be no inner states. In fact, even though we would be leading productive lives, perhaps even writing functionalist philosophy, we would be no more aware of them than we are aware of an operation while under general anesthesia. Life without pain might be appealing, but life without mentality would be utter oblivion.

I suggest that Chalmers' conceptualization of the conscious mind offers the best chance we have ever had of assembling a coherent, human-centered account of mental disorder. There is no mention of mental disorder in his book, *The Conscious Mind*, which is subtitled simply: "In search of a fundamental theory." Admittedly, an account of mental disorder is not fundamental, but I believe it is a crucial test for any theory of mind. If a theory of mind cannot provide an explanatory framework for mental disorder then, regardless of its other successes, it fails the ultimate test. Perhaps philosophers should pay a lot more attention to mental disorder.

<table>
<tr>
<td>

11

</td>
<td>

The Effable and the Ineffable: Property Dualism and Self–Control

</td>
</tr>
</table>

11-1. Introduction

The experience of the past one hundred and forty years should leave no doubt that practicing psychiatry without a firm grounding in a theory of mind is like sailing a ship without a compass. Thus far, I have been relying on principles that dictate the form of a theory suitable for psychiatry. These greatly narrow the field of available theories—effectively, to just one. It is worth reiterating these principles, as some of them present a considerable departure from psychiatric tradition:

11-1(a). We are working within a naturalistic ontology using an empirical methodology. This denies a supernatural element in human behavior, meaning everything is open to rational explanation except a few brute facts.

11-1(b). Because of the operation of a controlling element, human behavior is non-random. Attempts to explain the nature of the controlling element using naive forms of materialism have all failed. The concept of materialism therefore must be expanded to include the manipulation of information within the natural realm.

11-1(c). A substantial part of human mental life consists of the silent, rapid manipulation of information. Information enters the CNS, is processed and behavioral instructions are sent to the peripheries, entirely without leaving the natural realm. But information cannot be reduced to its substrate; therefore, the control of behavior cannot be reduced to matters of mere biology. There is no such thing as a non-mentalist psychology.

11-1(d). Mentalism is open to a naturalistic explanation. The most interesting differences between humans derive from their mental lives. Psychology is a subset of mentalism, and beliefs are irreducibly psychological in nature.

11-1 (e). Normal mental function falls quite readily into two distinct realms, the phenomenal or experiential, and the psychological or knowledge-based. These are intimately but not causally related. What we see of each other's behavior is determined in the psychological realm.

11-1(f). There cannot be an adequate functionalist account of both aspects of mental life. The whole point of functionalism is to sidestep the experiential realm. Since the pain of mental disorder cannot be gainsaid, the phenomenal mental life must be taken seriously. The ultimate test of any theory of mind is its capacity to account for mental disorder. Functionalism fails this test.

11-2. The Phenomenal and the Psychological

We need to look closely at the differences between the two realms of human mental life, the phenomenal and the psychological (to use Chalmers' term [1]). For the present, these can only be defined ostensively; it seems that, apart from our experience of these realms, we have not even the means of beginning to grasp them.

11-2(a). The Phenomenal Realm. This is the feeling, experiencing aspect of life which, for most of us most of the time, dominates existence. Ordinarily, when people speak of the mind, they have 'in mind' the constantly active and interactive internal video set or arena that is so full of vital experiences. Experience is so much part of us that we take it for granted. Yet the very act of experiencing something seems like one of the great miracles of the universe. That there is life is remarkable; that we can perceive it and reflect upon it confounds us.

It is important not to confuse the various elements of the experiential realm. Firstly, we have the classical senses of sight, hearing, taste, smell and touch. With large, forward-facing, color-sensitive eyes, we are well-adapted for binocular vision by day but poorly suited for conditions of low light intensity. Hearing forms the basis of normal human communication and is therefore critical to our existence as a species. Besides their role in communication, our ears serve to alert us to non-specific warnings in the environment.

Taste and smell do not appear to be so highly developed in humans as in other animals, but life would be very dull without them. Touch and pain, however, are especially acute. We can detect light touch, deep pressure, joint position, vibration and muscle stretch, as well as a range of pains, both cutaneous and interoceptive. Temperature sensation has obvious significance in a warm-blooded creature. In addition, we can detect position and movement of the head in a gravitational field. Various other, important sensations are mediated by central mechanisms: nausea, breathlessness, weariness, malaise, etc, not to forget the sexual sensations.

The experiential realm also contains the emotions. Emotions can't be defined, they just are what they feel like. Even though their neurophysiology plays a critical but largely unknown part in their generation and experience [2], emotions are not to be identified with their physiological concomitants. Firstly, there are the experiences that are widely accepted as true or core emotions—anxiety and fear, anger, sadness and grief, affection, happiness and warmth. Other inner states are sometimes not considered emotions, but they can't readily be separated so I put them here: the sense of security that underlies trust and mistrust, boredom, apathy and excitement, jealousy, drive and ambition, wonder, curiosity, self-satisfaction, etc. It might be argued that these are not so much emotions as cognitive sets or frames of mind. There is a case to be made for this point but I suggest their similarities with the core emotions outweigh the differences.

Finally, there are some important experiences that appear to have a strong base in physiology, but which are primarily related to the cognitive state. These include the senses of novelty and familiarity, of belief or conviction, bewilderment and that amorphous but crucial set of senses known collectively as the body image.

This list is not exhaustive, but it can be seen that the inner, experiential realm is full, vibrant and of central significance in our awareness of ourselves. This realm is what functionalism, behaviorism, reductionism and other attempts to bypass the "really hard questions of consciousness" (Chalmers) would have us believe is either trivial or nonexistent.

11-2(b). The Psychological Realm. In one part of our mental lives, we experience while, in the other, we know. If aliens arrived tomorrow, they would be impressed by public human artifacts, our arts and sciences and our technologies, but not the private senses and emotions that we seem to have in common with many other creatures on earth. Yet while our experiences will die with us, the knowledge we acquire can survive our passing, a feature unique in the animal world.

However, the communicable element is only part of our knowledge state, the easy part. To people raised in the age of computers, there is now nothing mysterious about the bulk collection, storage and transfer of information. But in each of us, beyond our public knowledge, is a vast, constantly active but silent realm of knowledge. I know so much; in fact, I have no idea just how much I know. Given the right receptor, be it human or machine, I can convey vast amounts of information without knowing how I know it or how it comes to me. You point to a tree and I name it: it is *Eucalyptus camaldulensis*, the red river gum, the most widespread tree in Australia. I know that. I don't need to force my tongue around the words, the sounds just happen. Once, when my daughter was about fifteen months old, I buckled on her shoes, saying: "There." She looked at them happily and said, recognizably: "Dere." How did she copy the sound? How do infants know which sound to make? We can't say how we know it, we simply do it. The Thai vowel written in English as -eu- (such as *deum*, to drink) is not like any English vowel. Thais cannot tell anybody how to shape their vocal cords and mouth to make the sound, but with a little practice, anybody can copy them. We don't know how we copy sounds but there would be no speech without this ability.

Without thinking about the movements of my fingers, I type these words. When I play the piano, I don't have to sit and recite "short A-sharp, long E-flat, pause...," but my fingers simply reach the correct keys (most of the time). I drive slowly along a rough bush track, changing gears every few meters, perhaps 200 times per kilometer. If you were to ask me about my 94th gear change, I couldn't tell you because I didn't think about it yet, while an unthinking action, it was correct but not a random event. In this crucial respect of being an "unthinking" capacity, language is much the same. I can walk down some stairs with you, talking about a film we saw while looking for a particular car in the street, yet there will be no mistakes in the performance of any of those very significant achievements. Many people are not familiar with the rules of English grammar, but they can produce and understand an infinite variety of original English sentences with no hesitation. When I am speaking, I do not know just what will be the third next word I will use, but it will be correct and in context—and you will immediately understand it. All of this takes place in the psychological realm, but at a speed we cannot apprehend.

If we play with a ball, I do not need to know the rules of ballistics to know how to run for a ball, to jump and catch it. In fact, monkeys can do it too, so ballistics has nothing to do with it. I once had a dog that never failed to catch a flying Frisbee (it was nothing much: she never learned to throw it properly). I know where things are even without thinking of them, and can walk into a dark room, reach for the light switch and flick it on without giving it a thought. I know how to make things, how to take them apart, who invented the telephone, how to find a number in the phone book, how to find the government department that deals with lost llamas, what a llama is, why it isn't an alpaca, a lama or a lemur, and so on, but this is all silent, only active when I need it and I don't have to ask myself what I know. I ask the library if they have a book, but I never have to ask myself: I wonder if I know anything about vicunas?

The differences between what we know and what we experience are exclusive: knowledge is acquired gradually and can be conveyed to another person, whereas the phenomenal contents arrive immediately and are wholly private experiences. While at present, we have no means of further analyzing the experiential realm, the psychological realm can readily be subdivided. Whatever I may be doing in the knowing, computing, calculating psychological realm, I know what I know but I cannot know how I know it; I am apprised of the contents of my knowledge state but its inner workings are utterly silent. Knowledge is conscious or reportable, but the mechanisms subserving my knowledge state are entirely unconscious and unknowable. So I can tell a square from a circle, but I will always bump into brute facts when I try to go beyond that. I can say that two plus two equals four but I cannot say how I know what '2' is without resorting to brute facts. I know injustice when I see it; how I know it is a mystery. What I know is thrust upon me, just as brutally as a green experience.

Two aspects to the psychological realm now declare themselves. Firstly, there are the very obvious contents of our knowledge state. From theories of mind or ethics to gossip and dirty ditties, we acquire and retain information as long as we are alive. Secondly, there is the silent and high-speed manipulation of the contents of knowledge. If I see you across a crowded room, I recognize you almost immediately; I don't know how this happens but the knowledge is thrust upon me and I accept it as my own doing. I suggest that if the term "unconscious" has any significance, it must surely apply to this silent, high speed "decision-making" level of the psychological realm of the mind. I recognize you "unconsciously" but I recall your name so fast and so effortlessly that it isn't fair to boast "I recalled it myself." It is recalled for me, presumably by my brain. I say "Good morning" without even knowing how I say the words. The difference between what I know and how I know it is profoundly important for a theory of mental disorder.

For convenience, I will call the overt, reportable level of the psychological realm the cognitive contents, and name the silent, unreportable level of the apprehension, storage and manipulation of information as the cognitive analyzer. These terms are used advisedly and will be modified in due course. It must be understood that this is not a case of building a homunculus because the processes are being broken down. I am taking one complex function and decomposing it into its constituent functional elements according to Dennett's concept of the "dumb homunculus." In epistemic terms, this is diametrically opposed to, say, the Freudian model of the ego defenses.

11-3. The Psychological Realm in Action

We now know a great deal of the physiology of perception. and detailed reviews of the function of different sensory modalities are readily available. The eye is well-known and is often used as the archetype of sensation. Light strikes the retina and is intercepted by a range of different receptors, leading to a barrage of coded information in the optic nerve. It must not be forgotten that the process of analyzing visual data begins at the level of the retina, where it is entirely unconscious in all possible senses of the term. Colors are detected by color receptors, lines and edges by edge detectors, movement by arrays of on-off detectors, etc. The detectors are all perfectly simple, straightforward and utterly mindless, tiny neuronal machines. We share this equipment with all other mammals and, quite likely, many other creatures. In fact, most of our knowledge of human visual systems comes from cats.

As the data flow from these very peripheral detectors is relayed back to the brain, it is further analyzed at each junction. What reaches the brain is not a flood of raw data, but a highly derivative assessment of what the eye and its supporting structures can detect of the world "out there." Essentially, this is what evolution has deemed important for our survival. This data flow moves through the brainstem until, eventually, it is lost in the cerebral cortex, but it is at this, the highest level, that the experience of seeing is generated. How, we can only guess but what we do know is that we humans see just what the eye and the brain tell us we need to see, and no more.

Thus, if we see a green square on a blank field, the data flow achieves two ends. Firstly, we gain an experience of something green and squarish "out there" and, secondly, we acquire two items of knowledge, Green and Square. The same optic data flow affects the two mental realms, the experiential and the psychological, such that two totally different mental events are generated, the cognitive contents (Green and Square) and the experience ("something greenish and squarish out there"). These are intimately related such that there cannot be truth in one and falsity in the other (as, for example, I experience a red circle but judge the event a green square), but neither causes the other. Both events are derivative. I do not see the green color then name it by matching it against a spectrum; that decision is done for me by the cognitive analyzer about whose workings I know nothing. The cognitive analyzer, in turn, does the bidding of the rods and cones in the retina. Until I apprehend the information, it is all handled silently and mechanically. There are no rewards for effort in realizing "Green."

Again, there are two further aspects to the information entering the psychological realm. Firstly, it may remain silent and simply be used as part of the information on which I base my daily life. If I am eating, I do not measure the distance my fork must travel to my mouth, but this information is processed silently and effectively to control the movement of my arm and wrist. If I 'say' to myself: "Piece of steak hiding behind the potato at 11 o'clock," I already know exactly where it is. In fact, I don't need to 'say' anything to myself because, before I can do so, I have already decided just where it is. Except I didn't make the decision, it was made for me. Monkeys are just as good at feeding themselves as I am and they don't have language. The great majority of the decisions on which I base my daily life are fully automated. If I try to interfere with them, I will probably start to make mistakes, an important point in a theory of anxiety.

I am not in any way suggesting that the cognitive analyzer presents its results 'to' anything. Its results are simply incorporated into the train of events known as mental life. The entity called "I, me, myself" is the sum total of these experiences and knowledge to the extent that, if and as they change, so do I. Take away half my mental contents and there will be a very restricted "I", as, for example, when I am half asleep, intoxicated or suffering a brain injury. Take away all my mental contents and there is nothing left, not even an I to note the absence of experience. When my mental life comes to a halt, I cease to exist. If the halt is temporary, such as during deep sleep, coma or an anesthetic, then a new sense of I will reassemble on waking, one incorporating a memory of a discontinuity, a join in the fabric of memory with no awareness of anything in between. If, however, the cessation of mental life is permanent, then there is no further sense of I. Before I was born, there was nothing, not even an awareness of nothing, and that is our destiny. Thus, there is no "pure consciousness" or "consciousness devoid of its contents," any more than there can be a symphony without sounds or a banquet without food.

The notion of a silent but causally-significant psychological realm is hardly new and does not present any particular difficulties for a cognitive psychology. There is also nothing conceptually novel about rapid, high-speed data processing exerting effects on the material world through dedicated transducers. There should be nothing novel about this taking place in the head. So we can fairly quickly assemble a model of causation for the sort of unreflective action that characterizes 99% of human activity.

Consider an everyday example: We see a group of animals standing in a ragged crowd and pressing forward slightly at an unseen barrier. The animals could be rats or humans, it matters little. Their eyes are fixed on a pole some eight meters away. Suddenly, a green light appears near the top of the pole. As one, the group surges forward, rushing directly towards a similar group heading the opposite direction. Surprisingly, the two groups pass through each other and continue on their separate ways without any collisions.

If we fit one of the individuals with suitable instruments, we will see a little burst of activity in the optic nerve just as the light changes to green. The impulses travel back to the brainstem and thence, via a series of nuclei, to the occipital cortex where they are quickly lost, at least to currently available tracking methods. Shortly after, an electrical potential gathers over the anterior cerebral cortex, Impulses are then generated in the motor cortex and proceed via the brainstem and spinal cord to the anterior horn cells, and thence to the motor endplates of the skeletal muscles.

The data input to the brain is in the form of a flow of digital impulses and the output is in exactly the same form; it would be economical to propose that the information coded in those data flows does not change its form at any point between input and output. I suggest that decisions such as walking on the green light are made at the level of data manipulation by the neuronal architecture of the brain, and that this manipulation of coded information is rapid and silent, i.e. utterly unreportable. If our specimen pedestrian 'says' to himself: "Ah, there's the green light, I'd better be off," then he is simply announcing what he already knows. Regaling himself in this way is entirely after the fact of deciding to walk. A laboratory rat could act in exactly the same way and on the same physiological basis as a human without being able to 'say' to itself anything like "Let's go!" I am not saying, as the behaviorists did, that humans and rats necessarily use identical processes to initiate behavior but I am saying that, in rats, we already have a proven principle that yields the same results as humans, so there is no *a priori* reason to invoke a new entity in 99% of human activity.

The results of all decisions in the cognitive analyzer are sent directly to the effector organs; by some sleight of brain, we can also feed the information through some other circuitry such that it is perceived in a similar, if not identical, way to other implicit knowledge. For example, I know that I know what 12x12 gives, even without saying it. I know that I know the National Anthem, without needing to sing it. Sometimes, my decisions are led through another brain system such that I 'hear' the answer as an external voice (although, in normal states, it lacks the conviction of a veridical percept). This notion will be used to account for the phenomena of hysterical conversion reactions and certain aspects of schizophrenia.

For the present, I emphasize that a very large proportion of human activity is in principle open to explanation as the outcome of silent, high-speed data-processing without there being any intervention by an immaterial spirit. Our decisions are largely automated, so a soul would only get in the way and slow things down. There isn't time for a spirit or Self to poke its ghostly fingers in the cerebral pie in the manner Eccles proposed. The decisions: "Circle, green, eight meters ahead and three up, nothing moving on the road!" are all made below the level of the cerebral cortex, as blind-sight experiments show. These types of decisions are quite as fast in rats as they are in humans. The next decision: "Let's get going, legs!" is neurologically more complex, but still doesn't require any sort of deliberation in the sense of 'mental speech.'

In support of this suggestion, I propose that the neuronal architecture of the cerebral cortex as currently understood [3] is ideally suited to the requirements of a high-speed digital data processor in which the input and output are of essentially the same form. Perhaps it would be better to say that those authors' conceptualizations of the functional organization of cortical cytoarchitecture are not incompatible with the suggestions above. If they had shown that the cerebral cortex were an amorphous syncitium, then it would be necessary to abandon this approach, but they didn't. The essence of their model lies in the complexity of the interconnections between discreet processing units and their modular organization. Thus, what we take for granted in computers is not in principle excluded by what we know of the brain's structure and function.

All that has been said so far applies to just one aspect of mental life, automated decisions. If I pick up an egg, I handle it differently from a similarly-sized rock, yet I never need to 'say' to myself: "Careful, stupid, this is an egg, not a rock." The decision "Egg" is thrust upon me and, without further ado, my right hand moves towards it at the appropriate speed, etc., just as a monkey's would. These types of decisions are made for us: we have all stumbled when we thought we had reached the last step, or spilled a near-empty jug through thinking it was full. This mechanism is interesting, but it does not offer any explanation for the creative aspect of human life. Creativity demands further development of this approach.

I am doing a crossword and reach clue 6-across. Without knowing how, I recognize an anagram of nine letters. All I know is that it should be an anagram. Why? Don't ask me, I will always say, "Because it looks like one."

Almost as soon as I read it, the answer comes to me, far faster than many computers could process the 362,880 combinations involved. This is creativity in action, but it must be automated as there is only one sense of 'I' in which I could claim responsibility for the answer, namely, that it arose in my head. I am using the word "automated" in the specific sense of rule-governed activity, although the claim that this process is automated doesn't yet rest on strong grounds. It is said that Mozart couldn't explain how he composed his music, so he believed it must be through divine intervention; I don't know how I solve an anagram, so I take it as evidence of mere, automated computation. So far, all that proves is that I am the product of my generation.

Language offers a better view of the possible processes involved. As Chomsky [4] is fond of saying, even after very limited exposure to all possible sentences in their language, people can produce and understand an infinite range of grammatically correct sentences. The most interesting cases are where people can't explain why they habitually say things a certain way: why do English speakers put the verbs after the subject, whereas German speakers put them at the end of the sentence in reverse order? How do people do these things without even knowing what verbs and nouns are? They do so under the influence of some sort of organizing principle, which I will call a rule.

Sentences are generated by rules that often are not explicitly known to the speaker. Children provide very clear examples of this. Small children soon learn to generate the past tense of verbs just by adding '-ed' to stems. Thus, as every parent knows, they will use words such as bited, catched, bringed, thinked, sleeped, etc. They can't explain why they do this, but they have acquired the pattern by experience of other verbs. At the age of two, my son had dozens of words like these. He had never heard these terms (we know this because we never used baby talk; we had no neighbors; most of the children he met spoke Indonesian and because we spoke as much Indonesian at home as English), yet he was entirely consistent in his usage: always as the past historic tense. Later, he added the present participle to produce a rough past perfect tense, again without any instruction whatsoever from either of us. Intuitively, he mined the language environment and extracted general rules.

Human language is a rule-governed activity. So is human work, human sport, human research, and even human warfare. Aha, you ask, what about humor, which relies on surprise for its laughs? Yes indeed, but the exception proves the rule: there must be cultural rules in place generating an anticipated outcome before a joke can surprise us with its unexpected conclusion.

I suggest we make our myriad daily decisions by the complex interaction of a range of data inputs processed according to pre-existing rules coded in the brain. While some of these rules are explicit, i.e. they can be reported, many others, if not most, are implicit. The inability to report a rule does not imply that it does not exist: the behavioral facts speak for themselves. Young children can show acquired patterns of behavior which definitely antedate their development of any recognizable language skills. They are not acquiring rules in the sense of memorizing the road traffic code or the rules of croquet, but clearly have pre-linguistic organizing principles governing their behavior, and I want to include these with the rest of the rules we use to control behavior. Normally, incorrect rules acquired at a tender age are corrected by further experience but, if subsequent experience is confirmatory, then there is no reason for implicitly-acquired rules to change.

We do not know how these "organizing principles" are invested in the brain, nor do we know how they are coded, how they are activated and interact, etc. Nonetheless, the fact that they exist is unassailable. That human behavior is non-random proves that some such organizing principles are operating during the generation of behavior.

11-4. The Phenomenal Realm in Action

Chalmers is quite blunt about the status of cognition. While "...cognition is an ontological free lunch ... (that) is governed entirely by the laws of physics...," the phenomenal realm is completely different: "Consciousness is ontologically novel..." [1, p 172]. Beyond our immediate experience, we do not seem to have any means of grasping the nature and impact of phenomenal experience. While decision-making now appears mundane, and we can even decompose the lofty processes of logic and mathematics, how can we possible begin to dismantle the experience of, say, utter darkness? We don't even know where to start.

We can, however, make progress of sorts simply be clarifying the relationships of different types of conscious experiences. As mentioned above, there appear to be at least three types, the ordinary senses, the emotions and those experiences related to cognitive function. I believe their similarities far exceed their differences, and they ought to be considered as but different forms of the same basic process or processes.

It is evident that the classic senses serve to notify us of the state of the physical world, outside and inside. Sensory receptors are activated by specific forms of energy that allow information to flow to the CNS, e.g. the eyes are only activated by light energy, the taste buds by chemicals, etc. By some unknown means, we experience the outside world under the compulsion of that information flow. Emotions are somewhat different. Again by some unknown means, we experience a diffuse and unlocalized but indisputably mental event that can vary in intensity from barely perceptible to overwhelming. These are accompanied by well-known physiological changes but every attempt to reduce emotion to those associated biological changes has foundered. My suggestion is that, as mental events, emotions are very similar to external perceptions in that they derive from activity in a specific receptor. This time, however, the causative event and its receptor both lie within the brain substance itself. There is no a priori reason why this should not be the case. There are many receptor functions in the body that respond only to internal stimuli, even though most of them are extra-cerebral. The carotid baroreceptors are a good example, and there are many other examples in the endocrine system. For emotions, I propose only that they are perceptions of a particular type, as different from ordinary perceptions as pain is from sight, but otherwise essentially the same class of events.

For the ordinary senses, the triggering events are normally external but, in this view, the triggers of emotions are events in the psychological realm, i.e. ordinary decisions. One set of decisions in this realm is of the form: "2+2 = 4" while another is of the form: "Snake+bare foot = danger." The former has no emotional impact, i.e. it does not activate any of the emotional circuitry, while the latter is highly emotional. By classing an event as dangerous, all we are saying is that it activates certain emotional systems. The single word "danger-ous" means: "Simply knowing this information will immediately activate all the neurological machinery involved in generating a sense of risk and prepar-ing the body to respond to it."

The decision that something is dangerous is made for us at a silent, unre-portable level. The first we know of that decision is a jolt of fear, a point of fundamental importance in the anxiety states. I don't have to think about it, merely seeing the snake is enough to activate the complex neuronal circuitry underlying the fear response. By classing another event as, say, humorous, we are saying no more than that it activates certain other circuits whose activ-ity is perceived as humor in (probably) much the same sense that activity in the visual circuit is perceived as light. If an event fails to activate the anxiety circuit but activates instead the humor circuit, then we would say it wasn't frightening but was funny. Thus, the eventual explanation (if any) of ordinary sensory experiences should also explain emotional experiences.

The remaining phenomenal experiences are intimately related to cognitive events in that they are only triggered by specific classes of information. For example, seeing a familiar face provokes just the experience (the sense of fa-miliarity) which compels us to say it is familiar. Conversely, seeing something for the first time fails to activate the "familiarity sensation," so we call it novel. Perhaps there is more to novelty than just a failure to establish a familiarity response, but the details are empirical. We often take this group of experi-ences for granted (it is surprising how few people can even name them) but there are neurological and psychiatric conditions in which they are disor-dered, with quite devastating effects on the individual. The harmless experiences of *dèja vu* and its opposite, *jamais vu*, are simply random events where one or other system is activated with no typical stimulus.

While the sense of familiarity is conceptually straightforward, the body im-age is more of a problem. The term refers to a highly disparate group of functions, some of them reportable, some not. A lot of what is termed body image is simply motor memory, some is somatic memory (for example, we know where our feet ought to be or how our mouths ought to feel), but some are more complex, e.g. two point discrimination and other somesthetic senses. The point is that these functions should not be regarded as separate from other experiences, but simply as variations on a theme. That they are mostly triggered and detected intra-cerebrally is of no more than passing significance: a wholly internal contribution to the phenomenal realm does not alter their fundamental nature as experiences, not cognitions.

In Chalmers' schema, phenomenal judgments are statements about or as-sessments of phenomenal experiences. I suggest that even inner speech is part of the experiential realm, in that the moment I convert some implicit or silent knowledge into the type that I 'hear' with my 'inner ear,' then, despite its informational nature, it has become part of the phenomenal realm. While driving, if I look at my speedometer and, without any deliberation, almost im-mediately lift my foot from the accelerator a little, then the information has not caused a phenomenal judgment. But if I 'say' to myself, "Too fast, slow down!" even as I lift my foot, then it has crossed the boundary.

While I am typing this, I 'hear' in my head the words spoken somewhat more slowly than normal speech. Nobody else can hear them. The decision to type the word 'and' is made before I 'hear' myself 'say' anything; inner speech is always *post hoc*. When I am reviewing what I have written, I 'read it aloud' in my head, at the same speed and with the same intonations as if I were giving a lecture. This way, I get a better sense of how it reads than simply by scanning it 'silently,' the way I normally read. The visual information enters the psychological and the experiential realms more or less simultaneously but the phenomenal judgment is a little slower than either of these.

All this is unremarkable: it offers an explanation of a great deal of human behavior, but not of the really interesting bits. Practically all of the above could be mimicked by rats, so where is the difference between rats and humans? Speech is often taken as an interesting difference, but I think the first point to remember about speech is that it is not particularly interesting. Speech, which physically conveys information from my inner realm to yours, is wholly neurological and therefore doesn't require anything new to explain it. Similarly, the neurology of the muscles involved in playing tennis is of very much less interest than the means by which the rules were formulated, communicated and learned. In understanding speech, we are mainly interested in the processes that activate the speech centers. Technically, the speech centers themselves represent nothing conceptually new even though their details are, unfortunately, almost entirely unknown. What takes place within them is largely mechanical. However, the really interesting part of speech, the functional organization of the brain that generates the instructions to the speech centers, is conceptually beyond us.

Speech is non-random; that is the difference between information and noise. I propose only that the organizing principles that generate its regularity consist of information coded in the neurological substrate of the psychological realm. These principles are therefore part of this realm. For convenience, we can call them 'rules.' Some rules are acquired explicitly, others implicitly, but, whatever the case, they function very quickly, silently converting incoming information to the sorts of instructions that allow the speech centers to activate the organs of speech. Somebody might like to call these instructions thoughts but I doubt very much that they would satisfy the ordinary meaning of this word. Thoughts are much more like "inner verbalizing" than the unreportable activity I have described. We are apprised of the outcome of this activity, which then becomes 'thoughts.' If I say "Did you see K?" then the decision to ask the question has already been decided. The psychological decision to ask a question and its informational content antedate any phenomenal events such as my 'saying' to myself: "I should ask him if he saw K."

Again, I do not see anything conceptually novel in the notion of the high-speed manipulation of data leading to activation of an output device, whether that device is the tongue, the arm or some largely unknown central function subserving emotion. The general principles are simple and well-understood. The everyday experience of 'mental speech' is sometimes a bit confusing. It exists, but there is no reason to believe that mental speech is either necessary or sufficient for activating ordinary speech. The silent world of information processing does that particular job in accordance with rules I may not even know. I certainly don't plan the jokes and puns I like to make; sometimes, even I have been appalled by the things I've said.

11-5. The Psychological and the Phenomenal in Concert

An example may clarify some of these notions. Consider Mr. Smith, our pedestrian anxiously waiting for the walk signal. The 'Walk' sign flashes green and its light strikes his retina. Almost immediately, a particular barrage of signals travels through his optic nerves. Even within the optic nerve, these signals are already highly derivative. The information traveling through his optic nerves has two jobs to do. Firstly, it must provide the basis for action in the informational or computational aspect of mind, the psychological realm. Secondly, it has to give rise to the experience of green marks glowing on a post. There are at least two ways this may be achieved.

One possibility is that the data flow may split, activating two quite separate circuits in the brain. One circuit, subserving the psychological realm, manipulates the information on which his subsequent behavior will be based. This will be processed in accordance with pre-existing instructions, such as "Green=Go," whereupon his right leg will swing forward just as his left leg throws his body weight forward. In the ordinary sense, there is no thought attached to this but it is nonetheless a willed action. If Mr. Smith were waiting on the corner for a friend, then he would have prepared a different response for the green signal. Simultaneously, the same data flow activates some other brain circuits which, by virtue of their organization, ultimately give rise to the experience of green light.

The second possibility is that the experience of green arises by a higher-order manipulation of the same data flow as gives rise to the behavioral decisions. That is, while the data are being processed in the rather pedestrian way described (and studies on rats yield nearly everything we need to know about humans), a further and simultaneous reprocessing of the same data by more complex "programs" will generate a "virtual machine" which is or gives rise to the experience of green. Now I don't want to stand accused of using unspecified (and probably unspecifiable) brain programs as a latter-day *deus ex machina* ("And then a miracle occurs..."), but I am using the term advisedly to indicate that, by means that are conceptually within our grasp, natural data processing has the potential to produce an outcome which, given its material substrate, is unpredictable and insubstantial yet is capable of influencing the material realm.

It may be that there is just one virtual machine although I prefer the idea that there are many, which, by sequentially flashing into and out of existence, generate the impression of something real, somewhat akin to the little lights flickering over the local fish and chip shop. By this or a similar means, the brain produces the illusion of an inner self, the only unexpected point in the process being that there is no 'I' to be deceived by the illusion. Rather, I just am the illusion. I can't see my sense of self, but I'm sure it's there because it feels like me. You are part of it but, when I die, my solipsistic cinema will collapse and my sense of self will cease to be. I am the ultimate illusion.

Returning to our pedestrian in the morning rush hour, Mr. Smith is keen to reach his office on time. What this means is that, while waiting for the light to change, other circuits in his brain are being activated that give rise to the experience of being tense and nervous. When the green light flashes, he 'hears' in his head the words: 'Thank heavens for that!' and feels his tension abate a little. As yet, we cannot answer the question of how the information that he may walk is converted to inner speech, but I suggest the process will be similar to how olfactory nerve activity is perceived as smell. The question of why it should happen just then will have to wait. As the information activates his motor circuits, it also deactivates or suppresses activity in his emotional circuits, which he experiences as relief.

It might be argued that this is all terribly mechanistic, just a case of a robot granted an inner life by fiat. My response to this criticism is that it is not a criticism. Anything with a rational explanation seems mechanistic just because we reserve the word for processes we understand. It is not an adjective for things that seem beyond comprehension. The process by which, while I sleep, my computer 'searches' a virtual library spread over the entire world is, I suppose, mechanistic, but this does not deny it is a remarkable achievement. Similarly, the processes of reproduction are indisputably mindless and mechanistic, but they work very well and babies are undoubtedly a joy.

Any well-known process can be described in simple terms of "A leads to B, which evokes C and causes... Solution P." In this work, my fundamental assumption is that all events in the universe will ultimately be understood in these terms. If that is mechanistic, then so be it, but I don't believe that demystifying human function converts us into robots. It is not my intention to write a theory for psychiatry that overlooks the fact that humans love to sing while marching to war.

11-6. The Sense of Self

Because everything flows from it, the question of how Mr. Smith decides he needs to hurry along just this road at this time is critical: this is what theories of human behavior are all about. Rats can be made to hurry but only humans can decide they had better hurry because today is an important day. The simple answer to Mr. Smith's anxiety is this: given his particular set of beliefs and his current informational status, then the decision to be anxious is made for him as the logical outcome of an entirely natural computational process (I am using the word 'computational' in its broadest, generic sense). But remember that a lot of Mr. Smith's beliefs and the processes leading to his decisions are beyond his awareness.

This calls into question the concept of self, the 'I' that has littered these pages. The terms Self, I, soul, spirit, mind, etc., have a lengthy history but, oddly enough, or perhaps sensibly, nobody wants to define them. They are all taken as ineffable, as beyond definition: Chalmers [1], Dennett [5] and Popper and Eccles [6] all dodged defining minds, consciousness and Selves, respectively the central words in their titles. I suggest the reason these terms are considered so difficult to define is because there is nothing to define. All of them refer to something that doesn't exist, mere reification of a disparate group of processes. I certainly see these terms as more or less synonymous. The properties of the one are the properties of the other; only their mortality changes.

"Everybody doubts his memory but nobody doubts his judgment." Well over three centuries have passed since the reclusive Duc de la Rochefoucauld wrote these words yet, still, they define the sense of self rather better than the clichéd efforts of many modern writers. They force a change in our view of the concept of self, diverting attention from a thing to a process or series of processes involving beliefs and attitudes. The essence of this epithet is that there is a basic sense of self which, to a very large extent, equates with an unquestioned core set of beliefs, opinions, attitudes, etc. These in turn inform our decisions, and it is by our decisions that we are recognized as individuals (there will never be a psychology of ants).

People may object to a circular element here, since I could say that I judge a belief to be correct and, since it is correct, I will believe it, i.e. my beliefs are necessarily correct and what is correct becomes my belief. However, I think the objection misses the important point that beliefs are often accepted en bloc without being judged. People believe certain things very strongly, even to the point that they will die protecting those ideas, but this does not imply that any critical thought has been applied to them. The individual has been unable to consider those beliefs separately from his self simply because they comprise such a large part of his core concept of self. They are the framework, as it were, around which his sense of self has accreted. Without my beliefs, who am I? Nobody I would recognize.

I suggest that the critical elements in the sense of self comprise a cognitive framework consisting of a set of beliefs and attitudes whose functional significance rests in their ability to influence behavior. These cognitive elements are clothed, as it were, by a continuous memory sequence based in the privacy of one's sensory experiences, by the fact that all of this happens to me. Take away my current experience and my memories of all that has happened to me, and what is left? Just beliefs: in a materialist system, there isn't anything left and, functionally, there is no need for anything more. The critically important beliefs are acquired gradually; the sense of self doesn't pop into existence on one's fifth birthday. They are acquired by the same processes, both explicit or implicit, by which one acquires any other belief, attitude or rule. Broadly speaking, they consist of a set of propositions about the nature of the world, about one's physical and mental attributes and their worth, and about the interactions between the two realms. Without the concept of non-self, the sense of self as an entity with boundaries has no meaning.

It is now possible to avoid the essentialist trap that Popper [7] disliked so much. He had the strongest distaste for the question: "What is....?" for the simple reason that this is very often the wrong question to be asking. So, rather than ask: "What is the Self?" I suggest we should ask: What are the processes leading us to believe that some *thing* is doing them? This way, we can break down the sense of self into a set of functions. For example: "How does the sense of self function as the central executive element in human life?" This is a very much easier question to answer: the core sense of self is not a thing, but is an experience of something constant derived from a lifetime of decisions effected by a relatively constant set of beliefs. Given a system of beliefs, decisions are easy to automate. If, without any particular effort, I decide that this tastes wonderful, that writer hasn't a clue or this sentence has too many examples, then I know I exist. It shifts the emphasis in the sense of self from the experience to the decision that the experience amounts to something. I believe that dogs have experiences; whether they can decide that the experience amounts to something is moot, but I suggest they cannot.

However, it must not be forgotten that the 'Self' is merely a sense of selfhood, not a thing. It is not a sense in the way we say "the sense of smell," but a more allegorical sense as "a sense of fair play," or "a sense of humor." These are functions or processes, not things residing in the head. A sense of fair play is a tendency to do things fairly, a tendency derived from a set of rules that the person takes as central to his sense of self. Without just those rules, he would not be himself but would amount to somebody else. A sense of fair play is not a thing but is an inclination, deriving from a cluster of rules, to act decently even when it is inconvenient. A sense of humor is an inclination to laugh a lot deriving from a complex set of rules governing how the world ought to be. My sense of self is just the set of rules that effect my tendency to make certain sorts of decisions based in a single view-point. Decisions are actions, not things: we cannot extract a common factor from a bunch of decisions and call it a Self.

Thus, if we demote the 'self' from the Executive Spiritual Thing implicit in Eccles' section of *The Self and its Brain* to the epistemologically simple matter of automated decision-making, then we avoid the infinite regress and all the other baggage that Selves bring with them. And because the sense of self is just a collection of beliefs and memories and the decisions they influence, the question of immortality doesn't even arise.

I believe the concept of automated decision-making must occupy a central role in the idea of self for several reasons. Firstly, there is the empirical matter of the speed at which decisions are made. I simply do not have time to judge a matter unfair: the sense of outrage wells up and possesses me, as it were. There may well be an evolutionary advantage in this: if I had to wait a long time before realizing a situation is dangerous, or I had to stop what I was doing to think about it, I wouldn't last long. As a matter of survival, fast decisions that err on the side of caution are better than slow decisions that are never wrong. Secondly, I don't know what it is about many situations that cause me to judge them unfair, but I know unfairness when I see it. I have no clear idea of my basic system of beliefs apart from one very important point: they're perfect. It's your beliefs that cause the trouble, not mine. Thirdly, there is the epistemological economy of dispensing with the problematic Self-thing and replacing it with a process, as processes never violate material principles. Finally, we have excellent models of automated decision-making already available to us. Everyday examples include mouse-traps, computerized chess, and the way baby's piece of bread and honey always falls sticky side down.

11–7. Conclusion

Many of the difficulties implicit in Self-things can be avoided by moving away from the idea of Things Residing In The Head, to using a model of processes as the effective elements in human behavior. While processes are not material things in themselves, they are, nonetheless, dependent on a material substrate for their instantiation. The search for a homunculus has led to more problems than it can possibly solve, e.g. how does the homunculus interact with the material realm? If we assume that everything attributed to the homunculus is in fact the outcome of perfectly explicable events in the material realm, then there is no problem with interaction: the substrate of the allegedly "immaterial self" is one and the same with the familiar, broader material realm. The manipulation of information within an immaterial realm amounts to a causally-effective "virtual machine" (or machines) arising from, but ultimately inseparable from, the physical realm.

The notion of beliefs is central to this work, and I concede, at present, it is essentially an irrefutable idea. We can never observe beliefs in action and can never in principle prove that what we believe to be the outcome of a belief is not the outcome of some other matter. A skeptic could therefore assert that my approach is non-scientific.

I would counter this as follows: If I promised to hand to you a million dollars in return for a glass of water but then, when you obliged, refused to pay, you would be within your rights to take me to court for my breach of contract. That is, you would accept that statements of intentions, beliefs, etc., are, or should be, binding in the real world, i.e. that they have a reality of sorts. My response is that any person who accepts that sort of reality cannot expect to be taken seriously if he objects to my reliance on beliefs to bridge the causative gap in my model. We don't need to fall into the trap set by behaviorists who believed that beliefs amount to naught, especially other people's beliefs. For the time being, beliefs exist as brute facts. If you tell me you don't believe that statement, I won't believe you.

<table>
<tr><td>**12**</td><td>## Interactive Dualism as a Partial Solution to the Mind–Brain Problem</td></tr>
</table>

12-1. Introduction

From the theoretician's point of view, the last twenty years have not been kind to psychiatry. One by one, the major theories on which we have based our claim to specialist status have been shown to be seriously deficient. The last broad attempt at a theoretical basis for psychiatry, Engel's biopsychosocial model, was empty (Ch.7). Since then, there have been sporadic efforts [1,2] but these are often little more than semantic manipulations. Oddly enough, and despite the need, there is nothing in psychiatry like the human genome project, a huge, coordinated attempt to overcome an intractable problem.

The end result is that psychiatrists now have nothing that amounts to an inclusive, integrative approach to mental disorder. At best, psychiatry is a protoscience, to use Kuhn's apt term [3]. I have argued that there cannot be a non-mentalist theory of mind. However, all mentalist theories suffer from the same failing, their inability to explain how the immaterial mind can interact with the material body. How can information about the physical world, which is perceived through the sense organs, be transferred to the soul for processing and then back again without breaching the laws of matter-energy conservation? At present, there are really only two starters in the race for a natural theory of mind, functionalism and dualism. In Ch.10, I outlined a case against Dennett's functionalism. In this paper, I will derive a hypothesis of interactive dualism that goes a long way toward filling the conceptual gap that Engel identified years ago.

12-2. Functionalism

Functionalism is the view that "mental states are defined by their causes and effects" (Baker LR, in [4]). That is, the relationship between the cause, the associated inner states and the effect defines a mental state. To a functionalist, a pain is the type of state associated with pinpricks, burns, etc., ("input"), which causes other inner states such as worry, and typically causes avoidant expressive behavior ("output").

Functionalism defines common, folk notions such as beliefs, attitudes, ambitions, etc., in terms of their association with certain types of behavior: "If two people, on seeing a ripe banana, are in states with the same causes and effects, then, by functionalist definition, they are in the same mental state— say, having a sensation of yellow." Needless to say, this does not endow a mental state with anything like the quality we would like.

One of the most influential functionalist philosophers, Daniel Dennett, has published a book boldly entitled *Consciousness Explained* [5]. In this, he defined the basic task of any model of consciousness as explaining the following phenomena:

12-2 (a): "Experiences of the 'external world' – such as sights, sounds (he included language), smells, slippery and scratchy feelings, temperature, limb position, etc..

12-2 (b): Experiences of the purely 'internal world' – fantasy images, day-dreaming and talking to oneself, recollections, bright ideas and sudden hunches; and

12-2 (c): Experiences of emotion and 'affect' – bodily pains, tickles, sensa-tions of hunger and thirst, intermediate storms of anger, joy, hatred, embarrassment, lust, astonishment and the least corporeal visitations of pride, anxiety, regret, ironic detachment, rue, awe, icy calm, etc.."

In the last paragraph of his work, Dennett conceded that he hadn't ex-plained anything at all: "My explanation of consciousness is far from complete. One might even say that it was just a beginning ... I haven't re-placed a metaphorical theory, the Cartesian Theatre, with a non-metaphorical ("literal, scientific") theory. All I have done, really, is to replace one family of metaphors and images with another ... It's just a war of metaphors, you say..." (p 455).

Given the task he set himself, it is my view that he could never have suc-ceeded. In the first place, his explanation of consciousness says nothing about cognition or intelligence. He might defend this omission by saying that intel-lect has nothing to do with consciousness but he had already indicated his theory was not just a theory of consciousness but a theory of mind. Part II is entitled *An empirical theory of mind*, while Ch.9 is *The architecture of the hu-man mind*.

By Ch.13, *The reality of selves*, his essay had degenerated into incoherence as he jumbled a huge range of mental functions into another, undefined in-tracranial entity called "The Self." I believe that this confusion led to his failure to explain consciousness. Quite clearly, conscious experience is merely a subset of all mental events, as are decisions regarding the boundaries of self and the disorganized range of mental functions he set as his basic task. The larger theory that will account for all of these phenomena is what we call a theory of mind.

There cannot be a stand-alone theory of conscious experience, separate from the phenomenologically distinct but closely-related mental events sub-serving knowing (cognition). Attempting this task is similar to offering a theory of locomotion for the left leg only: it might make the theoretician's task easier, but it won't explain why the body moves. In particular, there cannot be a stand-alone theory of conscious experience that mixes cognitive and experien-tial elements as though they were one and the same thing, yet ignores intellect, the mechanism of cognition.

His failure is brought about by the functionalist aim of "explaining con-sciousness away," of showing that it isn't really what it seems to be. Quite clearly, Dennett wasn't sure what he was trying to explain but, when he got there, he claimed it wasn't what it seemed to be. But sensory experience is *only* what it seems to be: take away the experience and there isn't anything left. It is that sense of *what seems to be* that a theory of consciousness must explain, but only as part of a larger theory of mind.

12-3. Natural Dualism

This point leads directly to the major objection to the functionalists, that they do not take consciousness seriously. Accordingly, at the other side of the philosophical arena, we find a modern version of one of the oldest of all concepts of mind. Following the failure of the supernatural dualism of Popper and Eccles [6], the most recent variant is in the form of what Chalmers [7] terms a natural dualism.

Chalmers starts with a materialist ontology, i.e. the notion that there is nothing in the universe beyond matter and energy and their interactions. A complete understanding of the particles of the universe and their associated energy states would tell us everything there is to know about the universe, its past, present and future. However, some material bodies have the capacity to know, to decide and to feel. And it is this internal aspect, this awareness of being something, that both requires and defies a stock materialist explanation. Difficult as it may be, this inner experience must still be taken seriously.

Within materialism, Chalmers argued, the only viable account of mind is a natural dualism, the notion that conscious experience is both real and natural. The mind arises from the brain by some constant and ultimately definable relationship, probably as a product of brain organization. He posited two aspects to mind, the experiential or conscious element, and the executive, knowledge-based or psychological realm. This formulation immediately leads to what he termed two mind-body problems and one mind-mind problem.

What Chalmers calls the psychological realm, the realm of non-conscious decisions, knowledge, action, etc., is conceptually nothing new. These days, every house has dozens of "dumb machines" that can make decisions based in vast stores of information and massive data flows. However, sensory and emotional experience, the "other half" of mind, remains an enigma: "The structure of experience is just the structure of a phenomenally realized information space..." (p287). What this amounts to in practice remains unexplained by the end of the book. Necessarily, experience is still a brute fact.

12-4. Tasks of a Theory of Mind

A basic theory of mind for psychiatry must explain a diverse range of mental phenomena:

12-4 (a). Exteroceptive sensations such as sight, sound, smell, touch, pain, temperature, position and vibration sense, pressure, sexual sensations, balance, etc.;

12-4 (b). Interoceptive sensations such as hunger, thirst, tiredness, nausea, loss of breath, etc.;

12-4 (c). Emotions such as anxiety, anger, joy, humor, sadness, etc.;

12-4 (d). Compound emotions such as triumph, despair, suspicion, guilt, familiarity/ novelty, yearning, etc.;

12-4 (e). Cognitive functions such as knowing that, calculating, deciding, working out, judging, recalling, being aware of, believing, intending, hoping for, expecting, realizing, meaning, implying, deceiving, getting a joke, detecting injustice, taking a hint, taking offence, etc..

These events fall naturally into two classes, the experiential (groups 1-4) and the knowledge-based (group 5). While the knowledge-based or cognitive functions can readily be reduced to their elements [8], experiences are irreducible. Clearly, a theory of the experiential element (wrongly named a theory of consciousness), is only part of the larger model of mental life. While the two classes of mental events have certain features in common, there are crucial differences between them that allow us to delineate a working model of mind suitable for psychiatry. What we need is a model where things go wrong but the malfunctions can be explained within the framework of the larger model.

In the first place, experiences are immediate, irreducible and ineffable, and have no communicable informational content. We simply have them or experience them but we cannot further analyze them. Sensations are thrust upon us, complete in every detail but are forever private. We talk about them as though they were public knowledge but they are not. Experiences can only be defined ostensively: "It's red, like a ripe tomato." Philosophically, they are brute facts or raw givens that cannot be explained to somebody who hasn't had them.

The other class, of cognitive or knowledge-based functions, is entirely different. These are not experiences but are processes or executive functions outside awareness. They are fast, silent (unconscious), reducible, communicable (as information) and have no experiential content. Thus, we can never catch ourselves in the act of making a decision. We can think about lifting an arm but the instantaneous decision is forever a mystery: we can never catch it in action. Similarly, I don't willfully decide something is familiar: that information is provided *gratis* by processes I cannot see in action. I will never know where my jokes come from, they are thrust upon me, complete, and I simply communicate them.

This is true of all cognitive decisions. I solve a puzzle but don't know how I do so. I jump to catch a ball but monkeys can do it, too. I drive a car along a bush track, changing gears perhaps every ten meters or more often, without ever once 'saying' to myself, "Engine straining, go down to second." Even if I say out loud: "Better change down to second," I have already made the decision before I say it. And so on. All of this takes place at a level I cannot introspect and, even though I can retrospectively reduce the processes to their sub-steps, I cannot catch myself in the act of actually doing them.

Some people object to this conclusion on the basis that, quite often, we consciously reflect upon what we will say and how we will say it, and that this therefore confounds my formulation of cognitive functions as non-conscious. My response is firstly, that the vast majority of human decisions are effected without any such "mental commentaries," that actual deliberation is quite rare and cannot be used as a general model of human decision making. Secondly, this type of reflection is unnecessary. If I 'say' to myself: "No, otiose would be better than unnecessary," then I have already decided to change the word. The commentary is otiose because the decision has already been reached.

As an intellectual being, knowledge arrives, answers are given, compositions are thrust upon me without my knowing where they come from. Knowledge is not random but is determined by organizing principles, or rules. The clearest example of a rule-based, cognitive process is speech. I speak without any idea of how I will say it. I know what I want to say (roughly) but the actual speech as it eventuates may surprise me as much as it does you. I do not yet know the third next word I will use but it will be in context, it will be grammatically correct (mostly) and you will understand it, all without any intervention of what might be called "consciousness." I believe this shows that the experiential and the decision-making or executive realms, while intimately related, are nonetheless profoundly different in nature.

When it comes to the informational or executive mental functions, we have powerful working models of automated decision-making, including very good biological models from animals. However, we have no models of conscious experience. When looking at the phenomena we need to explain, we are like a man trapped in a huge, greased glass bowl. He cannot even start to climb out as he can gain no purchase on his dilemma. No matter how he tries, he invariably ends up back where he started.

12-5. Turing's Automated, Non-Conscious Decision-Maker

To understand automated decision-making, we need to go back 55 years to one of the seminal papers of the IT revolution, Alan Turing's paper entitled *Computing machinery and intelligence* [12]. He showed that, as long as we can reduce the questions or decisions to an elemental form in which the machine simply has to answer yes or no, then a machine can mimic human intelligence. This established the concept of a universal computing machine but, conversely, he also showed that any human decision can be automated.

What this means, but doesn't seem to have been widely appreciated, is that any observable human output state can, in principle, be reproduced in a suitable machine. Therefore, and this goes beyond the argument in his paper, there is no *a priori* reason to suppose that such output states are anything other than strictly non-conscious, blind processes.

Needless to say, if we wish this statement to have any meaning, we need to define "human output states." Dennett was perfectly explicit: human output states that can be reproduced in machines include any and all conscious experiences: "If all the control functions of a human wine taster's brain can be reproduced in silicon chips, the enjoyment will *ipso facto* be reproduced as well" [5, p 31]. Is this logically possible? I can see no compelling case against it but I suggest that, for a working theory of mind for psychiatry, one that shows where things go wrong, it doesn't actually matter. With no derogation of our sentience, we can define the private, experiential realm out of the equation. Turing showed the way.

The essence of the difference between the experiential realm and the executive lies in the fact that, as argued, the experiential occupies no causative role in the generation of observable behavior, including emotions. The behaviorists noted this a long time ago, in, for example, the aphorism that we do not run because we are frightened, we are frightened because we run. They wanted to write the conscious realm out of the causation of behavior. The "decision" that something is dangerous takes place before the experience of fear can be generated. Behaviorists assumed this type of decision was necessarily a biological event, not mental in any sense of the word.

Here, I am using the term decision in its broadest sense that somewhere, somehow, the intact and healthy brain calculates that an event constitutes a risk and activates a series of neurophysiological output states (physiological changes, emotions) that we experience as the fear complex. Automated decisions generate the fear and motor reaction without so-called conscious intervention.

The crucial point of any output state, including behavior and emotion, is that it is immediate and unconsidered, i.e. the experiential realm has no primary or causative role. My brain decides for me what emotions I will experience but, in this context, we have to be very careful just what we mean by brain. I mean some executive decision maker that is at once fast, silent and forever outside awareness. Something automated.

This is where Turing's universal computing machine comes into its own. He reasoned that such machines with large memory stores have an almost infinite output capacity and thus, they can mimic any other discrete state machine. Given sufficient computing capacity and a large memory store, he concluded, the question of whether a machine can think becomes superfluous as we won't be able to tell the difference between a machine and a human. With the proviso that we don't deny our private, non-causative experiential state, there is no reason to suppose that, in making decisions, humans are doing anything more mysterious than machines or rats do. That is, all that counts in a working model of mind is that we humans follow rules while computing the myriad decisions that govern our output states (behavior, emotions, etc.).

This can be rephrased in practical terms. A Turing machine consists of an input tape, a memory, a read/rewrite head and an output tape. The input tape is simplified to the point of inanity, such that the data can be in one of only two forms, a one or a zero. All the machine has to do is read each datum sequentially, compare it with the memory store and decide whether to leave it as it is or change it. Needless to say, the memory has to be in the same form as the input data otherwise it can't be compared, and the output will also be in the same form because nothing has transformed it. As long as the questions can be reduced to a form where they can be manipulated by a yes/no machine of this type, we can compute any output state. Logicians agree that only certain recursive questions cannot be answered in this form, but they won't concern us here.

Is there anything of this form in the central nervous system? In brief, there is. The CNS is most definitely of a form that would support a universal computing function. I will go further: Nobody can ever show that the human central nervous system is not, in essence, a Turing machine.

Turing's model was purely hypothetical, but can we identify elements in the brain that support this model? Yes, but we must first separate the output states into causative and non-causative, otherwise the model will break down.

Turing's original model was only concerned with computing output states because it was on these that the features we class as uniquely human were based. Nobody can claim that seeing the color red is uniquely human, partly because we have no way of knowing whether we all have the same experience, and partly because birds seem to be pretty good at picking it, too. Thus, the experiential realm becomes a nuisance, standing in the way of a neat model that can explain everything we do without worrying about what we feel about it (which, of course, was the behaviorist ambition).

Psychiatry needs a model that explains what people do: if experience is private, universal and non-causative, an explanation of disturbed behavior can dispense with it. It doesn't matter whether or not we both experience red when we look at a tomato, all that counts is what we do about it, including what we say we feel about it. I experience the color red, but the experience is initiated for me by the color receptors in my retina, long before the visual input enters the brain: the decision that tomatoes are red is strictly biological.

In principle, the CNS meets the requirements of Turing's machine. It consists of receptors that receive energy inputs from the external world and convert them into a flow of digital data in the afferent nerves. The data flows are then manipulated at a series of points on their way back to the brain where further manipulation takes place but, crucially, always in the same form as they left the receptors. That is, there is no place in the CNS where the color of a tomato is physically reproduced. The entirety of human mental function is symbolically denoted. There is not an identity relationship between mind and brain just because mind is a symbolic function, and symbols, by their very definition, cannot be reduced to the substrate that carries them. There is therefore no conceptual gap between the input and output.

Since human memory is also in the form of coded impulses, we now have the essential elements of a universal computer within the structure and function of the CNS. There is an input state in coded form, a memory store that does not convert to a different realm (i.e., there is no breach of matter-energy conservation laws), a means of manipulating data in the same codes, and efferent tracts leading to effector organs which respond to exactly the same form of information, i.e. discrete impulses in nerve pathways.

The crucial feature here is that at no point does the data flow move from one realm to another, it stays wholly within the physical realm. This is not to say that the symbols are in the physical realm, because they are not. By their very nature, symbols are irreducibly insubstantial. If it can ever be shown that the data flow itself does move, that it somehow jumps from the natural to the supernatural, then this model will break down and Eccles will have the last laugh. I think I am on safe ground.

So far, what I have proposed is this: a split between the two great classes of mental events into a causative executive realm whose function is fast, silent and reducible but whose outcome is behavioral (public), and a wholly private, non-causative and irreducible experiential realm. We have excellent grounds for supposing that the executive realm follows a form proposed many years ago, one that has since provided the basis for one of the great revolutions in human history. We know that this model breaks no rules of the material universe and that it can achieve any definable human output (behavioral) state, including speech. We already have a model of memory in which the instructions for manipulating the data are coded in the same form as the input and output data and we have working models of unconscious decision making in every desktop calculator. In short, all that is missing is a means of accounting for the experiential realm. Once again, Alan Turing showed the way, although I'm not sure if he realized he did.

12-6. Generating Conscious Experience

In *Consciousness Explained*, Dennett spent hundreds of pages of diligent criticism panning the concept of the Cartesian homunculus, the soul, spirit or little man inside the man. He objected to this because he believed it necessarily involved ectoplasm or "spirit stuff" but, almost at the end of his work, he suddenly invoked a real, functional homunculus to complete his explanation (of mental function). In every respect, it functioned as a soul; it did everything a soul traditionally did as, without it, Dennett couldn't explain a thing. Of course, he didn't call it a soul or homunculus as that would give the game away; instead he called it a 'Self.' This Self-thing, he bravely insisted, was as much a biological secretion of the brain as a bird's nest or a beaver's dam and therefore was scientifically acceptable even when souls aren't.

The problem with the concept of the homunculus is not, as he supposed, that it necessarily invokes ghostly ectoplasm but simply that it explains nothing. In any theory of mind, the problem is this: we have certain mental functions to explain. If we cannot explain them in the physical realm, it avails us naught to attribute them to a little inner man because they still have to be explained in his little head. If we can't explain them in the first head, then we can't explain them in a second either, so we have to postulate a further little man inside the little man, i.e. we have started an infinite regress. This is the reason homunculi are non-scientific, not because they are a forbidden stuff that can't be localized in space. Unfortunately, Dennett's Self is non-scientific just because he endows it with the capacity to make the decisions that his theory was trying to explain. Eccles did this, too; he postulated a ghostly Self that poked its fingers in the grey matter, "read" what it wanted and then sent its decisions back to the brain. This is clearly an infinite regress. The only way out of this impasse is to propose, as I have done, that the experiential realm is entirely a causative dead-end, that it has no more executive powers than a cinema screen.

However, the cinema analogy is potentially misleading because there is no audience in the head to view the screen. Any model of mind involving a stream, field or screen that the mental elements occupy, float in or are projected on, is necessarily an infinite regress and, *ipso facto*, is non-scientific. There is therefore no place in a scientific model for a stream or field of consciousness, nor are the mental contents invested in consciousness in a particular part of the brain or by bathing them in chemicals or inner light or whatever. The experiential realm, Consciousness, the Self, soul or spirit, just has to be a functional dead-end otherwise it sets up an infinite regress. Necessarily, the conscious realm is pure experience with no capacity to observe or decide. Remove the experience, as in deep sleep, coma or anesthesia, and there is nothing.

Fortunately, we have suitable models for a non-located, insubstantial, non-causative entity. It is a mystery why Dennett proposed a biological, executive Self when he had already given an example of such a model, which he called a virtual machine: "Human consciousness … can be best understood as the operation of a 'von Neumannesque' virtual machine *implemented* in the *parallel architecture* of a brain that was not designed for any such activities. The powers of this *virtual machine* vastly enhance the underlying powers of the organic *hardware* on which it runs..." [5, p 210; his emphasis; see note].

I propose that the experiential realm is just one such 'virtual machine,' but not a machine in any other than the most general sense, because it doesn't actually do anything. The experiential realm adds a fascinating dimension to life, it is mostly good fun and life would be very different without it. However, as blind sight and split brain experiments show, we can still get by without it just because all that counts in observable (and therefore communicable) human affairs takes place at the fast, silent level of non-conscious decision-making. Somehow, by manipulating its informational input, the brain generates a sense that being alive is something that being dead is not, and that this sense is over and above decision-making. Remember that stuporous people will brush at their faces to remove a tickle, that sleeping people pull up the blanket when they get cold, we 'decide' to wake up to go to the toilet rather than wet the bed, and mothers sleep through the TV but wake when they hear their babies cry. The brain has subfunctions that do not cease even when the integrated whole we normally call consciousness has been interrupted. Some subfunctions are elementary or vegetative while others are highly developed and delicate.

This type of observation has always caused problems because people are so accustomed to thinking of decisions as something that only occur in full conscious awareness that they mistakenly assumed conscious awareness was essential for all decisions. Finding just one example of a non-conscious decision shows that it is not, that the mechanism used in the unconscious type could in principle account for all decisions. Somebody might object that I am suggesting that a driver could negotiate a highway in his sleep, or even that this book could have been written in my sleep. I would have to agree that this is logically possible but it wouldn't happen in practice because writing one hundred thousand words requires at least a hundred thousand decisions. What actually counts is not so much those decisions themselves but the prior intention to keep working at the task. But this decision requires memory, and there is no reason to believe that memory is fully functional in sleep, so the somnambulist driver would be no better off than a profoundly demented driver: able to make decisions, but not able to sustain an intention.

Decisions are made either immediately before or simultaneously with the conscious experience but quite independently of it. Granted, I am repeatedly going over this material to correct it but the errors are thrust at me from some inaccessible mental place, I don't find them in the experiential realm. Decisions are both causally effective and unconscious in every sense of those words. Experience is fully conscious (even if it's not remembered) and causally ineffective. Nothing of causal importance takes place in the experiential realm but it can certainly hurt, because that's what hurt means.

The next question is whether the CNS could generate a virtual machine of the type this model requires. For an answer, we need to go back to Turing. I don't know whether Turing explicated this point or it was done later, for him, but an important point of the universal Turing machine is that, with sufficient memory and computing power, it can simulate any finite or discrete state machine. That is, the computer can generate virtual machines, a property that has long been exploited. Most work on parallel computing, for example, is done on suitably programmed serial computers. The online auction house, eBay, and all internet banks are virtual machines. Remember, of course, that virtual machines are independent of their substrate, so Dennett's proposal for a sentient silicon wine taster is not as outrageous as it seems.

I propose that the experiential or conscious realm is just that, a virtual discrete state machine generated in the computational space of an extremely powerful universal computing machine, the human brain. I suggest this would satisfy Chalmers' hypothesis: "The structure of experience is just the structure of a phenomenally realized information space..." But does it *explain* experience? How can it explain why experience *feels like* something? How can a virtual machine create the sensations of green or bitter inside the squishy black of the brain?

The glib answer is that it is just that type of machine; it is an *experience generator*; that if it were not so, we would all be zombies, getting on with our one-dimensional lives with no awareness of anything, just as flowers and slime molds do. This is not entirely implausible. Architects routinely work with programs capable of generating an apparent three-dimensional model purely from a digital input. Using these programs, it is possible for people to "walk through" a model of their new home, seeing what it will look like from the inside. At the same time, other programs will generate a picture of the building in its new environment. Combining these two concepts would give an impression of something "in there" as well as something "out there." If they are realized at the same time, then there will be an illusion of being both "out there" and "in here." There is, of course, no observer: the whole thing just is an illusion which is totally dependent on the integrity of the brain for its realization. When the brain ceases to exist, the illusion dies with it. I don't find this kind of answer wholly convincing but, for the time being, there isn't anything better.

Could the form of the physical brain support such a mechanism? Most certainly, it is. Everything we know about the structure and function of the CNS supports the notion that it processes vast data inputs by cascades of stereotyped computation [10]. The basic cerebral unit, the cortical module, which is approximately 300mu wide and 3mm deep, contains about 10,000 neurons. There are about a million such modules, and each neuron has something of the order of 10,000 connections, so the concept of mechanized data processing is entirely consistent with our current views of the cerebral cytoarchitecture. I would suggest, however, that the cortical module is not the minimal functional element; rather, each neuron should be seen as a microprocessor in its own right (not just a single logic gate). With something of the order of one hundred trillion cortical connections, it seems unlikely that the brain doesn't have enough computing power to generate a virtual machine.

12-7. The Emergence of a Biocognitive Model

Since the collapse of the classic models (psychoanalysis, biologism and behaviorism), psychiatrists have been in search of a model to integrate the psyche and the soma. Indeed, so keen has their search been that they embraced the illusory Biopsychosocial Model without ever bothering to check its details. If, at any time over the past three decades, they had done so, they would have found it had none. This would have forced them into the embarrassing position of having to acknowledge that modern psychiatry is operating in a theoretical vacuum, that it has no scientific basis.

The model outlined in this paper offers a means of solving the conceptual gap between the mind and the body by postulating a split between a causally effective cognitive realm and an ineffective experiential realm. In a sense, this amounts to epiphenomenalism but not of the traditional type. Ordinarily, this term refers to models in which the mind is an epiphenomenon of the biological substrate. All effective activity takes place biologically and adherents of these views are, in the main, dismissive of the mentality of human mental life.

My model is totally different. It states that the mind has two irreducibly mental components, cognition and conscious experience, which together account for the whole of human mental life. In this model, "mere biology" does not generate output states. One mental component, conscious experience, is a real but ineffective byproduct of the same processes that led to the other. Only this way can we avoid the trap of the infinite regress implicit in all models in which the conscious element has its own decision-making capacity. Above all, it allows us to rely on known principles of physically-based data processing in accounting for the ability of the mind, including animals, to make the near-infinite decisions on which daily life is based.

This model is diametrically opposed to the biological approach that has gained the ascendancy in psychiatry over the past twenty-five years. Biologism was perhaps a necessary reaction to the unrestrained psychologism that gave psychiatry such a bad name but it has its limits. Just because of its inability to account for the central elements of human mental life, it cannot comprise the basis of a general theory for psychiatry.

The notion of a non-causative experiential realm makes some psychiatrists anxious but I believe this is due to a misconception of the nature of mental causation. Previously, "scientific" theorists dismissed all mental life as fanciful just because they could not account for it within their narrow concepts of science. But they still had to account for decision-making, so they split it away from mentalism, trying to reformulate it as "mere biology" or "mere reflex." On the other hand, those who believed that mental life counts for something resisted the split because it seemed that if they lost control of decision-making, they thereby lost their claim to relevance. In human affairs, decisions count whereas even the most devout mentalist has to concede that deafness or color blindness does not diminish humans. The older generation need not fear that by accepting a non-causative experiential realm, they are consigning mentalism to the epiphenomenalist rubbish bin. The mental sphere includes everything that counts as a decision in human terms and yet does not set up an infinite regress.

In suggesting that we can build a model of mind (and thence of mental disorder) without formally explaining the nature of experience, I am not implying that conscious experience doesn't exist or is irrelevant, nor am I slipping it off the table while nobody is looking. I am saying that disordered conscious experiences, which comprise the core of mental disorder as we define it, are secondary to disturbances in the cognitive realm. While we will use drugs, etc., to try to reduce the impact of those experiences, we don't need a theory of conscious experience to be able to explain the causation of mental disorder. I do not need a theory of perception to know that this experience is pain, its pattern indicates appendicitis and it should best be managed this way. Similarly, I do not need a theory of perception to know that this experience is an emotion, its pattern indicates anxiety and it should best be managed this way. Psychiatry is, after all, a pragmatic discipline.

In this approach, each person's explicit and implicit belief states govern his mental life. The model states that humans are sentient, rule-governed creatures, not id-driven and certainly not "mere organisms." Logically, we have to have rules before we can know anything: *Homo nomothetikos,* the giver of rules, came before *Homo sapiens.* By this means, we can readily account for personality and personality disorder, while our understanding of formal mental disorder moves beyond unknown "chemical imbalances of the brain." The application of this biocognitive model to practical psychiatry requires some reorientation of the current, categorical model. These points will be explored in the last section.

Nothing in this model breaks any rules of the material universe. There is no ectoplasm floating around to bridge causative gaps, there are no infinite regresses, no irrefutable elements, no question-begging pseudo-solutions, no slick redefinitions, no miracles and no hidden tricks. I haven't relied on any models that aren't already in use or other people haven't devised and implemented in other fields. This is not irrefutable, like psychoanalysis, nor does it test one's credibility by saying, as did the behaviorists, that consciousness doesn't exist. Unlike the biological psychiatrists, I haven't tried to reduce the mind to its substrate, nor tried to explain it away by legerdemain as functionalism tries to do.

Furthermore, I have indicated exactly where this model can break down. The critical element is that the coded information, including all the memory stores in which the rules are coded, flows from input receptors, through the computing machinery to the effector organs while remaining wholly in the physical realm as discrete nervous impulses, and it is at this level that all decisions are made. Conscious experience, however, arises from this level but does not act back upon it except secondarily. The effective data flow does not at any point jump from the material to the immaterial realm, except with this proviso: information is coded, so it is never "in" the physical realm. It is always "somewhere," floating in a private virtual space generated by the brain.

12–8. Conclusion

This is wholly and irreducibly a mentalist account of human behavior, yet it is firmly based in the physical structure of the brain. Unlike previous psychological theories, it takes account of the structurally defined limits of the CNS. It leads to an integrative model of mental function and dysfunction that can satisfy psychiatry's current intellectual vacuum. For the first time in the history of psychiatry, we have the outline of a model offering realistic solutions to a number of major problems. As a general theory of psychiatry, it restores the essence of humanity, our mentalism, to rightful primacy.

Part III: Toward the Future of Psychiatry

"All great truths begin as blasphemies."
Annajanska (1919)
—George Bernard Shaw

13 Personality Disorder

13-1. Defining the Problem

The orthodox position in psychiatry is that personality and mental disorder have nothing to do with each other. That, however, is a matter of definition: the criteria for the different categories are defined in such a way as to make them independent which, of course, begs the question. A better approach is to start with basic principles and see what emerges.

In Chapter 7, I argued that both the categorical and the dimensional approaches to personality are invalid. Since typologies are of no explanatory value (they describe but do not explain), where do we turn? The definition of personality is quite simple: it is the totality of interactions between the individual and his environment. Needless to say, this is an encyclopedic definition, and somewhat impractical, as it would never be complete until the subject dropped dead. We therefore abbreviate it to read: Personality is the total habitual forms of interaction between the individual and his environment, i.e., his behavioral dispositions. Now this would appear to be veering toward a dimensional definition but it avoids the trap by stating that the potential range of behavioral acts is more or less infinite; therefore, the distance or range between individual behavioral acts is infinitely small. Accordingly, any attempt to group them into clusters is artificial.

In practice, the scope of the definition has to be restricted to prevent it becoming encyclopedic. Matters such as culture, intellect, language, etc., are excluded because they don't help distinguish between individuals. For example, people of the same culture tend to have similar dispositions, while the same behavioral types can be seen in genius and in low intelligence. We also want to exclude temporary disturbances of behavior, such as are seen in illness or injury, intoxications and following major psychological stressors. In addition, behavior varies a great deal during childhood and adolescence, so the definition now reads something like: The distinguishing, habitual forms of interaction between the individual and her environment in the stable, adult modes of behavior.

At first glance, this doesn't seem very helpful. We want our definition of personality to say something valid, but to say it briefly and reliably. Above all, we want to anchor it in a theory of mind, because a *definition* of personality is not itself a *theory* of personality. A theory of personality is a conjecture, a hypothesis relating to the hidden mechanism that generates the observable behavioral events. That is to say, it explains them. Explaining is the act or process of making an event intelligible or comprehensible by showing how or why it occurred. Needless to say, the hypothesis must not beg the questions it is designed to answer, and must potentially be open to empirical testing. In fact, that is asking quite a lot of the model, but since worthwhile models of any sort are currently in short supply, we can be excused if the first draft doesn't satisfy everybody.

13-2. Solving the Problem

A theory of mind is a suggestion of an unseen mechanism capable of generating all observable behavior. Because it only has to explain the habitual behaviors, a theory of personality is a subset of the larger theory of mind. This is an important point, because a lot of people have spend a lot of time and effort conflating the two, thereby trying to make their theories of personality do too much – and failing. The most restricted account of personality simply looks at what a person has done in the past, and, on the limited evidence available, tries to predict how she will act in the future. As an inductive process, it is prey to the faults of all inductive systems but, in daily use, it can be extremely effective.

An essential test of a genuine theory of personality (as distinct from a description of types) is that it should entail an account of personality disorder. I suggest this is why orthodox psychiatry has been unable to come to grips with personality disorder: they never had a theory of personality order, because personality order depends in turn on a theory of mind.

Given the model of mind outlined in the previous two chapters, and the observations to be explained, can we connect the two in a meaningful sense? I believe this can be done quite readily. Behavior is an output state of the mind, and is therefore the product of the psychological realm. To account for the habitual modes of behavior, all we need do is propose that their regular occurrence is generated by rules encoded in the brain as part of its informational state. According to the model, they are in a form that allows them to influence the output state.

Can this be justified? By definition, habitual behaviors are not random. Their consistency or regularity allows us to conclude that they are being generated by some continuing or repetitively active state, and that state is what I will call a rule. Rules, as previously argued, can be acquired explicitly or implicitly; there is no implication that they are all acquired or retained in the form of language. As a simple example, take my accent. We all have an accent but very few of us can define it or say when we learned it, why we use it, how we generate just the tones we do, etc. (part of the reason is that I don't believe I have an accent; you do, but I don't). The accent is acquired implicitly at a very early age, and exerts a strong influence for decades at least. Its regularity and predictability means it is a rule-governed behavior and, of course, those rules are unconsciously effective.

In the case of personality, probably the great majority of rules governing the behavioral output are implicit (non-verbal, non-conscious) but that is an empirical matter. All that counts is that they exist. So the theory of personality devolves to the set of coded rules governing the distinguishing, habitual forms of interaction between the individual and his environment in the stable, adult modes of behavior. That's all. It is probably the most parsimonious explanation we can derive.

Personality just is a set of rules. As such, it is an artificial construct, a special subset of the much larger theory of mind. Since we've already defined certain sets of rules out of the process, e.g. common property such as the rules of language, the traffic code, the rules of golf, math, cooking, war, and so on, all that is left is the set of individuating rules, of which the possibilities are infinite. In fact, because everybody's experience of life is different, the conclusions they draw about the world and their relationship with it will also be different. This leads to a totally different conclusion from the existing approaches to personality.

In the first place, the standard psychiatric model has nothing to say about normal personality. Orthodox psychiatry is of the view that abnormal personalities exist (hardly contentious), but they are categorically different from normal people and from each other. This point is highly contentious. In fact, I am not aware of any evidence that could be used to support this view, and I believe it should be abandoned before it does any more damage.

The alternative model in psychology and psychiatry is the dimensional approach, which states that certain fundamental dimensions of behavior are distributed throughout the population and that every person can be given a score on each parameter. However, there is no evidence that human behavior is so tidy. What are called dimensions are in fact just loose clusters or clumpings of "rather similar behaviors." These are defined more to suit (the personality of) the researcher than to provide an accurate reflection of reality. There is no agreement as to how many dimensions there are, what they are, or how they relate to each other: Eysenck says there are three, somebody else says five, Cattell says there are sixteen... It depends entirely on how you choose to look at the problem. They are no more than descriptive typologies, classifying humans into predetermined types, which is about as useful as classing them into clusters according to height, race, blood type, etc.

This model says there are no dimensions, that an individual behavioral act (if there is such a thing) is the outcome of the interaction of an indeterminate number of rules and an almost infinitely variable current informational input. There is no discontinuity between individual behavioral acts: nobody can say where courtesy stops and rudeness starts.

This model is quite simple. Consider Mr. James Smith, a man of normal intellect and no compelling idiosyncrasies, who is sitting quietly on a park bench somewhere. He brings to his bench a personal background, a huge, rich history of events dating almost from the day he was born. His head is full of rules derived from his myriad life experiences, some of which he could tell you but most of which he couldn't. These rules amount to his personality (note I didn't say rules are identical with personality; a generative mechanism is not the same as its output, of which more later). When something happens near him, his reaction is determined by a high-speed and unreportable interaction between what he sees and his unique set of rules. Some of his rules are more or less fixed and won't vary much from one year to the next, but some are more fluid, even a little unpredictable. If, today, a man comes past and asks him for money, Mr. Smith may be inclined to smile indulgently and hand over a few coins. However, another day, he may have had an argument with his wife or his boss and not be feeling so chipper; this time, the same wheedling request may elicit only a snarl to get a haircut and a job. His personality hasn't changed, and the inconsistency doesn't mean he has a personality disorder, he's just being normal. Normality is a huge, multidimensional range and behavior is only disordered at the extremes.

The term normal personality has to mean something beyond mere statistics. We can apply the term to a person whose rules are such that they tend to generate responses that are fairly consistent from one day to the next. Since his "rules of life" give him rather mild and predictable emotional responses, and do not bring him into conflict with his social milieu, he is able to get on with whatever he sees as important. That is, Mr. Smith is a pretty ordinary, unremarkable citizen, which leads us directly to a definition of personality disorder.

I have outlined a case for what we call personality being no more than a subset of mind, a convenient fiction, if you wish. It is most important not to make the mistake of attempting to reify this cluster of mental bits and pieces. There is no such Thing as The Personality. Also, personality exists only as a set of rules that are necessarily coded in a form of memory. Therefore, anything that interferes with memory can affect the rules we call personality, and anything that affects current computational capacity will affect the application of those rules. That is, personality can change with, coarse brain disease such as tumors, infections and dementia, and with metabolic disorders and intoxications. In an adult, a non-traumatic personality change means brain disease until proven otherwise.

13-3. Personality Disorder

If the rules governing a person's life are internally inconsistent, or there are so many of them that he can't reach a decision, or they generate disabling emotions or cause repeated conflict with his neighbors, then we say he has a personality disorder. The type of personality disorder is of very little importance unless it leads to treatment, which most don't. Orthodox psychiatry agrees with this but adds the rider that eventually, biological research will explain all. The cognitive model says the exact opposite. It states that biology is not involved, that personality just is a set of rules, where rules are acquired psychologically and stored as symbols that cannot be reduced to their biological substrate. Biological psychiatry will therefore never have anything to offer in the field of personality disorder. Does this matter? I believe it does, because I see personality as crucially important, the pre-eminent factor in determining how a person functions in life. This will become clearer as we proceed.

Personality disorder exists where an individual shows a consistent pattern of interpersonal disturbance in adult life, such that he or she cannot reach full potential because of self-engendered constraints. We have to be careful here, because people with personality disorders are often very good at attributing blame for their own shortcomings on the social and/or natural environment. And the more aggressive they are, the less kindly they will take to attempts to pin the responsibility on themselves. At the other extreme, there are people who blame themselves for everything to the point where they are so burdened by guilt they can't move. In a proper assessment of personality disorder, all of this has to be teased out carefully.

It is the case that, because it doesn't see personality as causative of anything, orthodox psychiatry is very bad at assessing personality. People are given a formal diagnosis of mental illness first, and a personality assessment later. It does not encourage new psychiatrists to see human distress through the lens of personality. Indeed, some psychiatrists see personality as lying outside their field of interest, something to be left to psychologists and the other minor players while the psychiatrist gets on with the hard work of treating the mental illness by biological principles.

Part of the problem lies in the fact that psychiatrists only get paid for treating mental illness, so they have a very powerful interest in redefining personality disorder as mental illness and taking over the management. Unhappiness is no longer a reaction to life events, it is now a formal mental disorder, depression, for which drug treatment is *de rigueur*. This is certainly happening in Australia, aided and abetted by the rubbery American nosology that is so vague that practically any disturbance can be relabeled a mental illness and brought into the fold. For example, what used to be called a neurotic personality is now called Dysthymic Disorder and is treated with antidepressants and mood stabilizers. What used to be called a cyclothymic personality is now Cyclothymic Disorder and is treated with antidepressants and mood stabilizers. In particular, erratic and unstable men will acquire a diagnosis of ADD/ADHD and will be prescribed stimulants. Previously, a diagnosis of personality disorder was regarded as a contraindication for these powerful and addictive drugs but now they are handed out freely to anybody who isn't performing very well – which is, of course, the hallmark of the disordered personality. This is especially true now that the diagnosis of ADD/ADHD can be made much later in life, or even on a family history. Women showing a similar pattern of disturbance will be classed as Bipolar Affective Disorder and prescribed large doses of heavily sedating antidepressants and mood stabilizers.

In many parts of this country, psychiatrists no longer diagnose personality disorder. The reason they don't diagnose it is because they no longer see it; they have become so accustomed to looking at people through the microscope that they no longer see the "bigger picture." For example, the DSM-IV diagnosis of Cyclothymic Disorder is made in the presence of a "chronic, fluctuating" disturbance, in which there is "clinically significant distress or impairment in social occupational or other important areas ... e.g. the person may be regarded as temperamental, moody, unpredictable, inconsistent or unreliable." This just is a definition of personality disorder but, if the psychiatrist diagnoses personality disorder, he can no longer see the patient for exclusively psychiatric reasons. He is saying that the patient has a disorder for which psychiatry has notoriously little to offer and may be managed better or more cheaply by another discipline. That won't pay the bills in private practice but, even in public practice, may well result in psychiatrists defining themselves out of existence.

However, in this context, psychiatrists are not operating in a social vacuum. There is enormous pressure on psychiatrists *not* to make a diagnosis of personality disorder, especially in adolescents or young adults. School teachers, parents, lawyers, probation officers, the patients themselves... Everybody wants little Shane or Kirsty to be seen as suffering a genetically-determined brain disturbance rather than be classed as naughty because that way, the demanding, obstreperous adolescent can be sedated and nobody can be blamed. Psychologists are certainly part of this web of disservice because, if the nominated patient sees a pediatrician once every three months for another prescription (nowadays up to the age of 24), somebody must deal with the endless crises in between, and since upset parents and hostile teachers aren't mentally ill, they also need to talk. With respect to his "illness," of course, Shane has nothing to talk about but needs years of CBT and Anger Management on how to deal with the taunting at school, at huge cost. Even audiologists, physiotherapists and opticians get a look in, to overcome the 'Auditory Processing Disorder' or the 'Primary Motor Dysfunction' or the 'Central Visual Data Processing Deficiency.' Teachers, of course, need lots of seminars to learn how to deal with sedated children. Reclassifying personality disorder as illness has now become an industry with its own momentum.

On a behavioral level, we tend to classify people according to their most obvious characteristics, not one of which is unique to personality disorder. Every factor seen in a disordered personality can also be seen in normal people, albeit in minor form. This is because each of us, normal and abnormal, is using much the same mental rules most of the time; we normals simply apply them more flexibly. There is no categorical difference between ordinary tidiness and rigid obsessionality. We can all be aggressive when the occasion demands; it is merely the case that the psychopathic or antisocial personality sees more occasions than you or I. We can all feel frightened but if we habitually respond to neutral environmental events as though they were a threat, then we have an anxious personality. There is no cut-off point between pathological dependence and pathological independence; there is a range from low dependence to high and we all sit somewhere on the range, but dependent behavior also blurs across to other factors such as caring and nurturing.

If abnormal personality is simply a matter of mixed up rules, why can't we send these difficult people to school and teach them the normal rules of social intercourse? Part of the reason is the same as when your parents couldn't convince you to speak properly or get a decent haircut: you didn't think you were doing anything wrong. But, for the rest, even when people are extremely distressed and demanding help, they still show a bizarre resistance to change, as though something is actively preventing change. People whose self-destructive behavior has brought their lives to ruin a dozen times will pick themselves up and immediately set to work on their thirteenth disaster, walking examples of Freud's neurotic repetition compulsion. This is where the descriptive system of personality disorder breaks down entirely, because it can never explain these phenomena. The only "explanation" in modern psychiatry is that tired saw, Chemical Imbalance of the Brain. Thus, the personality disorder is a chemical imbalance of the brain, and resistance to change is also a chemical imbalance of the brain. However, I have already argued that this is a pseudo-explanation. In its place, we need an unseen mechanism that both explains and can itself be explained.

My suggestion is quite simple: that the distorted rules that give rise to the disordered behavior generate an output state which serves to reinforce the rules. That is, either directly or indirectly, the individual's behavior or emotions are such as to convince him that his beliefs or rules are correct. Of course, he doesn't refer to them as rules; he simply knows what is right: "I know I'm going to make a mess of it," or "I know you people don't like me."

Others might be: "I've got to tidy this place, I'd hate to get into trouble," or "Nobody's allowed to tell me what to do." A very powerful but unfortunately widespread one is of this form: "I'm stupid, ugly and worthless. I hate myself." It leads inexorably to: "If my girlfriend looks at another man, she's probably thinking of leaving me."

Of course, these types of rules aren't regarded as alien intrusions, they are simply accepted by the individual as part of the wallpaper of his mental life.

In some cases, the rules may generate emotions that serve to reinforce the individual's belief state, of which anxiety is by far the most powerful and most common. Otherwise, the rules may generate behavior that affects the social environment, thereby feeding back to the individual a reinforcing behavioral or emotional response.

So, in brief, we have a model of personality that satisfies a clutch of criteria. In the first place, it is consistent with a larger model of mind to the extent that it is a subset of mind. We do not have to invent a theory separate from or adjunctive to the broader theory of mind. Secondly, the theory is probably the most parsimonious concept available. It does not multiply the entities to be explained, nor does it invent more, which then require explanation themselves. Thirdly, it does not rely upon promissory materialism to complete the explanatory chain. Fourthly, it offers a model of personality disorder that uses the *normal* mechanism of personality to show how disorders develop. Finally, the theory immediately offers a rational explanation of a major clinical feature of personality disorder, the resistance to change, without invoking more entities.

Having said all this, it needs only be mentioned that, in the everyday setting, we still need to have a shorthand for talking about the various types of personalities because they will require different management. As long as everybody knows this is what we are doing, that it is like, say, talking about cars as small, medium and large, then it is justifiable. So, for example, today I saw a man with an anxious-obsessional personality, another with a well-concealed paranoid personality, then a very insecure man (low self-esteem) who covered his agitation with aggression, another with an anxious preoccupation with his health (hypochondriasis), and a very cheerful man whose inability to say no repeatedly brought him into financial problems and depression. Of course, their true personalities were vastly more complex than this but, as summaries, these vignettes don't do them any great injustice. Normal personality is a vast, multifactorial range spread across time, one that influences and, in turn, is influenced by, the environment.

The last consideration is that this model dictates treatment. If personality disorder amounts to a set of distorted rules, then treatment will consist of isolating the destructive rules and replacing them with more adaptive standards. This not only means a specific form of psychotherapy, but it also excludes a huge range of so-called therapies that have been used over the years. Chief among these is the Freudian model in its many avatars, which focuses attention on just one of the output states of the rules (emotion) rather than on the rules themselves. Thus, talking about one's past is largely a pointless exercise compared with the actual work of isolating the pathogenic rules; not infrequently, people will talk about how badly they were treated as children, just to avoid the hard work of taking responsibility for personal change.

Similarly, the huge behaviorist industry selling relaxation in its endless variants aims to suppress the output without changing the pathological factors generating the output. There is practically no limit to the variations of relaxation training, massage, audio tapes, books, ashrams, yoga, sex therapy, floatation, group awareness, QEEG, magnetic therapy, crystals, rebirthing, plastic surgery, success and motivational training and so on, that people are willing to pay for.

Least meritorious of all is the ancient idea that there is something that can be added to or subtracted from the diet that will turn the quivering, the mournful, the lonely or the enraged into bounding paragons of mental health. This includes special diets of inclusion or omission such as the tiresomely persistent Feingold diet and its many variants, megavitamin therapy, liver cleansing diets, minerals, powdered crystals, colonic irrigation, allergy therapy and so on, *ad nauseum.*

A great deal of the commerce that accretes around formal religions is also of no value. The endless rituals, blessings, amulets, incantations, pilgrimages, etc., are not doing anxious or guilt-ridden believers any favors. Rather, they assuage temporarily without actually showing a path to personal change. All of these things are a complete and utter waste of time and money, convincing the fearful, the gullible, the dim-witted or the lazy that there is a quick, pain-free fix.

No, there isn't.

13-4. Conclusion

This model of personality disorder derives directly from a model of normal personality. In turn, this flows from the larger model of mind developed from elementary principles in Part II. To my knowledge, this approach is unique in the history of psychiatry.

At no stage have the fundamental laws of the universe been strained; there are no new explanatory entities requiring account; there are no gaps in the chain of explanation; it does not rely on promissory materialism to 'save the day'; and all the processes invoked are already in use elsewhere. There is, indeed, nothing new in this model, just a different way of looking at an old problem. But really, it isn't new at all: people with disordered personalities surely do "march to the beat of a different drum."

14 | Anxiety

14-1. Introduction

Of the non-psychotic states, orthodox psychiatry places enormous emphasis on depression, almost to the point of dismissing anxiety. Indeed, the various anxiety disorders are commonly excluded from the list of "serious mental illnesses" (SMIs to the *cognoscenti*). Anxiety states are the province of the "worried well." The implication, of course, is that anxiety is not a serious mental problem, and therefore not the sort of thing that serious psychiatrists would bother with (and does anybody know a psychiatrist who isn't serious?) There is no rational reason for this: by any definition (of prevalence, standard measured disability, complications, careers and families ruined, early death), anxiety is a very serious disorder indeed.

I suggest this view arose because depression is more like a "real illness." To a certain extent, this was historical, in that anxiety was long seen as a matter of personal failing (e.g. the inadequate personality), while a biochemical "model" of depression (reserpine) was available many years ago. ECT and tricyclics, some of the first relatively effective treatments in psychiatry, brought depression firmly into the medical fold. In addition, psychologists made a powerful theoretical claim on anxiety, although they had less to say about depression. Without too much difficulty, psychologists could provoke fear in their favorite experimental animals, the laboratory rat and psychology sophomores, but they could not ethically induce states of depression.

My view is that anxiety is a most serious disorder, probably the most common single disorder in the world, and that it is directly or indirectly responsible for a very large part of psychopathology at all stages of life. Psychiatry's obsessive interest in disorders that might conceivably have a genetic origin has blinded us to the extent, severity and complexity of the anxiety states and, above all, to their nature. In this chapter, I will show that we need to reappraise anxiety itself, and its role in precipitating and maintaining a range of "SMIs."

14-2. Explaining Normal Anxiety

14-2 (a) Defining Anxiety: Anxiety is an emotion. As such, it is a brute fact, a raw given that cannot be further defined or explained. It can only be defined ostensively, e.g. "Anxiety is the combined mental and physical state experienced after a threat has been perceived. It ranges from the slightest awareness of apprehension or alertness, through concern, foreboding, fear and dread, to disabling terror and panic."

There are two components to the anxiety response, the mental and the physical, which, acting together, prepare the organism to respond to the perceived threat. I used the term "organism" advisedly, to warn that anxiety is a normal part of the animal world. All creatures above jellyfish have some sort of threat response, and plenty of jellyfish have elementary forms. For the next few sections, I will be talking about humans as primates, to emphasize that anxiety is *normal and adaptive*. Animals that can't respond to threats become breakfast.

14-2 (b) Describing Anxiety: In the physical body, the one we more or less share with chimps, the anxiety response shifts the body from a torpid state to a state or readiness or alertness. Picture a troop of baboons or chimps quietly grooming each other while munching on their favorite food. Around the edges of the troop are placed sentinels who, while eating, are not drowsy. They are watching the peripheries of their little range. If a sentinel sees something spotted slinking through the bush or something writhing along the forest floor, it will give a very characteristic call that has an immediate effect on the whole troop. Almost instantly, the troop is galvanized. With a variety of hooting and barking sounds, the males jump up and assume a posture of jittery watchfulness. Females grab their infants and leap for the trees. Youngsters wail and demand to be picked up while adolescents scream and hurtle to the nearest tree, where they rock branches or tear them off and throw them around. The picture is absolutely typical. Any text of primate behavior, such as the work of Jane van Lawick-Goodall, will describe it in fascinating detail.

If we look at the physiology of the alerting or "fight or flight" response, we see a series of changes that vary little from one species to the next. Their net effect is to ready the body for action. Blood is shunted from the viscera to the heart and lungs and thence to the brain and skeletal muscles. The heart rate increases, as does the efficiency of contraction. The respiratory rate increases and, typically, the animal takes a few deep, gasping breaths through the open mouth. The skeletal muscles tense and show a fine tremor. The pupils dilate and the eyes tend to dart in rapid saccades. Also very typically, the hair on the back and neck stands up (piloerection) and sweat prickles the body. Where possible, the ears are erected and move around, scanning the environment even when the threat is directly in front. In fact, there is hardly a part of the body that isn't involved in this response. Even the bowels may evacuate. At the same time, the brain shows very typical changes in activity. From the slow pattern of drowsiness, the EEG tracing swings to a sharp pattern, typical of the alert state.

These changes are mediated by a highly complex and poorly understood part of the brain, situated deep in the temporal horns. These systems, which are remarkably similar in all higher primates, are very closely associated with the deep nuclei associated with the rage response – an aroused animal can flicker back and forth between fear and rage with practically no discernible change in its physiology. All primates, including humans, have the machinery of anxiety hard-wired into the brain, and all respond to threats in a highly standard form.

In humans, the physical changes of anxiety affect the body from the scalp to the feet. In the scalp, we still show residual piloerection that is experienced as a creeping sensation of the hair and of the back and arms ("My hair stood on end!"). At the other end, on the soles of the feet and on the palms, there is sudden, profuse sweating that is quite distinct from the sweating of high temperature. This is often associated with a muscle tremor, so that people talk about "cold shivers." In between these bodily extremes, we can start with the eyes and ears. People report a hyperacuity of sight and sound, so that colors seem very bright and every sound seems to crackle with a preternatural significance. Because the person is usually breathing through his mouth, he gets a dry mouth and may tend to stumble over his speech. His throat seems tight and he may have trouble swallowing or speaking as his voice becomes tight.

Almost invariably, an anxious person reports that his heart starts to race. This may be simply a very rapid pulse, commonly up to 150 beats per minute, or may be experienced as a violent thudding of the heart with a slower rate. Almost as commonly, there is a very unpleasant, hollow feeling in the upper abdomen associated with a churning sensation in the stomach area, or maybe a hungry, knotted or butterflies sensation, it varies from person to person. Very commonly, people report that in this state, they cannot stand the sight or smell of food; they feel that if they eat, they will immediately vomit. A sense of nausea is very common and many people will begin a violent and noisy attempt at vomiting in the hope that it will relieve their discomfort. If anything does come up, it is usually just some acidic froth and bubble, although, if they have been doing it for half an hour or more (well-known in casualty or emergency departments), they may bring up some yellow or green stained slime. A fine tremor of the limbs is extremely common although it may be experienced more as a jelly-like sensation in the limbs, as though all the strength has been drained out.

Mentally, anxious people report very typical changes in both the emotional and in the cognitive states. The emotional changes consist of the sudden eruption of the sense of apprehension, fear or terror that characterizes the anxiety response. This may be disguised, as will be described later, but it is always there. It isn't possible to have all the changes listed above and not feel an emotion of this type. Cognitively, the frightened person reports a series of changes entirely consistent with what we presume a frightened chimp experiences. The thought processes seem to accelerate, to the point where the person describes an inability to keep track of them. Thoughts seem to pop into the head unbidden, usually thoughts about escape and perhaps only marginally connected with the threat. In addition, there is a narrowing of the attentional processes, such that the threat seems to loom larger to the point where he doesn't notice what is happening around or behind him. Everything seems to focus on the threat and he may not even hear voices behind him or see avenues of escape. Frightened people sometimes "forget" to escape.

As the level of anxiety rises, the physical signs and symptoms tend to plateau but the cognitive features continue to intensify. The terrified person may report that the world seems different (derealization), that it is "closing in" or that his eyes are playing tricks on him. He may feel time has changed, either accelerated or slowed, that he can't extract the meaning of words or that they are full of hidden meanings. Familiar things seem strange and *vice versa* and, in severe cases, he may report that his body has changed, that it no longer seems his own (depersonalization). Unexpected sounds make him jump badly as they assume a peculiar, frightening significance.

In the extreme reaches of terror, a person is almost unable to function. He can hardly walk and may need to be supported upright. He can barely string two words together and doesn't appear to understand what is being said to him. He will be trembling violently with the pulses in his neck plainly visible. Sweat drips from his body, his feet and hands will be pale and cold, perhaps even faintly purple; he will be panting wildly, may dribble and vomit but won't seem to know to wipe his face. The most innocent movement or remark may seem to terrify him further and he may suddenly break loose and run with no plans, even to the point of endangering his life.

14-2 (c) Responding to Anxiety: The experience of anxiety says that the subject, be it human or otherwise, has perceived a threat. Therefore, there are only certain things it can do. Assume a large and dominant male baboon is sitting on the ground near his troop when he sees a couple of hyenas approaching. He immediately jumps up and barks a warning, sending the young and the females to the trees or rocks for protection where they will form a wavering group, clutching each other and peering around in fear. That's one perfectly standard response to a threat: run away, although humans prefer to call it avoidance. The second is what the male baboons will do, bunch together and advance toward the threat, ready to fight. They will be highly aroused and, in this mood, will attack anything that gets in their way. Offence, as they say, is the best form of defense: a group of angry male baboons represents a formidable enemy and even large predators will leave them alone. Another response to a threat is also seen in many other species, submission. Thus, the puppy lies on its back and piddles; an older dog lowers its head, exposing the side of its neck to the aggressor. Young male baboons may present their rear ends for sexual penetration by a dominant male. Avoidance, submission, attack: in this respect, we are prisoners of our phylogeny.

Avoidance is the time-honored way of dealing with a threat ("Discretion is the better part of valor"). People who are scared of snakes do not live near tropical swamps. A child is taunted or beaten at school, so he truants. An employee is frightened of an authoritarian supervisor so he reports sick. Finally, he uses all his sick leave so he resigns and finds another job where he starts the cycle again. A lady resigns from her tennis club rather than accept the job of chairing the meeting. A youth joins a church group rather than join his mates looking for casual sex. **Displacement**, in which the frightened individual occupies himself pointlessly on something completely irrelevant, is a form of avoidance.

Submission is the basis of the totalitarian state. Most people will hump their backs and go along with something unpleasant rather than speak up and bring the forces of the state down on their shoulders. Submission invites bullying; the bullying will not stop until the victim declares: "Enough is enough." A direct **attack** on the threat is the other half of the flight or fight response.

Humans also have another response to a threat, which is to do exactly what the assailant wants, to the point of becoming the aggressor, or what Freud called "identification with the aggressor." Thus, young men in occupied countries joined the Nazi or Communist parties, often becoming more brutal than the invaders. This is also seen in socially marginalized groups such as biker gangs or frankly criminal groupings, and, of course, in dysfunctional families. In its most extreme form, it is known as *folie a deux* or Shared Psychotic Disorder in newspeak, where a submissive person assumes the bizarre beliefs of a dominant but psychotic partner.

14-2 (d) Explaining anxiety: The question "Why are you anxious?" can be answered at a number of different levels. Firstly, there is the evolutionary question, "Why do humans have the capacity for anxiety?" Next, there is the ontological question, "Why does anxiety feel so frightening?" or its corollary "Why do threats make us feel frightened and not hungry?" Answers to these questions explain normal anxiety. Then there are the questions of pathology: "Why are you anxious when everybody else is cheerful?" "Why is it so intense?" and "Why are you still anxious when the threat has gone?"

14-2 (d) (i) Evolutionary explanations of anxiety: Why do humans have the capacity for anxiety? The simple answer is the same as for the appendix: because our ancestors had it. But why did the capacity for anxiety arise and then persist? In brief, it has very powerful survival value. Anxiety as an internal alarm system saves our genes, so you could say (if you like glib answers) that anxiety is merely our genes looking after themselves. Animals without something like anxiety, such as swarms of jellyfish, are like grass. Their genes have to rely on another mechanism to avoid being eaten.

The anxiety response has two functional components; it alerts us to a threat and forces us to respond to it. The alerting response is very much a physiological matter. All higher animals show it, the sudden change from a drowsy creature stretched out in the sun to an edgy, jittery animal prowling around, scanning the environment warily. As mentioned before, huge numbers of physiological changes are involved, both somatic and cerebral. These responses are very fast, the whole body can change from torpor to racing agitation in a fraction of a second. And, of course, they have to be fast. What people call the "adrenaline rush" would be useless if it took as long as, say, digestion, or even waking up. We would be dead if it didn't get us ready for action in the order of tenths of a second. These are the obvious, physiological changes of anxiety that are often studied in cats, because they are cheap and the parts of the brain involved are large and readily accessible. This part of the anxiety response is almost entirely a brain function, not a matter of psychology.

The parts of the brain involved in the alerting response are buried deep in the temporal regions of the brain. They are the same in humans as in the other large primates and are part of our evolutionary heritage. Functionally, signals are sent from the frontal or thinking regions of the brain, directly to the complex nuclei of the midbrain. Subsequently, a shower of instructions descends on the body, mostly through what is called the sympathetic nervous system. The part of the brainstem that carries the alerting signals is complex and diffuse, a network of tracts and nuclei called the descending reticular activating system. Descending, as there is also an ascending system. Reticular means a network, as it is poorly localized, and is therefore relatively protected, and it activates the body. Above all, it does not function at anything we might call a conscious level. We do not need to identify a threat before responding. Signals from the environment are detected by the sensory system (perhaps a faint, scratching sound, or a slight movement on the edge of the visual field) and are processed extremely fast. The "decision" to respond to something brushing your ear in the darkness is not conscious in any sense of the word, even though you will accept it as your own. It can even happen while asleep.

So far, we are still creatures of the Pleistocene veldt, ever-alert for signs of the proto-leopards that roamed the Rift Valley.

The next thing to remember about the evolutionary anxiety system is that, once activated, it takes time to settle. It is not like, say, the visual system, which responds immediately to changes in light levels, or humor, which can die with the first glimpse of the policeman's cap. A person who gets a fright doesn't settle back to his somnolent state just because his tormentor laughs and says, "Ha ha, it was just a rubber snake." Once frightened, the agitation persists. The evolutionary advantages are obvious: if our fear died just because we could no longer see the crocodile, we would go swimming. Our internal alarm system is like a bell that has been struck once; the sound keeps coming and slowly, only very slowly, fades away. A single jolt of fear can ruin your whole afternoon.

14-2 (d) (ii) Ontological explanations of anxiety: Why is anxiety such a powerful and unpleasant emotion? It is powerful and unpleasant because otherwise, we would ignore it, with disastrous consequences. To save our lives, anxiety has to over-ride everything. It has to be more powerful than humor (fear kills laughter), rage, hunger, weariness, any sense of comfort, curiosity, sexual arousal, pride, everything except perhaps bonds such as affection and loyalty. Anxiety is the only emotion that does not reach a crescendo and fade away. Even laughter can become painful but anxiety builds up until we give in and escape the threat. This is terribly important in understanding the pathology of anxiety. It is the only emotion that can keep intensifying until we can no longer function. In this sense, its power can be its own undoing because it can render us incapable of responding. We will come back to this point shortly.

Why is anxiety unpleasant? For the same reason that bad smells are not attractive, they tell us something is wrong, the food should not be eaten. Why are the experiences of guilt and anxiety not just swapped over? Guilt is far too slow, and it inclines us to introspection, so it probably wouldn't work as an alarm system. These are ontological questions, and I doubt we can ever answer them. Why is red so very... red? Something to do with our photoreceptors and our brains, but it is probably a matter of cerebral coding, and perhaps forever be out of reach. I'm not sure that a complete understanding of our brain codes will tell us why red is just that rich, vibrant sense and not vongrish, but I don't mind. As long as it does the job.

14-2 (d) (iii) Sufficient explanations of anxiety: Essentially, that is all anybody needs to know about anxiety. To summarize, as an emotion, anxiety is a raw given or brute fact that cannot be further analyzed. A person who feels anxious has perceived a threat. A threat is an awareness or knowledge of an impending danger, a looming crisis to which we must respond or suffer an insult, injury or loss. The threat is the external stimulus; anxiety is the first-line internal response that brings us to a state of alertness and compels us to respond constructively to the threat. Just remember that people use the word "fear" either for the threat itself or the subjective response to that threat.

As an internal alarm system, anxiety is most needed during childhood. Neonates have almost no capacity to respond selectively to danger. By the age of six months, infants can respond with alarm to separation from the parents but, by the age of two, it is powerful, dominating the child's interactions with the world. Thereafter, it fades until, by the age of about sixteen, it appears to be at low ebb (especially in boys). That's not quite true: teenage boys are re-markably blasé about the natural world but can be paralyzed by the social world. The very rare individuals who are apparently born without a capacity to experience anxiety do not survive early childhood. Autistic children, whose emotional capacity is severely restricted, are also at grave risk.

In adulthood, anxiety again becomes more intrusive, partly as a result of experience but I would also allow an evolutionary component, as the individ-ual approaches the age of reproduction, and has to start to think of risks not only to self but also to spouse and offspring. All adults can get frightened; the neuronal machinery of anxiety is hard-wired into the brain as the result of many millions of years of evolutionary experience. Anybody who says he has never felt anxious in his life is either a fool or a liar, more likely both.

I believe it is important to talk about anxiety in this rather dispassionate or objective sense because an understanding of the processes involved in normal anxiety leads directly to an understanding of abnormal or pathological anxi-ety. There is nothing mysterious about a panic attack: anxiety is a rule-governed mental process whether it is functioning adaptively or maladaptively. It is important to see anxiety as the predictable outcome of perfectly explicable mental imperatives that can be teased out to provide a rational basis for treatment. The worst thing is to talk about anxiety as though "It" were some sort of slavering, primeval monster, breaking free of its chains in the bilges of of our psyches, ready to engulf its unwilling host. By the same token, the bio-logical approach, which says that an anxiety state is a chemical imbalance of the brain, is both inaccurate and destructive. It removes the sense of control that is essential for any anxious person who wants to lead a normal life.

14-2 (d) (iv) Why anxiety is not stress: The alert reader will have noticed that, in some 4,000 words about anxiety, I have not mentioned the word "stress." This is deliberate, because the word has no meaning in human af-fairs. Is that shocking? Well, it's correct: it was originally an engineering term, defining the external force acting on a structure to produce a deformation, or strain. The Austrian-born physician, Hans Selye (1907-1982) borrowed it for his "general adaptation syndrome" but, because his English was a bit scratchy, he used stress where he meant to use the word strain. Thus an in-dustry was born.

For the rest, forget it: the word has now become useless, for which we can largely blame the American Psychiatric Association. This august body forgot to distinguish between stress as the external threat and stress as the internal response, between stress as a noun, an adjective and as transitive and intran-sitive verbs: "Work is such a stress, I'm always stressing about it. My boss stresses me to the point where I'm so full of stress that I'm about to have a stress attack. I'll have to destress on somebody before I go out on stress."

Expressions such as Post-Traumatic Stress Disorder contributed mightily to the confusion. Most people think it means there is something called stress you get after trauma, like you could get a bruise or perhaps a Post-Traumatic Depressive Disorder (I made that up), but that's wrong. Post-Traumatic Stress Disorder actually means "The Psychiatric Disorder That Comes On After Ex-periencing an External Stressor of Traumatic Intensity." The terms Stress Disorder and Depressive Disorder are horses of a totally different color; they don't name or nominate the same class of events. The former identifies the cause while the latter nominates the nature of the condition. Using them as though they were the same is a category error. There is no place in science for words with at least five separate meanings.

So much for stress. It's not worth getting stressed about it.

14-3. The Psychophysiology of Normal Anxiety

Some people might regard the idea of normal anxiety as a solecism, but it is similar to normal death or normal grief. The suggestion that all anxiety is abnormal confuses normal with desirable.

As mentioned, anxiety ranges from the slightest apprehension, through concern, fear, terror and panic, with as many points between as poets can invent. Consider a normal person (or chimp, or rat) sitting against a rock under a tree, calmly chewing on the nuts dropping around him. We can measure his basal physiological state and then watch what happens to it following a variety of stimuli.

14-3 (a) Minimal acute anxiety response. A nut falls from the tree and bounces off his shoulder. He jumps slightly, recognizes what it was and picks it up to eat. For a few seconds, his heart rate accelerates slightly, his breathing rate increases and there may be a barely perceptible flush of sweat on his palms. He will feel a slight *frisson* of apprehension but it quickly settles. This is the mild, acute anxiety response, and we can graph it as follows. Note that in these graphs, I will use the biological term "arousal" in place of anxiety. We can measure the physiological parameters of arousal but we can't measure anxiety because it is a subjective experience. Note also that the word acute means "of sudden onset." Its antonym is chronic. Neither of these words relates to intensity or severity. In each graph, the dotted line at a nominal arousal level of 6.5 indicates "clinical significance."

Fig 14-3 (a) Minimal Anxiety Response

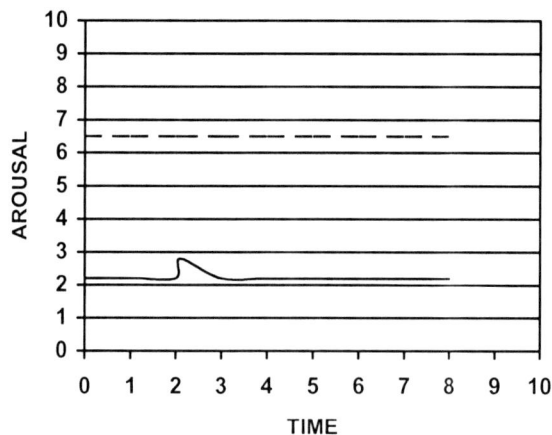

14-3 (b) Mild acute anxiety response. The same man, chimp or rat is sitting under the same tree. Suddenly, he gets a glimpse of something slithering through the grass near his foot. Before he has time to think what it is, his body is activated. An array of neuronal impulses is projected down the brainstem to all parts of the visceral body, changing his entire physiology. With a yell, he jerks back and rolls to his feet. Within a few seconds, he will show the characteristic physical concomitants of a fright. His heart is pounding, his hands sweaty and slightly tremulous, he will be breathing quite fast, and so on. That is, his arousal level is moderately high. However, after a few seconds, he realizes the intruder was nothing but a harmless lizard looking for crickets. With a bit of an embarrassed laugh directed at his startled neighbors, our hero pokes at the lizard with his foot and tries to make a joke of it. However, he knows he got a fright and is too edgy to sit down again and resume his lunch.

Typically, the duration of the response is not proportional to the intensity of the stimulus. For every unit increment in the stimulus intensity, the fear response lasts longer and longer.

Fig.14-3 (b) Mild Anxiety Response

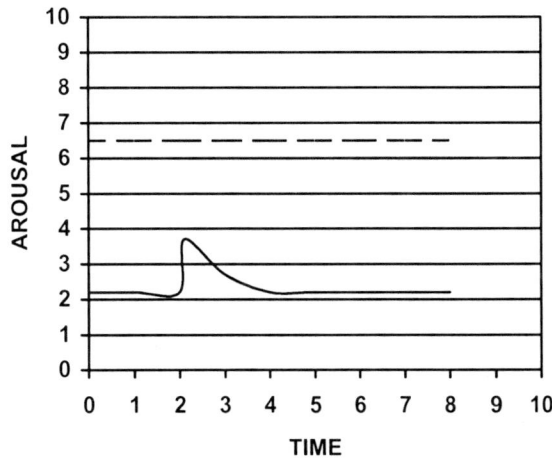

14-3 (c) Moderate acute anxiety response. This time, our unwilling subject is right. A large and very poisonous snake lifts its head just where he had been groping for a nut. For a split second, he watches in horror as it draws itself up to strike then, with a cry of fright, he jerks away and leaps to his feet. Startled, his neighbors jump up and grab sticks to chase the intruder away. This time, he is really shaken. He shows quite intense agitation, with shaking, sweating, pounding heart, churning stomach, shortness of breath and so on. In addition, his cognitive function is disturbed. Even though he doesn't try, he would be unable to stop thinking about the danger he had been in. He would be inclined to forget other matters (that he has to collect nuts for his mother in law), and he might react irritably to somebody suggesting he had been mistaken (I know rats can't suggest error, but they can nip each other and start a fight). He would be most unlikely to go back to the same spot and may want to leave altogether. Half an hour later, he would still be unsettled, his heart rate considerably above its level before he saw the snake. He might still be a bit sweaty and would not feel like eating. In the case of humans, we would say that the symptoms of his anxiety response almost reached clinical significance. What is clinical significance? That's a good question but the essential point is that, if nothing further happens, he will get back to normal fairly soon. Even if the symptoms do reach that blurred line called clinical significance, the only management is masterly inaction, sitting on one's hands. Nature will look after its own. Humans can't speed that up but we certainly can delay it, and there's nothing like an eager amateur to make a mess of a normal recovery process.

Fig.14-3 (c) Moderate Anxiety Response

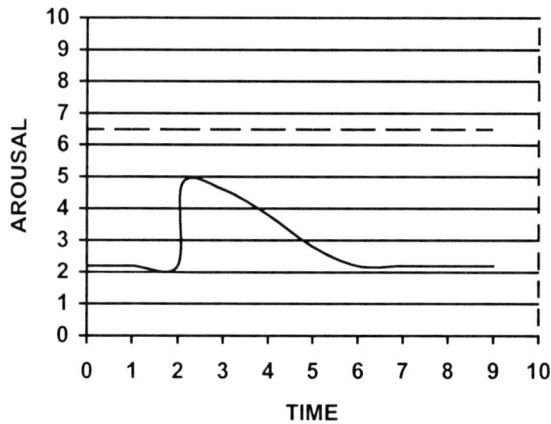

14-3 (d) Severe acute anxiety response. This time, the player in our little drama sees the snake and jumps to his feet but sees he is trapped. He can't get past it but it is rearing to strike. Too late, he realizes he is standing in front of a hole in the rock, that the snake clearly wants to get into the hole and he must be standing between it and its eggs. Hypnotized by the deadly creature in front of him, he can do nothing but press against the rock wall. He is too frightened to move as he knows it will probably strike at any movement, but he has to move to let it past. His frightened neighbors gather around, yelling advice. Slowly, the animal tightens its coils. He screams in panic for somebody to do something but nobody has any weapons. Its mouth gaping, the snake hisses furiously. He can see its huge fangs bare in its mouth. From the corner of his eye, he sees somebody but is unable to make a sound. Suddenly, a stick thuds down and the snake writhes in its death agony.

Sweating and shaking, our friend slumps to his knees. His heart is pounding violently, his breath is rasping in his throat, his mouth is dry. Suddenly, he turns aside and vomits, a ragged, noisy heaving that brings only a few chewed nuts and some yellow-stained froth. To his embarrassment, he realizes he has wet himself. Twitching and shaking, he manages to get past the dead creature and collapses on the ground while his friends crowd around. As soon as he can, he gets to his feet and tries to make his way home. For hours, he is weak and shaking, unable to eat, unwilling to be alone. He can't think of anything but the threat he survived. Every time he tries to close his eyes, he can see the deadly creature swaying in front of him. That night, his sleep is delayed and he jerks awake several times before settling into a restless, broken slumber. Next day, he is better but still unsettled. He does not want to go back to the same place and is easily agitated by reminders. If nothing further happens, he will return to normal but he will be unable to acquit his normal duties for much longer (unable to cope, in common talk).

Fig.14-3 (d) Severe Anxiety Response

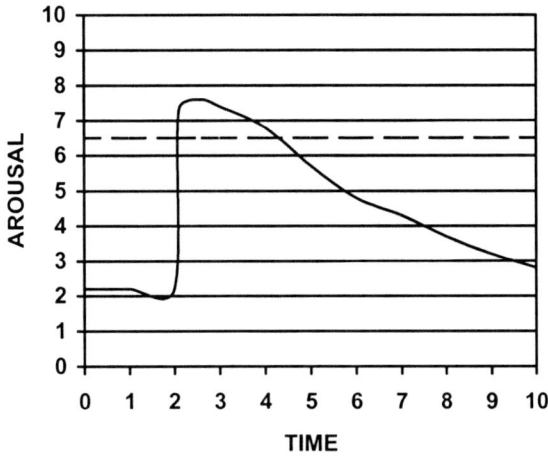

14-3 (e) Extreme acute anxiety response. The word extreme doesn't mean rather unpleasant or even very unpleasant. It means *in extremis,* the furthest point or the point beyond which there is no return. In human affairs, it means "at the limits of human experience." Nobody should use the word more than once a month; ordinary people shouldn't use it at all because they will never approach the limits of human experience.

14-3 (e) Extreme Anxiety Response

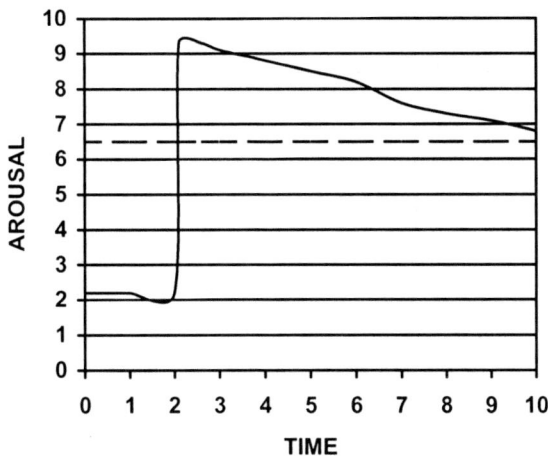

A person who experiences a protracted and overwhelmingly terrifying event will show clearly defined physical and mental changes sufficient to prevent any approximation of normal function for days, and a pattern of disturbance that might continue for many weeks before he returns to normal. The most common cause by far is warfare but violent crime isn't far behind. The noise and upheaval of war pushes the individual's level of arousal so high that he is unable to eat, drink or, care for himself, to think, plan, remember or do anything but stumble along in a trancelike state. Natural disasters might be equally violent but people seem to adapt somewhat better to them. For most people most of the time, these types of anxiety states are caused by other humans.

14-3 (f) Generic anxiety response. The previous sections illustrate an important point about anxiety, namely, that it not only gets the frightened person ready to fight or flee, but it may also be so bad as to stop him doing either. It may in fact lead to his downfall. The reason is simple: if the threat persists, the response it generates does not plateau or fade away, it becomes more and more intense. Thus, as the muscle tension needed to make rapid responses intensifies, it leads to a faint tremor, then to a more obvious tremor, then to violent shaking that can be so bad as to stop the person defending himself. The over-breathing may lead to dizziness, the churning stomach may lead to vomiting, and so on. This peculiar feature of anxiety has been known for a long time but it was first formalized about a hundred years ago by two American psychologists. They graphed the relationship of performance and arousal, describing what is now known as the Yerkes-Dodson relation. It is fundamental to an understanding of pathological anxiety.

Fig 14-3 (f) Yerkes-Dodson Curve

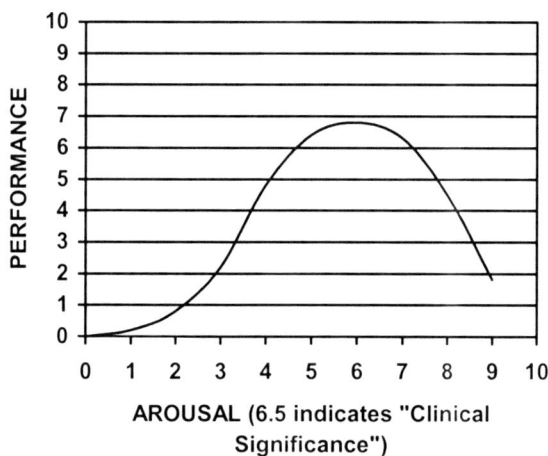

AROUSAL (6.5 indicates "Clinical Significance")

The curve of the Yerkes-Dodson relation plots the changes in performance as the level of arousal rises (see Note 1). When the arousal level is zero, say when the subject is asleep, performance is clearly zero. However, when the level of arousal goes up one unit, performance lags. Anybody with teenagers at home can see this each morning. When they wake up, these organisms are largely incoherent for a considerable time. Their arousal level has to rise a long way before they start to make sense (usually, they only come to life when everybody else is ready for bed). Thus, the first part of this curve rises slowly, then it starts to accelerate. However, it can't keep rising for ever. There comes a point when further rises in arousal do not lead to much improvement in performance. Finally, the arousal becomes so high that it is actually counterproductive. Performance deteriorates, and this stage is what people commonly call mental breakdown. In fact, it isn't mental breakdown at all, merely performance breakdown, but that is splitting hairs because performance is breaking down just because the mental life is becoming disorganized. I cannot over-emphasize the importance of this relationship in human affairs. It explains more about mental disorder than any other single function.

If we give tranquillizers, including alcohol, to a normal person, his performance deteriorates. If we give them to an over-anxious person, his performance improves. It all depends on his arousal level when he takes the drugs. The objective of what is variously called sports psychology or personal motivation, etc., is to get the person to his optimal level of arousal and hold him there. If his level of agitation rises further, or if he starts to become tired or bored, his performance will drop. In professional sport, irritating the opposing team to upset their performance is considered fair game. In military terms, the objective of psychological warfare, including terror raids, is to push the enemy soldiers into the upper reaches of arousal so that they can no longer function effectively.

This was the *modus operandi* of the Allied forces in the First Gulf War (1991) and it was brutally successful. For a month, the defending Iraqi troops were subject to round-the-clock ground and air bombardment with the objective partly on destroying their infrastructure and material but also on preventing them sleeping. When the attack came, they were incapable of defending themselves and simply fled. At the extremes of agitation, including acute catatonic schizophrenia, a person who has become mute and rigid can be "brought around" by giving him an intravenous injection of an anesthetic agent such as sodium amytal. It's a bit of a party trick to impress new trainees in psychiatry.

14-4. The Descriptive Psychophysiology of Abnormal Anxiety

The problem for any theory of anxiety is simply that most people suffering from anxiety are not in any sort of threat or danger at all. They are anxious in the face of tranquility, and their distress does not fade with time. Something is keeping it going, something is continuing to serve as a threat. A proper understanding of normal anxiety shows where this essential defensive system can start to malfunction.

14-4 (a). 'Excessive' anxiety response. If a person who is already at his optimum level of arousal gets another minor fright, his agitation will increase and his performance will deteriorate disproportionately. Observers who didn't know he was already at his peak performance might think he had "dropped his bundle," i.e., that if he tried, he could "pull himself together and stop carrying on." Quite often, people use a bright and effervescent exterior to conceal the fact that they are on edge. At the first sign of additional pressure, they may burst into tears, complaining that they "can't cope" because nobody gives them "a fair go" or perhaps rush out in a state of intense agitation, complaining of dizziness, choking sensations, the walls closing in or any of the huge list of anxiety symptoms. Others maintain an air of sullen irritability, flaring into rage after the least upset, then, shaking, flushed and sweating storm out for a cigarette.

In the following figures, the solid line indicates normal response to standard stimulus. The dot-dash line indicates 'excessive response' to standard stimulus in a previously anxious subject.

Fig. 14-4 (a). 'Excessive' anxiety response.

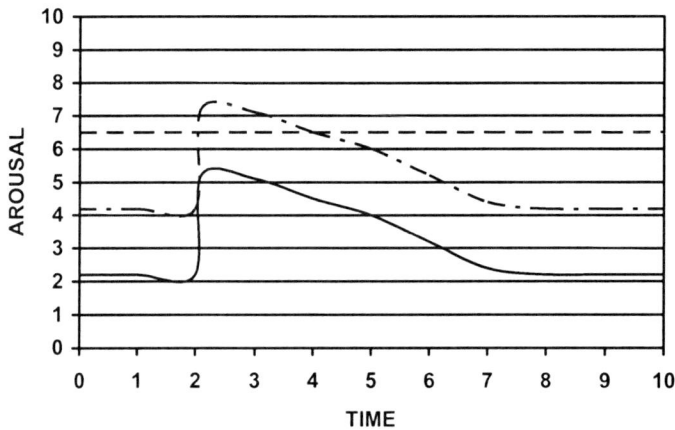

14-4 (b). Cumulative anxiety response. Normal people who experience an everyday fright will react in a fairly predictable manner (see Figs 15-3b and c). There will be an immediate elevation of arousal level followed by a slow return to normality. If, during the recovery stage, somebody experiences a similarly frightening event, then his arousal level will be pushed much higher, just because it started higher. A person who has experienced a number of relatively minor upsets in rapid succession may appear inordinately disabled, just because he hasn't had time to settle between the blows.

14-4 (b) Cumulative Anxiety Response

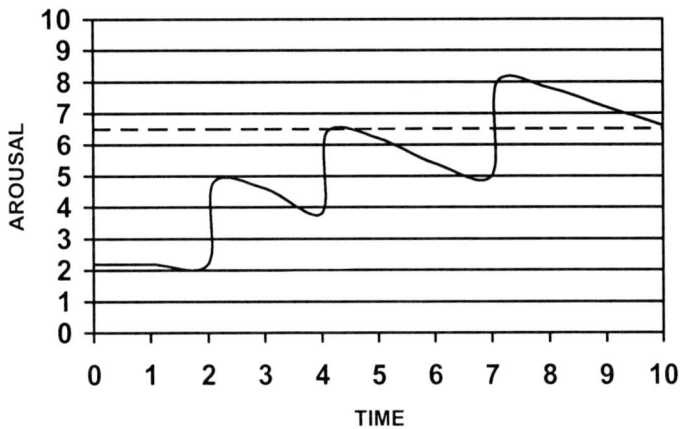

This is very common in warfare, in disasters and emergencies, but also in the work environment and among emergency personnel. Graphing arousal against time shows this more clearly. This leads to what might be called a cumulative anxiety response, i.e. the cumulative response to a series of external stressors. With this concept, we are moving toward a psychophysiological theory of anxiety.

14-4 (c). Chronic anxiety response (Chronic stressor). We run into problems with the word "chronic" because, in this context, it can have two meanings. It can either mean the response to an external stressor that has itself become chronic, i.e., the stressor goes on and on and the response never has time to settle, or it can mean an anxiety response that continues long after the stressor has abated. I will argue that, on pathological grounds, these represent two quite different conditions and have to be treated differently. It is similar to saying that, even though viral pneumonitis and bacterial pneumonia are clinically very much alike, they differ at the causative level and must therefore be managed differently.

To start with, a low-grade stressor that continues to exert its malign effect day after day, week after week or longer, can cause a cumulative anxiety response as outlined above. This is extremely common, not just in the military setting such as jungle and urban fighting, but also in the ordinary workplace where it can have a devastating effect on perfectly healthy workers. In civil life, examples include unpredictable working conditions such as emergency recovery work or where there is a covert element of danger such as threatening supervisors, danger from the general public, etc.. Since these types of reactions commonly result in major disability (and compensation claims), they need to be taken seriously.

14-4 (c) Chronic Anxiety Response (Continuing Stressor)

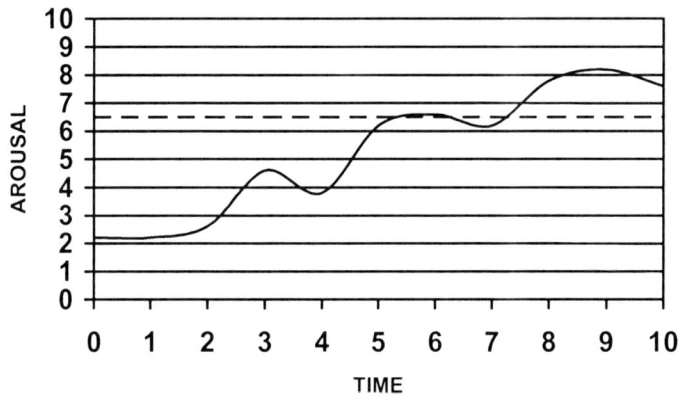

AROUSAL

10
9
8
7
6
5
4
3
2
1
0

0 1 2 3 4 5 6 7 8 9 10

TIME

14-4 (d). Chronic anxiety response (Chronic response). In this type, there is a discrete traumatic event (that may continue over a period, such as war) but, one day, it stops. However, the sufferer's travails don't stop with it and may even get worse. A single, massively traumatic event can cause severe, lasting disability, which is not what common sense dictates. For many years, this caused major problems for psychiatry as it was obvious the sufferers were in a terrible state (see Sassoon's poetry, especially *Repression of War Experience*), yet everybody knew that real men didn't go to bits just because they were blown up.

This devastating disorder has had many names in the past century, including shell shock, war or battle neurosis, anxiety-hysteria, effort syndrome, DAH (Disordered Action of the Heart), character defect, malingering and, most recently, Post-Traumatic Stress Disorder. In simple terms, the disruptive symptoms of a high arousal state continue indefinitely, even in the absence of further stressors, to the point where the individual cannot function. The anxiety symptoms soon become complicated by depression, by substance abuse and paranoid ideas but the primary disorder remains a disturbance of arousal.

14-4 (d) Chronic Anxiety Response (Single Massive Stressor)

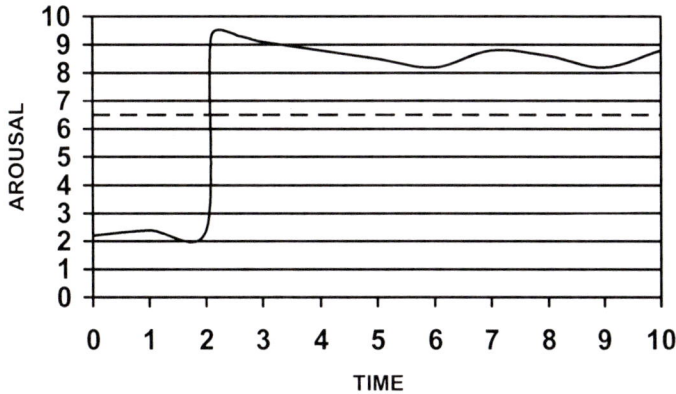

The most protracted case I have ever seen lasted 68 years, in a veteran of the Battle of the Somme. Starting from 1922, his symptoms were recorded in considerable detail about every ten years until I saw him in 1984. During this time, he lived a very quiet life in a small country town, carefully protected by his wife from any undue pressures, but his symptoms did not settle. He had a classic post-traumatic state but, persistent as his symptoms were, I'm sure he didn't hold the record.

14-4 (e). Phobic anxiety response. Everybody knows about phobias, the Greek term meaning fear, which describes the crippling levels of anxiety some people experience on even the slightest exposure to certain objects. In the context of the subject's life, there reactions are violently excessive and almost always irrational but, to qualify as true phobias, they must lead to avoidance. If the subject does not attempt to avoid the feared object, it isn't yet a true phobia. Quite often, there are rituals to overcome the exaggerated fear but these are not central to the diagnosis. Typically but not diagnostically, phobic fears are silly and pointless, such as a fear of snakes in a city dweller, fear of frogs, a person who fears geckos but not snakes, people fear cockroaches but never flies or mosquitoes, birds (including a lady who had an isolated fear of emus, of all things) but not fish, a doctor feared hairy caterpillars but not maggots, thunder but not lightning, and so on. However, the most common and disabling phobias relate to social life.

14-4 (f). Panic states. Everybody also knows about panic states. Symptomatically, panics are identical to phobias, the only difference being that they have no single or definitive cause so there is nothing the subject can avoid. From the sufferer's point of view, a panic attack "comes out of the blue." This isn't quite true, there is always a cause but it may be very minor and escape attention. Graphically, the reaction is the same except there is no obvious external stimulus. Some of the most persistent and disabling panic states result from preoccupations and rituals, the obsessive-compulsive disorders.

14-4 (g). Hypochondriacal states. This group of fear states has always infuriated psychiatrists because we can't even name them properly, let alone assign them a cause or treat them effectively. They blur with other conditions on the border of psychiatry and general medicine and it isn't always clear what we are dealing with. I reserve this name for the condition in which, in the absence of a definitive physical cause, the sufferer shows a persistent anxious preoccupation with bodily health (including neuropsychology) to the point of impairing his daily function. We have to be very careful here, of course, because it is far too easy to label a querulous patient as a nutcase and ignore the complaints, until the autopsy report arrives.

14–5. Explaining Abnormal Anxiety Responses

Each form of anxiety reaction must have a specific explanation to show why it is different from the others. The model being developed here allows a precise formulation for each disorder without begging questions or stretching credibility.

14-5 (a). Excessive anxiety response. There are two reasons why a person might overreact to minor environmental pressures. Firstly, he may just have experienced a quite severe pressure and be on the cusp of the Yerkes-Dodson curve. For example, somebody may come to work after having heard from his wife that she wants to leave but he is too embarrassed to tell anybody. More commonly, he may always be on the edge of an outburst, tense, jittery and irritable. This is personality-based, where personality is the set of rules by which a person is distinguished from his neighbors. In this model, a person who becomes agitated in response to what are objectively neutral events in the environment is presumed to have a system of rules that leads him to misclassify non-threatening events as threats. As a result, he is consistently on edge, always apprehensive that the next minute will bring disaster; i.e. given his set of beliefs, his emotional response (high levels of anxiety) is quite appropriate. In simple terms, he sees the world as a dangerous place. Anybody who lives in a dangerous place will be on edge. Anybody who is on edge will react badly to minor upsets ("catastrophizing").

This does not imply that these people are "weak characters" or that they have Cyclothymic Personality Disorder or Bipolar Affective Disorder. It simply means that they normally function so close to their maximal performance level that even a slight elevation of arousal necessarily leads to a deterioration of performance. This has very considerable forensic significance. In insurance claims, defense lawyers will often try to claim that nobody could be so silly as to misjudge an innocent event as a major threat; therefore, the claimant must by lying. This is a false argument.

Some of these people will be excessively bright and cheerful, everybody's friend, buzzing around in a shower of little laughs, always so helpful, always organizing things, nothing is too much trouble, until, at the age of forty-five, they develop a depressive state unresponsive to the usual drugs and then, sadly, at fifty, they retire. Others are rigid, obsessional creatures of habit who want everything just so and maintain iron control over their little worlds by the ever-present threat of an explosion. Some are distant, humorless people who bury themselves in work and politely decline invitations to the office Christmas party, others are chronically miserable and wander around from desk to desk, telling whoever will listen of how the world is treating him so badly and why doesn't anybody recognize his talents and give him the break he deserves?

The point is that the external manifestations of the problem are protean; what counts, what determines treatment, is what goes on underneath. Classifying people into types just by their external behavioral manifestations of disorder misses the point of what is generating the behavior that needs explanation. A person who is breathless from asthma doesn't get the same treatment as a person who is breathless from pneumonia or somebody else who can't breathe from anxiety.

If the sufferer's view of the world is distorted to the point of causing him distress, why doesn't it automatically correct itself? Why does this disorder not only persist but also intensify with the passage of time? The answer is simple: the outcome of the abnormal beliefs (intense agitation, distress, perhaps depression or alcoholism) reinforces the beliefs. That is, a person who expects every interaction with his supervisor to lead to trouble is proven correct every time he deals with the supervisor just because he becomes so agitated that all he can recall is that it was terrible. Next time he receives the summons to the supervisor's office, he is trembling before he has replaced the phone. He is caught in a system of self-fulfilling prophecies, an endless nightmare of interlocking vicious circles of anxiety. People selectively recall scary incidents, which may have an evolutionary basis.

14-5 (b). Cumulative anxiety response. At first glance, there is nothing remarkable or unexpected about the psychophysiology of a cumulative anxiety response; plotting the rising level of arousal seems to say it all. Because the resolution phase of an acute anxiety response is slower than the initial response (it can easily be hours or days), there is plenty of time for a further insult to compound the injury. There doesn't appear to be need or room for an intrapersonal contribution.

However, under normal civilian conditions, the history of this type of response usually indicates that the consecutive stressors haven't been hours or days apart, but very often weeks or months apart. This isn't what the graph indicates. A normal anxiety response should resolve quicker than that, so what happens? A careful history will show that the frightened subject has been rehearsing the original stressor in his head, such that he remains in a state of agitation long after it should have resolved. The problem was that the original event scared him badly. He did not win, and losing may cause a burning humiliation, or an intense fear that it may happen again. Each day brings a dozen reminders, and each reminder sparks a semblance of the original stressor, such that he cannot settle.

Now this isn't invariable; plenty of people who experience a bad fright will settle quickly enough and nothing more will come of it. However, anybody who feels at risk from a further incident will automatically be on edge, i.e., will be at a higher level of arousal than otherwise. Every reminder maintains the anxiety, so what seems to have been just a single incident will actually be a bad one followed by dozens or even hundreds of minor ones. Continuing apprehension perpetuates the original reaction, keeping the arousal level above normal, which explains why this type of reaction is more common in people in unhappy marriages, who are feeling bullied or pressured at work or who are in financial trouble, etc.

14-5 (c). Chronic anxiety response (Response to a chronic stressor). In physiological terms, this is very similar to the cumulative anxiety response, except there is a single, unremitting stressor. The physiology is perfectly straightforward: effectively, a healthy person suffers a train of minor upsets without having time to recover fully between them. Gradually, his arousal level is pushed to the point where his performance is beginning to break down. Just to complicate matters, because the problem arose slowly, he often doesn't recognize the changes himself (although his family certainly will). He may well feel under pressure but he will never sit down to write a list of his symptoms and will therefore not realize he is unwell. Indeed, he may object strenuously to suggestions that he is unwell, particularly as he is not able to recall a single incident that pushed him "over the edge." That's because there was no single incident. If there had been, such as a disaster, Blind Freddy could have seen it but workers, especially men, are often loath to admit that they "can't hack it," and hang on long after common sense dictates they should have walked out. Perhaps they need the job, perhaps they don't want to admit defeat, there can be many reasons but, in compensation cases, the lack of an overtly traumatic incident does not mean the claim can be rejected.

14-5 (d). Chronic anxiety response (Chronic or post-traumatic response). A single, massively traumatic event causes severe, persistent psychiatric symptoms in a previously healthy and well-adjusted person with no evidence of brain damage. When the young officer in S.14-4 (a) (iv) enlisted, he had the world at his feet. The only son of the owner of a flour mill, he was a very pleasant, industrious and intelligent young man. In August, 1915, he was studying engineering but interrupted his course to serve. In just five minutes, everything changed. At approximately 9.15am on the morning of July 1st, 1916, he watched in horror as nearly ninety percent of his company, many of them his schoolmates, were mown down by machine guns. He himself wasn't injured and he continued to serve but, slowly at first then faster, his mental state deteriorated. Finally, he was discretely sent home and allowed to resign his commission but he never recovered.

Can this be explained by invoking cryptic changes at the level of cerebral neurochemistry? I don't believe the idea of a psychologically-induced "chemical imbalance of the brain" has any merit whatsoever. I cannot imagine how simply watching something could cause such widespread and enduring disturbances of cerebral neurochemistry without also impairing intellect or causing other disturbances consistent with diffuse brain damage. It would be impossible for just one chemical change to induce this, it would have to involve dozens of neurotransmitters in widespread areas of the brain, affecting some centers but not others, in a pattern that could not approximate anything biological. However, I can readily imagine how a person's coded rules could be changed by a profoundly traumatic event, and how these rules could then exert a malign effect enduring for, as we have seen, a whole lifetime. In any event, if a chemical change were found, it would indicate the mechanism, not the cause.

Assume that, at the time he enlisted, his system of coded rules was internally consistent and did not bring him into conflict with his social or physical environment. He could "cope" because he wasn't scared of his world and didn't under- or overestimate his capacity to deal with it. Essentially, he was a normal personality. The slaughter changed all this. From seeing the world as a rather pleasant place for a chap to have a laugh (and I imagine rural Western Australia in 1914 was a pleasant place), he came to see it as brutal, unpredictable and uncaring, and himself as the man who did not stand by his troops in death as he had sworn to do.

Everything became dangerous, everything was a reminder of his dead mates; he couldn't talk to their families without dying inside from the guilt. At every chance encounter in the street, he panicked, his heart went wild in his chest, so he stopped going out. His wife did everything for him; he simply stayed home and attended their little business out of sight. He became depressed over his guilt, over the burden he placed on her, over his failure to raise his children properly and so on. Every ten years or so, his fear and guilt became too much and he approached the Department to see if he could get treatment but his heart was clearly fine and, in his crowning humiliation, he was publicly labeled a malingerer.

Because he could no longer expect the world to be a nice place and his body to behave itself, he lived in fear of trouble. However, the trouble he expected simply was his own anxiety. Because he lived in fear, his arousal level was constantly elevated. Because his arousal level was constantly elevated, he reacted anxiously to trivia. Because he reacted excessively to trivia, such as medical interviews, the authorities were convinced they had worked him out. The response compounds itself but, in those days, nobody could see this possibility. His case notes from 1935 stated: "Only a truly guilty man would act like this ex-officer. Application rejected." He was indeed guilty, but it was survivor's guilt.

We can account for all his symptoms by a single explanatory entity, a change in the coded rules by which he ran his life. Five minutes of horror on July 1st, 1916, overwhelmed the pleasant rules he had garnered during his early years, forcing them to become disorganized, internally inconsistent and self-defeating. They created anxiety where there should have been none, and convinced him he was a weakling who didn't deserve to live where better men had died. He feared his neighbors' contempt but, above all, he feared his own symptoms. For sixty years, he loathed himself and longed for death but he couldn't bring himself to the final betrayal of leaving his wife to raise his children without a war widow's pension.

14-5 (e). Phobic anxiety response. A lady takes her seat in my office and, with some embarrassment, explains why she has come. "I know it sounds silly," she apologizes, "I know they can't hurt me, but I am terrified of frogs."

In tropical Darwin, this is something of a handicap but I set her mind at rest. "No, you are not scared of frogs."

She looks at me in some perplexity: "But I have lived here for twenty years and every Wet (monsoonal) season is the same, frogs everywhere, and I'm terrified of them. I can't go outside and they even swim up the toilet."

"Adventurous little souls, aren't they," I sympathize, "but the truth is, you are not scared of frogs. You are scared of how you will feel if you go near a frog, which is a totally different thing."

This causes some consternation as she struggles to adjust her view of her own mental state. Finally, she succeeds and the treatment can start.

There is no such thing as an isolated phobia. Every anxious person has some feared objects, and every person with a phobia also gets anxious or panicky in other settings. There are many paths to a full-blown anxiety response but the neurotic ones (i.e. anxiety without an adequate external stimulus) all have a common mechanism: the subject is terrified of his or her anxiety symptoms. In the case of the classic phobia, the person has set up a prediction: 'If I go near/away from X, I will feel very bad.' Predicting a bad feeling automatically results in a sense of foreboding, otherwise known as anxiety. However, if the bad feeling he predicts just is the sense of anxiety, then the unhappy subject is caught in a true vicious circle, or negative feedback loop. That's all there is to phobias.

I expect to feel bad if I have to give a speech, but the bad feeling I expect just is anxiety. The closer I get to it, the more apprehensive I become, just because I know with absolute certainty that the bad feeling is about to engulf me and matter of fact, here it comes right now, I can feel my heart starting to race, my hands are starting to sweat and shake, my stomach is about to turn over and I might vomit in front of all these people and they'll think I'm a complete fool, I think I'd rather die than have everybody sneering behind my back...

Classic learning theory taught that the subject has simply learned to fear the phobic object and only needs to learn that it isn't dangerous for the symptoms to go away. Older people might remember what was called flooding, when the lady in my example would have been locked in a room full of frogs until she was so exhausted from being frightened that she simply stopped being frightened. Nobody does that now because people get sued for scaring somebody witless and not curing them.

There was also systematic desensitization, when the subject was gradually exposed to the feared object until he could touch it without fear. It took a long time and the results were rather unpredictable, because it didn't focus attention on the mechanism of phobias. This is why the symptoms often didn't go away but simply popped up again somewhere else. The subject is mortally afraid of his own mental state, which is like being afraid of your own shadow: there's no escape. In order to cure a phobia, the subject must see the mechanism involved and must also learn that anxiety isn't dangerous: uncomfortable yes, but not dangerous. The good news about anxiety is that nobody ever dies from it and it always goes away – if it isn't stirred up again.

Social phobia is not a separate condition from any other phobia, nor is it different in nature from other anxiety states. Anxiety itself is always the same, it just means the person has perceived a threat. If the threat is simply the symptoms of his own anxiety, then he is neatly trapped.

14-5 (f). Panic states. The temperature caused by a bacterial illness is the same as the temperature caused by a viral illness. There is only one sort of temperature, the hot type. The panic of a panic attack is exactly the same as the panic of, say, a bad phobia. There is only one sort of panic, the scary type. It is said that a full-blown panic is the worst sensation that a person can experience and still stay alive. In a panic state, the feared object just is the panic state itself. A person who has experienced one panic lives in mortal dread of another. He need only feel the first stirrings of apprehension to believe he is about to be thrown into another maelstrom of mind-melting, bowel-watering terror.

Anybody who reads the endless popular books on anxiety will start to think that panic is some sort of mental coronary that strikes its victims randomly, even whimsically: "I was walking to work when suddenly It struck me. I thought I was going to die from It, I had never felt anything so terrible. My heart was beating so fast I thought it must stop, I couldn't breathe, my legs turned to jelly and I couldn't even think who I was or where I was going. It was the worst thing I had ever felt. I wouldn't wish It on my worst enemy"

This is crude alarmism of a low order: panic doesn't "just happen." Everything has a cause, including panic. Panic is a state of terror that can only be generated if the person gets the idea he is in mortal danger. In recurrent panic states, the dangerous idea is just this: I am going into another panic. This explains why it keeps happening, but not why it started in the first place. The answer is usually revealed by a careful history. Of course, some people have been panicking for so long that they can't remember how they started but others have the clearest recollection of the first one. There has to be a stone to start the avalanche but, as with real avalanches, finding the offending stone may be impossible. However, we can usually tease out the contributing factors.

Most people who develop panic states are primed for them. It is common for the person to be unwell, often with some sort of febrile illness that weakens but doesn't really declare itself. Typical illnesses include post-viral states, malaria, hepatitis, diarrheal illnesses, especially anything chronic such as amoebic dysentery, and so on. The person may be recovering from an illness such as pneumonia or from an operation, especially on the bowel. Anything that debilitates a person and inclines him to develop low blood pressure, palpitations, nausea and dizziness is a prime candidate. Over-tiredness is also a common factor, but most important is a pre-existing state of apprehension. People often have their first major panic while troubled by work or marital problems. The ushers in law courts are accustomed to people collapsing while waiting for their cases. Panic is more likely to occur when the person is hot, perhaps from the weather or more likely being in a crowded and airless place. Unpleasant smells are significant, including the smells of hospitals. Other factors include a sense of being trapped, such as in dentists' chairs, aircraft and lifts, by an aggressive person, etc.

Our victim is already feeling unwell from a cold. He argued with his wife the night before and slept poorly. He oversleeps and rushes out without eating breakfast but he is caught in a slow and overcrowded bus. By the time he gets to work, he is feeling pretty terrible but gets worse when he is told to see the boss immediately. Suddenly frightened for his job, he starts to run up the stairs but gets dizzy from the exertion. Halfway up the stairs, things start to go black. He slumps to his knees on the stairs but there is nobody around and he can't get help. From somewhere comes the idea that he must be having a heart attack and is about to die. At this realization, he panics. In a moment, fear overwhelms him. He develops the full book of somatic and cognitive symptoms of anxiety, drowning in a sense of overwhelming dread at what will happen to him and his family.

So it happens that, next time he feels a slight sense of dizziness or he tries to climb stairs, or he develops a mild fever, his first thought is this: I'm going to have another turn like that last one. Oh no, that was the worst thing imaginable, I need help, I've got to get out of here. The more frightened he becomes, the worse he feels; the worse he feels, the more he is convinced he is having a heart attack; the more he is convinced he is having a heart attack, the more frightened he becomes. In theory, it is very simple, so simple that some psychiatrists have difficulty believing that anything so simple could cause the overwhelming experience of a true panic.

The first panic attack starts mildly as a fairly ordinary sense of unwell or dis-ease caused by a combination of factors, physical, psychological and social. It quickly spins out of control because the person fears what is happening to him and can't stop it: of course he can't, because the way to stop it is to stop fearing it. Panic is more likely to happen in somebody who is already inclined to be anxious but that's not essential. It is also common in people (mostly men of the butch or macho type) who think that illness is caused by weak minds and who can't understand why their bodies let them down when all they've got is a touch of bronchitis. Their first experience of fainting terrifies them; if they've never really felt frightened before, the first time is so scary that they live in dread of another attack.

Panic is a negative feedback loop or self-reinforcing cycle of fear of fear. The symptoms become the stimulus for further anxiety which, in turn, impels the symptoms. There is nothing wrong with the brain. Just like an amplifier with a feedback loop, it is amplifying and replaying exactly what it picks up. Panic should be understood as a two-stage process. In the first or initial stage, the fear reaction has a direct cause but, with time, the feared object shifts away from the initial cause to fear itself. That is, in the second stage, the panic reaction itself becomes the new feared object.

14-5 (g). Hypochondriacal states. There is nothing conceptually difficult about what used to be called hypochondriasis. The term indicates a person with an unhealthy preoccupation with matters of health, illness, etc., who is convinced he has an illness, but who has no evidence at all of physical illness. That's not quite right: he has plenty of signs he takes as signs of illness (nausea, dizziness, palpitations, tremors, numbness, etc.) but we see them as inconsequential. However, in dealing with these patients, we have to be very careful because if the psychiatrist doesn't take a patient's complaints of illness seriously, then the next person to do so may be the pathologist.

The modern term for this group of disorders is Somatization. I don't like this word as it reifies the action of being preoccupied with health. It implies there is something the patient 'gets' or 'has,' but this is false. There is no *thing* called somatization, only people complaining about their health. Similarly, the term "cancer phobia" is a misnomer. It isn't a phobia at all, simply a state of dread.

The typical patient is seen at the cardiology outpatients clinic, or neurology or gastroenterology, complaining intensely of a range of vaguely-defined symptoms that are not in themselves serious (dizziness, unsettled stomach, odd palpitations, poor concentration, lack of energy, etc.) and don't amount to very much. After extensive and expensive investigations, he is given a trial of a drug that either doesn't work or causes nasty side-effects so he goes off to see somebody else, and so it goes. Why are they never comforted by the negative results and the great physician's reassurances?

Once again, the process is simple: for whatever reason, a person fears ill health. As a result, he constantly scans his body and his internal environment for even the most trivial departure from perfect normality. Now this raises a problem, because to the truly preoccupied, there is no such thing as a trivial departure from good health. Every abnormality, no matter how tiny, might be the first sign of a cancer, or a stroke, or a heart attack or whatever. The important point to note is this: these people all fear death or disability. Any deviation from inner perfection could be the first step on the road to the grave. Therefore they become anxious, which makes their bodies deviate further from normality, which convinces them they are right to worry as all the signs of incipient disaster are there for them to feel. They are scared.

This is why they become resentful when told there isn't anything wrong with them, not because they have been exposed as frauds. They don't like to be told they are worrying over nothing (who does?) but they can't just drop the whole matter and walk away whistling because they can feel their stomach churning/ heart pounding/ chest tightening/ head reeling, etc..

They are not easy people to deal with: "And if that doesn't mean cancer, doctor, you tell me what it does mean."

"It means you're frightened."

"Of course I'm frightened, who wouldn't be? I'll bet you wouldn't be so patronizing if it was your stomach/ heart/ etc."

The fear of illness creates the symptoms that reinforce the belief that there is a serious illness that the doctors are too lazy/incompetent/venal/malicious/ etc., to diagnose and treat properly.

This group of people is very large. They keep the "alternative health industry" alive and thriving, gleefully chasing everything from diet and massage to crystals and group rebirthing. The same cycle of self-reinforcing panic can be seen in opiate addicts. They are convinced they will feel terrible if they don't get their drugs and quickly develop disabling symptoms if their supply is interrupted. They believe that if they don't get their 'fix,' they will go into the most terrible withdrawals, which is, of course, a vicious circle: they fear withdrawal; the fear makes them feel bad, which convinces them they are going into withdrawal so the fear intensifies. Simply giving them an injection causes them immediate relief for which they are often pathetically grateful. It is the basis of the casualty officer's trick of giving a saline injection to a panicking person and telling him he will get better. The expectation of improvement relieves the anxiety that was causing the problem in the first place.

There is a cluster of nondescript symptoms such as irritability, lack of energy, dizziness, flatulence, poor concentration and memory, clumsiness, blurred vision, headaches, shortness of breath, aches and pains, poor sleep, loss of appetite, low sex drive and so on, which constantly pops up in the popular press as yet another mysterious syndrome for which a dramatic breakthrough is imminent, if only the noble research group could convince the chiseling, hidebound or jealous medical profession to hand over more research money. Some of the names for it are benign meningoencephalomyelitis (which is more benign than it sounds), total allergy syndrome or twentieth century allergy, chronic fatigue syndrome, adrenal exhaustion syndrome, and a huge range of poisonings and toxicities, not forgetting effort syndrome, Agent Orange and Gulf War Syndrome.

The symptoms of these protean disorders just are the symptoms of anxiety and the grumbling depression caused by chronic anxiety. The same symptoms are up for grabs for anybody who needs a label to conceal the fact that he is anxious. Just for completeness, psychiatry has retaliated with neurasthenia, Briquet's Syndrome, hysteria, inadequate personality, Factitious Disorder, Somatization, malingering and other unpleasant expressions. Each is based on the same set of symptoms, just anxiety in another form.

14-5 (h). Free-floating anxiety. This expression was popular in the 1960s and 70s but unfortunately seems to be coming into fashion again. It signifies a patient who is constantly anxious about everything, as though he had a Large Ball of Anxiety floating around freely in his inner space. The theory is that this quantum of anxiety latches on to different ideas as they present themselves, an anxious cathexis as they say in Freudspeak. It is a deceitful expression because it misrepresents the process of becoming anxious as a Thing or entity separate from and alien to the frightened person.

The patient's problem is that he fears the world in a generic sense. To him, everything is frightening just because he doesn't believe he can cope with it. Why can't he cope with it? Because he feels weak and jittery, his heart races and his mind skitters around and he can't learn anything or concentrate or keep an erection... But feeling weak and jittery and so on are the symptoms of anxiety, so why is he anxious? Because he believes he won't be able to cope, just because he is weak and jittery, his heart races and his mind skitters around... It is a true vicious circle, an endless cycle of self-fulfilling negative predictions.

Men often don't like to talk about being anxious. To them, anxiety is a moral defect, a sign of a weak character, not a trap they can't escape because they can't see it. They are more comfortable with the idea of a wicked, willful Thing floating around inside, one that sabotages their every effort, as it spares them the shame of being seen as weak.

When a psychiatrist says somebody has "free-floating anxiety," it shows he hasn't taken a proper history.

14–6. Conclusion

Untreated anxiety is a crippling mental disorder with a major impact on individuals, families and societies. The message from this chapter is that anxiety must be taken seriously: nobody gets scared for fun. Why can't I make myself nervous just for laughs? This is not a trivial question but goes to the heart of the concept of cognitive causation of anxiety. I can't believe anything I know to be untrue. Therefore, I can't believe there is a threat when I know there isn't one. This is the outcome of the modular system of brain function. It says that the affective module that is switched on when I believe something cannot also be switched on when I don't believe it. The two systems cannot function together, just as I cannot see myself surrounded by darkness when I see light all round. The two systems are incompatible.

For psychiatry, it is important to see anxiety as simply a normal emotion driven to extremes by the same sorts of mechanisms as trigger "adaptive fear responses." The current (obsessive) preoccupation with the surface manifestations of spurious chemical defects of the brain means that we miss the point of looking at the underlying processes to see where they have gone wrong. As an emotion, anxiety refers to the future. We can't fear the past, we can regret it or be angry or amused but not frightened. We can only be frightened of the future. Our capacity for abstract thinking gives us the capacity to fear our inner states. If we expect to feel bad, we will become frightened. If the bad feeling we expect just is being frightened, then we are trapped in a vicious circle. Anxiety is the only truly recursive human emotion. Sometimes, it would be easier if we didn't have any.

15 Depression

15-1. Introduction

Orthodox psychiatry is obsessed with depression. It is also obsessed with seeing depression as a biological disturbance of brain function, to the complete exclusion of a psychological account of the condition. Perhaps this arose because the ideal model or exemplar of depression, grief, is universal in its form and content, to the point where it is difficult to argue that it doesn't have a biological basis. In addition, depression was one of the first of the major psychiatric syndromes for which biological models and some sort of effective treatment were available.

On the first point, it is true that humans in all cultures and at all times have shown highly standardized emotional responses to certain kinds of events. Thus, anxiety is the standard response to an impending threat, laughter is the standard response to another type of incident, crying is certainly the same all over the world and grief is the unvarying response to loss. If the syndrome of grief occurs without an obvious loss, it is called depression.

On the second point, treatment, depression was very much an after thought. The original idea for the various kinds of "shock therapy" (chemical, insulin and electrical) came from the effect of epilepsy on schizophrenia, and the first patient treated by the inventers, Cerletti and Bini, was schizophrenic. It is highly likely that more people have had ECT for schizophrenia than for depression. In addition, the first relatively effective drugs in psychiatry were antipsychotics. Antidepressants came later.

In the 1970s, depression was thought to be the result of disturbances of a loose class of cerebral chemicals known (also loosely) as "biogenic amines." These were supposed to be concentrated in the hypothalamus and the walls of the third ventricle. This catchphrase eventually died for lack of any evidence and was replaced by the idea that the effective antidepressants influence certain of the cerebral neurotransmitters. They do, but not consistently (different drugs affect different transmitters), not reliably (antidepressants are only about 60% effective while placebos are 40% effective) and not in any pattern that leads to an understanding of emotional life. These days, orthodox psychiatry insists that depression is due to a "chemical imbalance of the brain." Where, how and why this is effected is not known.

I won't be arguing that depression doesn't have some basis in biology, because my whole thesis to date has been that human behavior is the outcome of a complex interaction between an emergent mind and the physical body. It would be like arguing that the physical structure of the brain does not have any role in determining the crying reaction or the alerting response. Rather, I will be disputing the idea that depression is necessarily a primary biological disorder and that the sufferer's beliefs and experiences are irrelevant. I use as my starting position the notion that the typical depressive reaction is a biologically mediated reaction to a range of psychological states, the final common pathway, as it were, just as the experience of pain is the outcome of certain classes of stimuli. In the case of depression, the events fall into the class of losses. Any biochemical changes are the mechanism of depression, but not the cause.

15-2. The Depressive Syndrome as Absence of Pleasure

15-2 (a). Defining depression. Depression is a sustained mood of sadness and despair associated with ideas of guilt and worthlessness, a reduction in psychomotor activity and a loss of appetites, including food, sex, social interaction, curiosity and dominance. Anybody who says, "I was so depressed on Saturday afternoon but then I was invited to a party and had a great time," was not depressed (and should not get antidepressants).

While discussing anxiety, I put the view that emotions have their own logic. In this sense, a sustained mood of sadness and despair is not inexplicable if it is seen as the psychologically-determined outcome of perceived losses. Thus, we can expect to see the depressive syndrome in people who have sustained major losses. Examples include people who have lost their houses in fires or storms, after the loss of a spouse, a business or fortune, loss of health such as amputations or a stroke, loss of a job, career, major interest, on exile or expulsion from a social group, loss of freedom, and so on. The standard grief reaction can be colored, as it were, by varying degrees of fear, yearning, suspicion or anger but these tend to fade as the danger recedes and then the true sadness and despair come through.

However, these obvious incidents don't explain most cases of depression. It is true that in the six months prior to the onset of a depressive state, there is an excess of adverse life events, of which losses are a major part, but there are still many cases who don't appear to have lost anything. They still have the same family, house, job, income, health, hobbies and pastimes, but they have lost interest in them; their various personal and social attachments are intact but no longer seem satisfying. This is the mystery of most cases of depression: at first and even second glance, there hasn't been a significant loss. Indeed, depression may follow happy events such as a marriage, childbirth or a promotion.

15-2 (b). Critique of the standard model. Insofar as conventional psychiatry has any model of mind, the standard idea is Jamesian, i.e. it assumes that a person's normal mental life consists of a train or stream of objects and events moving along to be inspected by an inner eye. In ordinary life, the objects are lit by a bright, warm light so the little man behind the Cartesian eye feels cheerful. Following a loss, the glow is abruptly switched off; the objects remain the same but the warmth has gone so that, where once there was joy and laughter, everything now seems dull and lifeless. It sounds crude but, taken to its logical conclusion, that's what their model amounts to.

The biological model is a variant of this crude approach. It says that the inner warm glow is a primary biological function which, for unknown biochemical reasons, flicks on and off whimsically, as though a "black cloud" had just covered everything. When the inner effulgence changes to blue, the little man inside becomes glum and morose. The dull color leads the little man to change his assessment of the objects in his life, from valuable to pointless. Classic psychiatric theory states that the mood disorder is primary and all other phenomena flow from it. Under the influence of unknown "chemical imbalances of the brain," the mood changes from cheerful to despairing, thereby driving the cognitive state to somber conclusions.

15-2 (c). Depression as an output state. The model I will develop here is different. We have to avoid any and all notions that need a hidden observer for completeness. To do this, I will use the concept of moods being an output state driven by the cognitive state which, in turn, is determined by a variety of inputs.

I start with the position that the normal mood state is one of moderate cheer, derived from a background sense that one's basic needs are being met, life is going somewhere and nothing much is going to change. The biological model is that the mood is primary: a person in a good mood sees the world through rose-tinted lenses. My model views this differently. It says that the knowledge that things aren't too bad, or even just tolerable, generates a moderate sense of happiness, neither too much nor too little. If I believe things are going my way, then I will feel happy. The knowledge state is primary, the emotional state is always secondary.

As an emotion, happiness is an end-product, an output state that cannot be further analyzed. I suggest that normally, we function about half way up the happiness scale. Depression is therefore defined as zero happiness but not as a negative quantity. Depression is not the opposite of happiness, it is the absence of happiness. This means we don't have to invent an extra mood called Depression. So far, this is only a simpler way of looking at the same phenomena.

Depression arises, not from a different color shining on the same objects, but if the mood of happiness is switched off. When the so-called "happiness circuit" shuts down, nothing can give pleasure, which is exactly what depressed people say. They don't say, "I hate my garden," but simply: "My garden gives me no pleasure." Looking at their lives, they say: "Nothing interests me, nothing excites me. Everything is gray."

In grief, as the archetype of depression, recognition of a massive loss, that something precious has gone, forces the person to give up on the lost object. I propose that it is the cognitive act of giving up that causes the mood of happiness to drop to zero. This is homologous with the anxiety response: recognition of a threat causes the arousal level to rise. Of course, in early stages of grief, people try to deny their loss. This may spare them the crushing enormity of the loss but, in its place, they experience an intense agitation as they struggle with the threat of loss.

In ordinary grief, no matter what the cause, the sudden loss of happiness seems to induce a cognitive distortion, in which the person reappraises his whole life as useless and pointless. I suggest we should look at the same facts from a different point of view, that the absence of happiness means that, for the first time in their lives, people see the objects in their lives completely neutrally. A grief-stricken man doesn't say his house is bad, but looking at his house generates the same mood as if he saw a suburban house in another city, i.e., nothing. It generates no mood because his normal, background sense of comfort has been switched off. His "happiness center" has been blocked; nothing can get through to stimulate it. It is perhaps analogous to local anesthesia, in which the nerves are blocked. Nothing can stimulate them and the arm feels useless and lifeless, as though it doesn't belong. Local anesthesia doesn't produce a negative feeling; it produces no feeling, a numbness that is so far from normality that it is profoundly shocking. Eating food after local anesthesia to the mouth doesn't produce a negative taste, it produces no taste, an experience that is so far from normality that it is profoundly shocking. Grief doesn't produce a negative feeling; it produces no feeling, a numbness that is so far from normality that it is profoundly shocking. We are in the habit of defining our normal moods as zero; anything higher is happiness, a positive quality, while anything lower is therefore a negative quantity, which leads to the impression that depression is a mood in its own right. It is not.

I suggest the block to pleasure occurs at the cellular level; a lasting chemical change induced by the sense of loss. The sense of loss just is the knowledge that whatever was valuable has been torn away and there is no hope so give up. Giving up is the mental state that triggers the essential neurochemical changes that, in true depression (as distinct from passing bouts of misery) persist for months.

There will certainly be objections to this suggestion. People, including biological psychiatrists, will say: "This is rubbish. The mood called depression is a powerful, crushing pain that is a negative thing and compels people to see their lives negatively. Things they previously liked, such as a job or a neighborhood, they now say they loathe." It is true that sometimes, depressed people take a strongly negative view of things but more commonly, they say: "Everything's going nowhere. The house is a burden, my job is boring, my friends are using me while everybody at the golf club drinks too much and only talks about sex or money. Even the flowers in the garden do nothing for me." That is, he suddenly sees things neutrally, a state that other, disinterested people would call reality. The dispassionate observer would say the depressed man's previous cognitive assessment was unrealistic. The loss of happiness forces him to see what other people would merely say is the truth.

"No," the biological psychiatrists will say, "it goes much further than that. Depression is an actual pain, haven't you seen depressed people cry?" Of course I have, but remember that tears are at least as common in fear as in grief; tears indicate distress as a non-specific emotional response. Too many people think they are an infallible indicator of despair and hopelessness, but distress and depression are not the same thing. Distress is a state of agitation whereas pure depression consists of a numbing and withdrawal. True, the act of giving up is distressing but it passes, leaving people in a state of numbness, walking through a colorless life feeling detached and disinterested. I'm not suggesting that giving up is just a short, sharp shock because it isn't; it takes a long time to give up on all the little things about a person that made a relationship. It is also important to remember that not every mood experienced during a grief reaction is depressive in nature. There is certainly fear ("How will I get by without her? I can't survive, I know"), and also a lot of anger clouding the picture. The emotion of yearning is also an intense discomfort. It is a powerful factor in any experience of loss, yet it gets remarkably little attention from psychiatrists.

In this model, acceptance of the cognitive assessment, "I have lost something important," causes the grief or depressive reaction, i.e. it forcibly removes all traces of pleasure and enjoyment from life. Just as acceptance of the cognitive assessment, "There is a threat," causes the anxiety reaction, so too the acceptance the fact of a loss directly causes the absence of happiness or humor. A depressed mood is not formally a negative thing but is simply the absence of a positive thing, although happiness is so pervasive that we take it for granted. The stricken person goes into a state of detached neutrality, which we see as withdrawal, during which he arrives at a new knowledge or awareness of his life. For example, a man must get used to life without his wife or the job he wanted, or a woman must accept that her husband will never stop drinking. She gives up the idea of a happy marriage. During the early stages, everything else seems hopeless and meaningless just because it can give no pleasure: "hopeless" means "no hope of enjoyment." The depressed person's capacity for pleasure is blocked. The usual daily state, of mild optimism, arises because whatever we have or do generates a sense of mild pleasure. That's what "meaning" means: as the hedonists argued, it means pleasure. The absence of pleasure means the absence of meaning, which is expressed as despair: "It will never work; I'll never get anything out of it, so why bother?"

This is the pure type of depression formerly known as melancholia, the apathetic, withdrawn and detached form in which the person shows no interest in food, activity, people, places, things, ideas or entertainment, including sexual activity. Melancholic people have no interest in life but may even be so apathetic that they don't even attempt suicide. Only when the depression starts to "lift," meaning they recover some capacity for activity, will they attempt to finish the life that has lost all interest for them. The pure apathetic depressive syndrome differs from the other forms, from the angry or paranoid types of depression, from grief itself, in which yearning is so powerful, or from classic agitated depression in which anxiety predominates.

Gradually, over a period of months, whatever cellular changes were blocking his capacity for pleasure wear off and he starts, slowly at first, to get some enjoyment from things. His wife is gone; at first, going to parties reminds him too poignantly and he avoids them but eventually, he can try one or two small outings and they don't go too badly. And so he adjusts to a new reality, severing himself from the old life because thinking about it rekindles the sense of loss until, one day, he feels sufficiently optimistic to find himself a new partner. That is, he is once again able to contemplate the future and see a real chance of pleasure.

15-3. Depression as the Final Common Pathway

15-3 (a). The mystery of recurrent depression. I have still not answered the objection flagged earlier, that most people presenting with a new case of depression have not suffered a recent adverse life event. This is particularly the case where people suffer recurrent depressive states. Some people may suffer ten or more discrete episodes of depression and it is just not realistic to keep claiming that they have suffered losses each time. This is why the Freudian model was so attractive, it indicated that one major early loss could predispose the individual to further bouts of depression just on the threat of a loss alone. But even this doesn't work because, in practice, most people with recurrent depression have not experienced even a threatened loss.

Biologically-influenced psychiatry has adopted a rigidly objective approach to its subject matter, rejecting all suggestions of mentalism just because it doesn't fit with the narrow definition of materialism. Thus, psychiatrists probing a depressed person's recent past will focus on the standard lists of major life events. Typically, the patient cannot recall such events, so the box is left empty. Because no life events can be elicited, researchers take this as evidence of the biological causation of depression. I suggest this is wrong because it overlooks the fact that humans not only have an external life, they also have an inner one.

15-3 (b). Demystifying recurrent depression. In line with the model being developed in this work, I propose that the great bulk of recurrent depression is precipitated, not by painful external events, but by painful mental events. This is actually a fairly safe position to adopt: some recurrent depression must be due to persisting adverse life events but, in the main, humans adapt to unpleasant circumstances remarkably well. People soon adapt to prison, to brutal regimes, poverty, chronic illness and disability. If the external conditions are painful, people adjust or go under.

For ordinary people suffering another bout of ordinary depression, I suggest that the cause is an unsuspected abnormal mental state acting back upon itself in a variant of the negative feedback loop. Assume that the person experiences years and years of mental *dis*-ease and distress that prevents him enjoying life, that something goes wrong inside whenever he tries to have fun or even lead a normal life. However, he may not recognize this as odd because it has always been there, or perhaps he does recognize it but he can't talk about it. Eventually, he reaches the point where he has to adjust or go under, but since he doesn't see his own distress is the damaging factor, he gives up on an aspect of himself or of life, thereby entering a depressive state. The cognitive act of giving up induces the core depressive state.

How do we know that he cannot recognize his mental state as the destructive agent? Because if he did realize it, he would change it, just as he would change his shoes if he decided they were too tight. The damaging element in the cycle is seen as egosyntonic, at one with the self, not something he likes but he believes he can't change it.

There is only one mental state that can cause persistent distress of sufficient severity to lead the subject to the point where he feels life is not worth living: anxiety. My proposal is that chronic anxiety *causes* recurrent depression. There are several reasons why I believe uncontrollable anxiety is the prime candidate as the "toxic emotion" in the causation of recurrent depression. Firstly, it is very common, more common than depression itself. Secondly, it is the only genuinely intolerable emotion. Wild rage can be bearable but profound fear compels the subject to escape it, he has no choice. Thirdly, it is the only emotion that does not spontaneously remit with the passage of time. Unlike anger or laughter, anxiety has no upper limit. Fourthly, not only does it not remit, but it is the only truly recursive emotion, i.e. it acts back upon itself, leading to self-reinforcing states of distress. Fifthly, it is commonly associated with depression, although the standard view is that it is "comorbid," i.e., not causally-related. Finally, orthodox psychiatrists will laugh in disbelief that anything so trifling as mere anxiety (which is not even a serious mental illness, after all), anything so damned... girly, as anxiety, could cause a serious, life-threatening, biologically-determined illness like depression. And so they beg the question, because the whole point of the discussion is this: can we assemble a convincing model of recurrent depression as a psychogenic disorder? I think we can.

15-3 (c). The explanation of recurrent depression. Assume a person reaches adult life with severe, personality-based anxiety that seriously affects the quality of his life. Perhaps his problems relate to the natural world, with fears of heights, blood, animals and the like, or maybe they relate to the social environment, such as meeting strangers, or he fears aggression, loneliness or disapproval. They might be performance-related, in that he fears failure at work or, worst of all, in performing sexually. The possibilities are endless. Whatever the cause, he does not recognize he has a problem that he can rectify. Anxious people often say: "But I thought this was normal, I thought everybody felt like this but they could simply handle it better." All he knows is that he becomes intolerably agitated at different times, that it interferes with his life and, above all, that he can never speak about it. Men in particular see anxiety as a moral failing. To acknowledge anxiety is to acknowledge being less than a man, the most frightening thing of all.

As a result of his anxiety state, his life goes badly. He loses one job after another; even if he can find relationships, he cannot sustain them; he is forced to conceal a large part of his private life and live a lie; he may start drinking or using drugs to feel better; he has to make excuses for avoiding things, on and on until he has practically no life left. Then, one day, he realizes that, if life goes on like this, it isn't worth living, so something has to go. He has to give up on part of normal life itself, like having a girlfriend or a decent job. That realization leads to depression. So he adapts and gets used to a restricted life but, sadly, things don't seem to get any better. Anxiety grows and spreads until it consumes his life. One day, he realizes that life itself has become worthless. Suicide becomes the only option. For a long time, he struggles against the idea until, in a state of wild rage, of grief or of profound detachment, or something in between, he ends his life.

Recurrent depression implies there is something wrong somewhere. A first bout of depression after about the age of thirty tends to indicate a normal personality reacting to abnormal circumstances. Recurrent depression, especially from an early age, strongly implies that abnormal personality factors, operating in the "here and now," are causing the disorder. Abnormal personality factors consist of inconsistent or self-destructive rules arising from early in life. These rules are coded at the level of brain languages and are not necessarily accessible to the subject. While he may recognize that he had a rotten childhood and is having a bad time as an adult, he can't tell anybody what is going wrong in his life.

15-3 (d). The treatment of recurrent depression. Recurrent depression is a major socioeconomic issue, and its treatment imposes a huge burden on health services, meaning a huge burden on the taxpayer. A recent paper by several of the country's most senior psychiatrists looked at the way ECT is used in Australian private psychiatric practice [1]. It showed enormous variations in regional and temporal usage of this form of treatment, with about 600% difference between the highest and lowest rates. The authors acknowledged that statistical analysis of the figures (mainly clumping) may have blurred important local variations. That's a pity, because my practice of psychiatry raises a question they did not consider.

Since 1977, I have practiced psychiatry in both private and public sectors, in the isolated North and in the urbanized South of Australia. I have worked as head of department in two teaching hospitals, one in Perth and one in Darwin, and in solo private practice. From 1987-93, I was Regional Psychiatrist in the Kimberley Region of Western Australia where I established a genuinely isolated psychiatric service for about 27,000 people, half of them Aboriginal, in an area of 420,000 sq km (i.e. the size of Washington and Oregon states combined). I had no staff, no dedicated facilities and practically no reliance on outside services. At the time, I was as much as 3,200km from the nearest available mental hospital, roughly the distance from London to St Petersburg, or New York to York Factory on Hudson Bay [2].

Since I graduated in psychiatry, I have personally assessed and managed something like 12,000 patients. Less than 1% of my patients are admitted to hospital each year, and very rarely for more than a week [3]. At both hospitals where I worked, ECT was used before and after my appointments, but not during. At all times, ECT was being used in private practice and in other public hospitals, even in the same area. For the last twenty years, I have practiced psychiatry in one of the rougher areas of this country, most of it with no support services whatsoever. I have not used ECT since June 1977.

There is no evidence that my patients have a substandard outcome. For example, in the past ten years, only two patients are known to have committed suicide during treatment. Neither would have been considered for ECT elsewhere.

The paper on ECT provided no evidence to suggest that any psychiatrist need use ECT. It appears to be little more than *façon de utiliser*, a convention or a habit. It has more in common with something like circumcision than with any genuine medical necessity. It would be ironic indeed if ECT actually led to an increase in costs. Given my experience, I think it is appropriate for psychiatrists who use ECT to show why it is necessary.

While on the question of costs, we should also look at drug prescription. In the case of recurrent depression, there are two groups of drugs to consider, antidepressants and mood stabilizers. Antipsychotic drugs are also prescribed but I don't have any figures for them. My rate of prescribing antidepressants is on the 8th percentile of the national rates and getting lower. That is, while most psychiatrists in this country are prescribing more and more antidepressants each year, my rates (scripts per patient per year and scripts per consultation) are actually dropping.

The other group, the so-called "mood stabilizers," is a disparate group of anticonvulsants and lithium used to prevent further breakdowns in people with recurrent depression. These are all toxic and mostly expensive drugs with a range of distressing side effects and a dangerously low lethal ratio. That is, the ratio between the therapeutic dose and the minimum lethal dose is low, so toxicity is common, including fatal overdoses. Despite the numbers of patients I see, I do not use these drugs in my practice. Anybody taking these drugs when referred to me will soon be withdrawn from them – to their great relief.

On the few occasions I have ever told this to another psychiatrist, it has provoked guffaws of disbelief followed by suspicious glances. They seem unable or unwilling to consider the idea that it is possible to practice psychiatry without these agents. My response is simple: my extensive and diverse experience in psychiatry demonstrates no need for ECT or mood stabilizers. If just one psychiatrist can practice this way for thirty years, so can every other psychiatrist in the world.

15-4. Conclusion

Confidence is not a thing in itself, it is simply the absence of anxiety. There is no mood called confidence. A man who climbs a cliff confidently is climbing it without fear. Similarly, depression is not a thing in itself, it is simply a sustained state of absence of pleasure. There is no mood called depression. It is not a different mood in its own right. A depressed man is living with no prospect of pleasure.

The mental act of giving up something important induces a profound and lasting change in the mental state, one in which the subject temporarily loses the capacity for any sort of pleasure or satisfaction. The absence of happiness is thought to be chemically-mediated, at the cellular level, by principles that are understood from other examples. Such chemical changes are the mechanism or agency of the depression reaction, not its cause.

Depression is a reaction to life events. Sometimes the events are outside but mostly, they are inside. Sometimes, observers can recognize them and sometimes they cannot. Sometimes the sufferer can recognize them and sometimes he cannot but, if he can, he may feel there is nothing he can do to change them and he just has to get used to an unpleasant or unrewarding life.

The most common and most powerful cause of persisting difficulty gaining a sense of reward in life is an unsuspected chronic anxiety state. Personality-based anxiety severely truncates a person's capacity to live life to the full. He has to make some sort of adaptation to it, either by using drugs and alcohol in a vain attempt to feel normal, or by giving up on important areas of life. Either way, he will suffer repeated bouts of despair until, one day, life itself loses all meaning.

Routine treatment of the primary anxiety state in recurrent depression brings about massive cost savings, not to mention a vastly improved quality of life and productivity for the sufferer.

The search for the depressive gene has blinded orthodox psychiatry to the real cause of recurrent depression which, in irritation, they have relabeled as "comorbid anxiety," i.e. a nuisance. Don't forget that Fleming wasn't the first person to see that *Penicillium notatum* killed bacteria, it was just that everybody else thought it was a nuisance that spoiled their experiments.

16   Psychosis

> "Everybody doubts his memory, but nobody doubts his judgment."
> —De la Rochefoucauld.

16-1. Introduction

Psychosis means any severe mental disorder in which the person has lost control of his mental state to the extent of being out of contact with reality. In practical terms, this means a person who is either hallucinated or deluded. A hallucination is a sensory experience, perceived as though through the senses but with no basis in reality, accepted by the subject as a veridical percept. A delusion is a fixed, false belief out of context with the subject's cultural or intellectual background. It is fixed, meaning one cannot appeal to reason or empirical evidence, and it is out of context, meaning it is unique and bizarre. These definitions are essentially subjective but, in practice, they are fairly reliable and valid.

Psychiatry has recognized two great divisions in the group of psychoses, those caused by physical or organic factors and those occurring in the absence of brain disease. In the organic psychoses, coarse brain disease, intoxications, metabolic disorders, concussion, post-operative states, etc., result in a typical picture of disturbance. To begin with, the patient is confused, meaning there is a disturbance of cognitive function with loss of short term memory, poor concentration and disorientation. Because of the loss of cognitive function, the patient often doesn't know where he is or what day it is. He will forget the people around him and often misinterprets names, sights, sounds, etc. Also typically, the psychotic symptoms are of a fleeting nature, with visual hallucinations predominating. This picture is common in the general wards of any big hospital, especially at night.

The other class of psychosis is called the "functional psychoses," meaning a disturbance of function in the absence of recognizable brain disease. At the end of the nineteenth century, this group was divided in two, dementia praecox and the affective or mood disorders. Not long after, dementia praecox was renamed the group of schizophrenias, comprising catatonia, hebephrenia, paranoid states and simple schizophrenia. These groups are descriptive only, have little predictive value and are not reliable. In most Western countries, about 1% of the adult population suffers schizophrenia which, because of its early onset and chronicity, means it is the single most devastating disorder in the world. Even today, some 10% of people diagnosed with this condition will commit suicide.

For many years, manic-depressive psychosis meant just that, people whose moods swung wildly between mania and profound depression, passing through varying periods of relative normality. More recently, the condition has been renamed Bipolar Disorder and broadened enormously by relaxing the diagnostic criteria. In Australia, this process has reached the point where television advertisements encourage viewers to diagnose themselves and to demand treatment from their general practitioners. Treatment, of course, means drugs. The advertisements are sponsored by a drug company. And why shouldn't they be? Doesn't everybody know that psychosis is a genetically-determined biochemical imbalance of the brain that can only be controlled (not cured) by a lifetime of drugs?

That's not entirely fair. There is still some dispute within psychiatry as to the exact nature of the biological disturbance in psychosis, but it is just a matter of time until powerful neuroimaging techniques coupled with molecular genetics reveal the precise causative link. In the meantime, a stream of new drugs is transforming the management of these disorders, opening doors where previously there were just walls.

I should point out that the foregoing paragraph comes from notes I took at one of the first lectures I attended in my psychiatry training. In April, 1974, the professor gave a stirring oration on the breath-taking advances of modern biological psychiatry. Unfortunately, events have shown he was speaking a little prematurely, but his palpitating prose would still inspire today's trainees as they wait in eager anticipation of the imminent breakthrough that will allow psychiatry to triumph over this dire condition.

This is the standard line. Only a churl would suggest it is mere "group thinking," the process whereby a group of like-minded but otherwise intelligent men can be catastrophically wrong. There have been many examples in the history of science where the orthodox view, accepted by generations of the great and impartial, has been overturned. The scientific establishment of the day had managed to convince themselves not only that they were correct but, more to the point, that they had no need to consider the possibility they might be wrong. It was a self-selecting, self-assuring, self-reinforcing exercise in intolerance. Just because their views were correct, criticism wasn't needed; therefore, anybody who presumed to question them was acting maliciously and should be dealt with accordingly. At the risk of being labeled a churl, I wish to question the received view.

16-2. The Category Of Psychosis

16-2 (a) Psychosis and normality. Given the definitions above, it would seem to be a fairly simple matter of deciding who is psychotic but, in practice, it is far from easy. In fact, it is so difficult that we have conventions to evade the issue. The reason is that every sign, symptom, observation, test result, historical event, etc. seen in psychosis is also seen in a very wide range of psychiatric disorders, as well as in complete normality. Not even delusions themselves pass this test, as the crazy ideas seen in a mental hospital blur imperceptibly with those held by extremist religious and political groups, as well as the cranky, the ridiculous and the obnoxious. If I want to believe that angels stand at the head of my bed when I sleep, nobody can stop me by appealing to experience or reason, which is the core definition of a delusion.

My case is that there is no sign or symptom that is both necessary and sufficient for the diagnosis of psychosis. Nobody can point to a sign or observation and say: "Every psychotic person has this sign, and no person who is not psychotic **has** it." This means there is nothing about psychosis itself that allows us to separate it from normality. Therefore, there is no true category of psychosis; it is wholly artificial, meaning the result of artifice. This conclusion is a matter of logic, not of practice. I am not suggesting we can't distinguish the florid cases, because we surely can, but the borderlands are often impossible to decide just because there is no empirical evidence we can bring to bear on the question. It is just a matter of judgment. Since human intellect ranges beyond the empirically verifiable, there is no independent standard by which anybody can say where sanity stops and psychosis starts.

If we class each person in the world on any one or all of the full range of psychotic symptoms, and line them up, it is an empirical fact that we will not end up with discrete clusters of people. We will find that our subjects distribute dimensionally from those with the least sign of madness, in an unbroken line to those with the most. Even on the question of psychotic symptoms, people distribute in just the same way as they do when graded according to height, weight, skin color, intellect, religiosity, political views and how much they like chocolate cake. The decision to diagnose psychosis is made by flimsy convention.

16-2 (b) Defining psychotic symptoms and normality. From an objective point of view, one of the core symptoms of psychosis, delusional belief, is probably the most unreliable. It is one thing to say, "I heard a voice," because there can be a degree of confirmation. But beliefs are not in the same class as sensory experiences; there are very many, firmly-held beliefs of profound importance that are not open to empirical confirmation. It is pure convention how we classify them. Throughout history, people have been tortured to death for their beliefs but died unyielding. That, surely, meets the definition of a fixed belief; its truth or falsity depends only on who holds the axe.

But the central point of the biological model of psychosis is that delusional beliefs are held just because of a defect of brain metabolism. They are not held through choice, as are political or religious beliefs: nobody chooses to be psychotic, and nobody can say, "I am deluded," as it would imply he knew it was wrong. But there is necessarily no biological test of the beliefs themselves that would allow us to distinguish between true belief and delusion. A biological psychiatrist would say that it isn't necessary, that the search is for a biological marker for psychosis (gene, enzyme, brain damage, etc.) rather than psychosis itself. This simply sidesteps the issue because nobody knows what the marker is marking until there is a clear definition of psychosis. Biological psychiatry therefore fails to give us a basis for determining its truth.

Hallucinations of various sorts are common in a wide range of functional and organic psychiatric disorders, including severe depression and severe anxiety states, both acute and chronic, and in culturally-determined states. Even the so-called Schneiderian first rank symptoms of schizophrenia occur in a wide range of disorders, to the point where they are more common in severe personality disorder and post-traumatic states than in schizophrenia itself.

The classic disturbances of schizophrenia, distortions of time, misperceptions of self, etc., are also common in all anxiety states, including the post-traumatic states, in depression and in personality disorders. Depression and elation, of course, occur in both psychoses and in all non-psychotic states.

Within the functional psychoses, the classic division between schizo-phrenic and affective disorders does not stand up to examination, as the category of schizoaffective psychosis confirms. In fact, the closer one looks at the symptoms, especially tracking them over time, the more the "line in the sand" is blown away. The old groups of psychogenic psychosis, schizophreni-form psychosis, reactive psychosis and the cycloid psychoses all describe brief psychotic states with a mixture of affective and schizophrenic features. Once again, there is no categorical difference between the two groups of psychoses.

16-2 (c) Biological markers and psychosis. Notwithstanding the epis-temic problem with markers, the search for consistent biological abnormalities in psychosis thunders along. Every day brings a new finding, a new clue to a major breakthrough, but nothing ever comes of them. First it was neurons, then neurotransmitters, then neuroimaging of damaged areas, then viral par-ticles and now genes have become the latest bet. Even today, there are half a dozen brain areas under suspicion, dozens of genes, swarms of neurotrans-mitters and a range of toxic substances in the environment including illegal drugs.

The problem of physical causation of psychosis is not a shortage of mate-rial, but the fact that practically everything can be associated with the onset of psychosis. Schizophrenic psychoses are four times more common after head injuries than in the general population. Typical symptoms can be seen in a very wide range of disorders, starting with Alzheimer's Disease, and includ-ing practically every other neurodegenerative disease known, while Parkinson's syndrome is traditionally associated with the affective psychoses. The genetic diseases such as Huntington's Disease, are a significant cause, but this is also true of a huge range of metabolic diseases, a variety of drugs and intoxications, including alcohol, amphetamines and cannabis, heavy metal poisoning, gassing and so on. There is hardly a disease state known that does not have a positive association with psychosis, so the problem is not a shortage of information.

This vastly expensive search is constantly turning up suspicious indices but not one of them survives closer examination. Every physical finding in psychosis is seen in only a proportion of the cases, and also occurs in normal controls. The search is driven by technology; it races ahead but leaves no signs of its passing. Yesterday's hot topic doesn't even rate a mention in to-day's footnotes, because psychiatry never looks back, it's too embarrassing. One review noted: "Although there has been no shortage of recent findings in the neuropathology of schizophrenia, hypotheses that can tie findings together have not been abundant." The authors were, of course, being coy: such hy-potheses pop up all the time, but they don't last.

Their own suggestion was a variation on the "neurodevelopmental" theme. This suggests that a small disturbance in a critical area of the brain early in life is magnified and amplified as the brain develops. The initial disturbance may be genetic, or the result of an intrauterine or perinatal viral infection or due to obstetric damage, etc., but it is small and critically located. The thesis depends on the actual mechanism of brain development. The brain isn't like a computer, which is built in modules and screwed together at the end of the production line. It builds itself, under the direction of the genome. Each step depends on what has gone before, so a tiny defect early in development can have a major effect later in life. This is the principle rather grandiosely known as chaos theory.

Embryonic neural crest precursors influence subsequent development in a cascading manner. Cell extensions are drawn out by hormonal influences emitted by target neurons; if the target isn't there, the axons won't reach out toward them, meaning the connection isn't made and, crucially, never will be. Once that phase of development is over, there is no going back. If, for example, a kitten's eyes are stitched closed at birth, certain essential layers in the primary visual cortex will fail to develop. Once the crucial stage of development is missed, the defect can never be rectified. Moreover, that small defect will induce its own defects in a spatio-temporal cascade, so the end result may be the loss of a small, vital tract that would otherwise exist as a series of steps through the brain. This approach has the potential to unite some of the disparate findings of a tiny loss of brain substance here, a disturbed transmitter there, or a subtle neuropsychological defect indicating damage somewhere else.

It should, however, be noted that this is not a theory of psychosis but simply a different way of looking at an old problem. It is an orientation, not a model, a principle that might allow a theory to develop. Without the proper way of looking at a problem, the theoretical solution will never suggest itself. Historically, Newton had to overcome his repugnance for action at a distance before he could recognize the evidence for gravity and build his theory. I am suggesting that the traditional biological approach of "a single lesion for a single disease," encrypted in the American nosology, is the wrong orientation for this question. How can there be a single physical cause for any particular psychosis when the overwhelming physical evidence is for a host of predisposing factors, but no single cause? In my view, this gives the clue to a new orientation toward psychosis that might just prove fruitful where the old approach has been so barren. But first, a word on treatment.

16-2 (d) Treatment of psychosis. Treatment of psychotic states has always involved physical methods, initially mere restraint but later involving diet, purgation, bleeding and iced water dousing. From about the mid-nineteenth century, opium in various forms was used to control excitement. Early in the next century, synthetic narcotics and hypnotics became available and from the mid-1930s, various types of "shock therapy" were devised. These included electroshock (ECT), insulin coma therapy and chemical convulsions (cardiazol). Only a modified form of ECT is still used. In the early 1950s, research in antihistamines led to the discovery of the phenothiazine tranquillizers, leading to the advent of the relatively specific group of antipsychotic drugs. In short order, antidepressants followed with the benzodiazepine tranquillizers arriving by the late 1950s. The tranquillizing effect of lithium was discovered in the late 1940s but did not gain wider use until about the mid-1960s. Since then, various anticonvulsants have been used as adjunctive "mood stabilizers." Discovery of effective drugs was entirely fortuitous but they accelerated the gathering process of "deinstitutionalization." Over the last forty years, the great Victorian asylums have closed as mentally people are no longer admitted to hospital for life.

Currently, drug treatment of psychosis is based purely on what works. However, people commonly extrapolate backwards from the known effects of the drugs on neurotransmitters to suggest that, if an antipsychotic blocks substance X, then psychosis must be due to an excess of substance X. This is fine until somebody discovers an antipsychotic with no effect on X. The ultimate goal of biological psychiatry is to develop specific gene replacement therapy for each mental disorder but, pending the discoveries to set this program in place, psychosis is treated with the group of major tranquillizers.

These drugs, generally expensive and with unpleasant, often toxic, side-effects, are widely used throughout the world. However, and despite anything their apologists may say, they are most definitely not specific in any way. They are tranquillizers in that they reduce arousal and thereby calm agitated people but they are less "magic bullets" than blunderbusses. Every antidepressant is also an anxiolytic while the mood stabilizers are primarily anticonvulsants and antalgics because they stabilize nerve membranes; their effects on mood are those of non-specific sedatives that do not habituate. Each of the antipsychotics can be used in a wide variety of disorders, meaning they treat symptoms, not the disorders themselves but, even then, their results are not very good. ECT, of course, was initially developed because of the well-known effect of seizures in calming people with schizophrenia but it is also widely used in the affective disorders. Once again, we find there is nothing specific about psychosis.

16-2 (e) Reorienting our view of psychosis. So far, I have argued that there is nothing unique or specific about the psychotic state. Psychosis can arise in the absence of any family history of the disorder, in the absence of any known brain disorder, and in the absence of any known trauma or anything like a "schizophrenogenic mother" or sexually-predatory stranger. There are no causative allergies, no guilty season of birth, no sinister viral epidemics and the worldwide, post-war epidemic of illegal drugs has had no measurable effects on the incidence of psychosis in any country.

On the other hand, psychotic episodes have been described in every known disturbance of brain function, genetic, intrauterine, traumatic, infective, toxic, neoplastic, metabolic and degenerative. How can we synthesize this? What orientation will allow us to view the problem in its proper light? I suggest the neurodevelopmental theory may not be far from the mark. However, we have to get away from the concept of psychosis being a unitary disorder with, thereby, a unitary cause. It is blinding us to the evidence that is there for all to see. My proposal is as follows:

16-2 (e) (i). We need to stop thinking there are categories of mental disorder. Since there is no demarcation criterion separating the psychotic disorders from everything else, there are no categories of mental disorder, only dimensions. Everything blurs into a huge, multidimensional field of human distress. Oddly enough, the editors of DSM-IV have already wrought this change for the affective psychoses. By widening the definition and by changing the name (from manic-depressive psychosis to Bipolar Affective Disorder), they signaled that there is no substantive difference between the mildest cases of affective disturbance to the most severe, that the old demarcation criterion (of psychosis) was a red herring. In what follows, I hope to effect the same service for schizophrenia.

16-2 (e) (ii). Schizophrenia-like psychoses are not uncommon in epilepsy, Huntington's Disease, lead poisoning and a wide variety of other injurious conditions, but they follow the same course. The person shows non-specific signs of disturbance which then coalesce into the classic picture of a treat-ment-resistant schizophrenic state. Gradually, the symptoms intensify then they seem to "burn out" as the primary (degenerative) disease process takes its toll. That is, the schizophrenic picture is a phase in the deterioration of the brain.

16-2 (e) (iii). If the neurodevelopmental theory is correct, a small change in the brain early in development can have catastrophic effects in later life. Yet this seems counter-intuitive just because the immature brain is actually re-markably good at reallocating damaged functions to intact areas of the brain. I don't believe this is such a problem for the theory because it need only pos-tulate that the impaired functions don't come become significant until later adolescence, by which time it is too late for the brain to adjust. However, no-tice that I have jumped, from talking about damaged areas to the notion of damaged functions. Because that's what the brain is, a function generator, and the most important function of all is the one that is most damaged in schizophrenia, the personality. I have argued that personality consists of the acquired set of rules by which the individual assesses the world and his place in it and determines his response. The functionally integrated implementation of these rules will depend on a healthy brain. Where there is brain damage, the personality will show impairment in just those functions subserved by the damaged areas. Personality, of course, is a subset of the mind, and mind is an emergent function of the brain. Therefore, any damage to the brain will be magnified as its effects work through to the full mental domain. In talking of brain damage, I said: "Each step depends on what has gone before, so a tiny defect early in development can have a major effect later in life." But what is true of the brain will *a fortiori* apply to the mind, and its subset, personality, just because these are of a higher order than the brain itself. If biological psy-chiatry accepts chaos theory as having any relevance to brain development, then it must further accept it in relation to the mind.

16-2 (e). (iv). Combining points (ii) and (iii) suggests that the symptomatic schizophrenic syndrome results when the brain can no longer generate the functions of mind in the normal, integrated manner. Subsequently, the syn-drome "burns out" when the damage becomes so extensive that cognition fails. That is, symptomatic schizophrenia constitutes a phase of a failing mind resulting from a failing brain. The declining brain causes the mind to start to disintegrate just because mind is far more complex, higher-order entity than the brain itself, and the brain is the most complex material thing in the known universe. However, the mind has its own reparative functions too, so the assumption is that something stops these coming into play.

16-2 (e). (v). Can this model account for cases of psychosis arising in a perfectly healthy brain? The principle is that the schizophrenic syndrome represents a phase of a failing mind. Therefore, can a mind fail in the com-plete absence of organic disturbance of the brain? The Yerkes-Dodson curve says that it can, that the level of arousal can reach such heights that all men-tal functions begin to break down. We would expect the highest order functions, such as judgment, affective integration, etc., to show impairment before the lower level, and this is exactly what happens in all psychoses, espe-cially schizophrenia. This must occur in the absence of massive external stressors, just because they aren't present in most cases of schizophrenia. However, anybody can be distressed, so but some other factor has to drive the level of distress to such a pitch that the mind begins to malfunction. I suggest the critical factor is what is commonly called insight, that the person inadvertently drives his own mind to disintegration just because, for one personal reason or another, he cannot accept there is anything wrong. This is universal, to the extent that there can't be psychosis if there is no loss of insight. Nobody can say: "I am deluded and hallucinated," because the definition is that, while these experiences are false, the subject takes them as reality. Claiming to be deluded would be akin to saying, "I believe a lie."

What about the cases who say: "I have schizophrenia. It is caused by a chemical imbalance of the brain. I have to take tablets for the rest of my life and go to rehab when my case manager tells me." I do not believe parroting what the doctor believes amounts to insight. The crucial point is that they evade personal responsibility for their condition. They are saying: "It isn't me, there's nothing wrong with me, it's just my brain chemistry." They know nothing of brain chemistry and, even when they study it on the Internet, they do so only with the intention of proving they cannot be held personally responsible.

16-2 (f). The synthetic or biocognitive view of psychosis. Combining both cases, I suggest the correct orientation toward the mystery of psychosis is to see it as a phase, not a state. The model of schizophrenia, which flows from that orientation, is that it is the highly complex result of a failing mind, where the primary disturbance can be a disorganized perception caused by evolving brain impairment, or it may be a mood or other disturbance resulting from innate personality factors but, in both extremes and in the huge, amorphous field in between, the crucial factor that drives the person to develop just this syndrome and no other is the refusal to acknowledge that there may be something wrong. Static brain damage does not cause the syndrome but it is the person's reaction to the damage, specifically, his attempts to compensate psychologically for what he cannot understand, that drives him to develop the full syndrome.

When a person's mind becomes chaotic under the influence of a drug-induced panic state, we call it a drug-induced psychosis. When mental chaos is the result of overwhelming external stressors, we call it a psychogenic or reactive psychosis. When it happens in the course of a degenerative brain condition, we call it a symptomatic schizophrenia. When he manages to reorient himself and recovers his mental balance, we call it a schizophreniform psychosis. When the chaos is dominated by affective symptoms, we call it affective or schizoaffective psychosis.

But when a fine personality based in a normal brain, with no external stressors, no drugs, no head injuries etc., slowly withdraws and declines into a self-sustaining or reinforcing chaos, one that does not get better, then we call it nuclear or process schizophrenia, the dreaded *dementia praecox*. Of course, we tell his parents something about brain chemicals and powerful new drugs but only to spare them the full horror of watching their beloved son descend into the pit of darkness from which there is no escape.

This means, of course, that any of our children could develop schizophrenia, which is a chilling thought.

16–3 Conclusion: Everybody is Right

All of the many physical changes reported in psychosis are probably right. This model predicts that there will be many more of them, that, as the technology of neuroscience advances, it will find more, and more subtle, changes in the brain state. They will, of course, be concentrated in those brain areas subserving the highest functions, of which personality is the pinnacle, but we will have to broaden our concept of the causation of psychosis to include such personality factors as lead to distress, especially secret distress. But I don't believe there will be any progress in understanding the world-knot of schizophrenia until we move away from the "state" approach, replacing it with the concept of madness as a phase in the disintegration of personality.

17 Other Myths in Psychiatry

17-1. Introduction

In this final chapter, I wish to look briefly at some smaller classes of disorders to show the scope of a genuinely integrative dualist model of mind. I choose these topics, not to write a general textbook of psychiatry, but simply to show how an organized approach based in a coherent scientific model can make sense of some of the untidiest topics in psychiatry.

17-2. Dissociative Disorders

17-2. (a) Introducing dissociation. The whole area of dissociation, post-traumatic states, stress, borderline personality disorder, childhood sexual abuse, dissociative identity disorder, conversion states, somatization and recovered memories, not to mention ritual satanic abuse and alien abduction, is complicated to the point of opacity. Anybody who claims to be able to make sense of it is deluding himself as it lacks even the most elementary basis in science. It is probably the most undisciplined welter of pseudoscience inflicted upon the general public since the collapse of Marxism.

The term Dissociation is now taken to refer to an area of scientific activity. It has the trappings of science, with conferences, professors, committees, learned journals, forensic experts, grants, research projects, public support groups and impassioned debates. Yet, bizarrely, no definition moves beyond the ostensive which is, of course, a solecism as there can be no ostensive definition of an unseen process. DSM-IV sidesteps the issue by giving only a descriptive account: "The essential feature of the Dissociative Disorders is a disruption in the usually integrated functions of consciousness, memory, identity, or perception" (p477). For each of the dissociative disorders, the authors provide lists of criteria to meet before the diagnosis can be made. However, this says only when the label can be applied: it does not in any sense name or define what it is being applied to. There is no link between the observable phenomena and the alleged causative process, so there is no way of knowing when the definition is being correctly applied. That is, the definition lacks validity.

Other writers grapple with the same problem but inadvertently illustrate an important point in the non-science that characterizes this field. One authority stated: "Dissociation is that process in which normally related psychologic experiences and events are detached from each other and result in a distortion of experiences with both subtle and profound alterations in interpretation of the meaning of personal and interpersonal events." Note how he has jumped from describing a group of disorders to an unseen process. Also, he assumes a formal psychological theory or model in which "experiences and events" are first attached to or associated with each other, then lose their attachments as a result of his cryptic process. There is, of course, no such model available to him.

17-2. (b). Clarifying dissociation. There is a profound epistemological problem with this whole area, which is that, using the alleged symptoms alone, nobody can tell what is the outcome of the actual process itself, and what is due to the brain's secondary or compensatory mechanisms. In addition, the "process-driven" symptoms can be either positive (an addition to human experience) or negative (a loss or reduction). All available lists of so-called dissociative symptoms give more or less equal status to each component, the only difference being that some are deemed more serious than others. The lists of symptoms do not, and can not, distinguish between causes and effects. In the absence of a model of the alleged process of mental dissociation, nobody can say what is primary in the "process of dissociation" and what is secondary. That is, the diagnostic lists do not distinguish between the primary functional changes and the mind's attempts to compensate for the putative disintegrative process. I will argue that if we organize the lists of symptoms into appropriate groups, then the solution to the vexed question of the actual "process" of dissociation becomes clear.

17-2. (c). Explaining dissociation. Using the DSM-IV approach, the symptoms of dissociation occur widely in adult psychopathology. In addition to the four formally-acknowledged dissociative disorders (Amnesia, Fugue, Depersonalization, Dissociative Identity Disorder) and the rest, the symptoms are also found in such diverse conditions as Acute Stress Disorder, Adjustment Disorder, Post-Traumatic Stress Disorder, Generalized Anxiety Disorder, Panic Disorder, Phobic Disorder, Conversion Disorder, Somatization Disorder, Obsessive-Compulsive Disorder and various personality disorders, especially Borderline Personality Disorder. The eating disorders, self-mutilation, ADD/ADHD, and various sexual disorders and paraphilias are also associated with these types of symptoms. Quite apart from the desired effects of intoxication, drug and alcohol abuse commonly lead to dissociative symptoms.

This list can be expanded when we include the various psychotic states, in which severe symptoms of this type are absolutely typical, and, as every clinician knows, the full range of depressive conditions. Finally, we should not forget intellectual handicap as a potent source of dissociative symptoms. That is to say, there is hardly a psychiatric condition in which these symptoms can not occur. After very lengthy experience, I don't believe I could name a single recognized psychiatric diagnosis in which, at one stage or another, I have not seen these particular symptoms.

Furthermore, classic dissociative symptoms are typically seen in non-psychiatric conditions such as overtiredness, the hypnoid states (going to sleep or waking up), intoxications, etc., as well as actual hypnosis. Such symptoms are absolutely typical of many physical illnesses, including any febrile illness; dehydration; hyper- or hypothermia; concussion or severe headache; metabolic disorders such as diabetic states, renal or hepatic failure; any brain affliction including epilepsy, early dementia, tumors, hemorrhages, infections and poisonings; severe pain; hypotension and hypertension and so on. To this very extensive list we must add the "normal" dissociative states of daydreaming, vivid fantasy, novelty, intense concentration and preoccupation, *deja vu* and *jamais vu*, as well as the culture-bound dissociative states of shamanism, religious excitement, possession and the like.

Now if we take the advocates of "Dissociation: The Entity" at face value, we are asked to accept that there is a single "process" (either psychological or biological, they're still arguing) to account for the enormity of these conditions. I contend that this is asking a bit much of any theory. Do they mean the dissociative state is secondary to all the above psychiatric conditions, or are they perhaps implying it is the primary causative disorder underlying the totality of physical and mental conditions listed above? That, patently, is absurd. As anybody who has had malaria knows, dissociative symptoms are extremely common in that condition. Nobody would suggest that the *Plasmodium* has the capacity to winkle its way into the "usually integrated functions of consciousness, memory, identity, or perception" and lever them apart.

In order to rationalize this mess, my suggestion is that we amend the definition slightly, to read: "The (group of) experiences formerly known as the Dissociative Disorders arise through a disruption in the usually integrated, *modular* functions of consciousness, memory, identity, or perception" (*pace* DSM-IV).

We have to be very careful of this word "disruption," because it carries its own baggage. It is a bit like referring to masturbation as "abuse": sometimes it is, and sometimes it isn't. Normally, the mental functions of cognition, conation and emotion function smoothly but I can readily "disrupt" them. Indeed, I can do it with such consummate ease that the marvel is that they stay together in the first place. We are so accustomed to everything mental slotting into place that we forget how complex it is.

So I suggest we stop getting excited about apparent "dissociation" and start to see it as just a variant of normal. Among the majority of the world's population, it is normal to function in a detached ("switched off," "zoned out," "fazed out") state for quite long periods. Anybody who doesn't agree with this can try planting a couple of paddy fields with rice seedlings, or take a long, third class rail trip through India, and see whether slipping into a zomboid state doesn't have its attractions. People at prayer dissociate themselves from their surroundings, as do people at very interesting conferences (and boring conferences). People at football matches, at political and religious meetings, anybody looking down a microscope or using an ophthalmoscope, and so on, are all "dissociated" for the duration. We do this deliberately and easily: remarkably, children never hear their parents say, "Turn off the television," while parents never hear their children say, "Can I have five dollars?"

All it means is that we have the capacity to switch off our emotional responses to events that, in other settings, would evoke a typical emotional reaction. We can choose what to note and how to respond to it, including not noting it and making no response at all. This is not contradictory and does not imply pathology. Mostly, it is the very practical matter of knowing that we can't respond to everything. Medical students do not mourn their cadavers.

The reason we can do this is because that is just how the brain functions: it assembles a verisimilitude of life from a huge range of subfunctions. However, while this type of "dissociation" is a variant of normal, simply a voluntary loosening of the mental ties, it also merges imperceptibly with the abnormal states. Accordingly, anything that can interfere with normal brain or mental function can induce these symptoms. Very roughly, we can group the symptoms according to their causes.

The first and greatest class of so-called "dissociative experiences" are the diverse borders of normality by which we slip into a state of detachment just because it suits us. What does detachment mean? It implies a self-serving state of reduced awareness of or responsivity to the surroundings. This might be failing to hear the neighbor's dog barking, or not responding to pictures of starving children on the television; it might be watching the traffic closely and not seeing your friend waving from another car, it might be entirely deliberate, as in yoga or trance states, or it might be "coming to" and realizing you have no recall of having driven the last half hour.

This last state is interesting, because it shows the modular function in action. When I was working as Regional Psychiatrist in the Kimberley Health Region of Western Australia's far North, I routinely had to drive 1000km along empty, straight roads through semi-arid country at night. "Coming to" was not uncommon. All it said was I had been driving without forming a memory of driving, just because I had been concentrating on something more absorbing (usually this work). However, for some reason, I had also forgotten the cue for whatever had been occupying me, so I had no way of recovering my memories of the last half hour. This says only that memory and concentration are separate, modular mental functions. Usually, they work together but this is contingent, not necessary. It is possible to drive along an empty road paying the road just a few milliseconds attention each second. These flickers of awareness are enough to keep the driver on the road but they need not enter memory. That's normal. After driving 1000km, I don't remember every corner, every tree or every gear change. Memory is highly selective; it has to be, otherwise the systems would overload. I can attend to something but not remember it.

Sleep walking is similar. My children (who were both highly accomplished somnambulists) were talking about it recently. "How can he walk from his bedroom through the living room, down the corridor and into the other room without banging into things?" asked the nine year old. "It's easy," her brother replied, "you're half-awake but you just don't remember it."

The second class of experiences to consider is the disturbance of normal, integrated mental function resulting from physical disturbances of the brain. If my computer is too hot, it starts to malfunction, but not in an "all or none" way. Rather, it starts to do odd things, a glitch here, a miscue there. The same is true of the brain. Because the brain is a collection of subunits (located in the head for embryonic convenience, but not by necessity), different routines will be more sensitive to physical changes than others. For example, in diabetic hypoglycemia, not all parts of the brain are equally sensitive to low blood sugar. Primitive parts, such as the motor system or secretomotor functions, are more resistant than more recent developments such as the neocortex. But our essentially human functions are almost entirely located in the neocortex, so confusion is the earliest sign of hypoglycemia, not paralysis or olfactory hallucinations in clear consciousness. Thus, the most complex and sensitive subsystems will malfunction first, generally, but not necessarily, those systems based in the neocortex such as the highest forms of judgment, concentration and the visual associative system (illusions, misperceptions, vague shapes and colors). Speech will decline before respiration, verbal memory will decline before motor memory, fine motor control of the fingers will be lost before spinal reflexes of the legs and so on. This makes perfect sense within the modular framework of mental function.

Now we come to the real test, the psychologically-determined disturbances of integrated mental function. Here, we see the greatest folly of the tradition of "Dissociation as a single process" that began with Janet and Freud. I have suggested that the smooth integration of normal (as ideal) mental function is rather remarkable. The wonder is that it stays together as well as it does, but there is no doubt that this requires a lot of training. Now the defendants of the reality of Dissociation, including the authors of DSM-IV, have stated it occurs in just about every abnormal mental state known. My model says this is not unexpected, because abnormal mental states not only amount to deviations from normality but they also induce a ripple effect of further deviations from normality, which are then mistakenly attributed to a mysterious "process of Dissociation." Is there any single abnormal mental state capable of inducing transient disturbances of the smooth integration of the diverse functions underlying normal mental life? There most certainly is, one that has been known since time immemorial as a powerful cause of mental aberration: Anxiety.

Looking at the lists of conditions in DSM-IV in which dissociative phenomena are found, it is clear that the most likely culprits are those states in which high levels of anxiety are found. In fact, any other condition that pushes mental life to the extremes (certainly depression does this) will induce a transient uncoupling of mental function. The whole point about normal, integrated mental life is that it occurs only within a narrow range of physical *and* psychophysiological parameters. We spend most of our lives within these limits and so regard them as fixed, secure and reliable when, in fact, they are easily breached. Indeed, they are so easily breached that we might be better to regard normal mental life as actively held together against centrifugal forces, as it were, rather than something that stays together by its own inertia, the default position, as they say. A quick look at the Yerkes-Dodson curve (Fig. 14-3 (f)) will illustrate the point.

If a physical model is required, then think of the difference between putting four marbles in a large shallow bowl compared with turning the bowl upside down and balancing the marbles on its base. In the latter position, the marbles would "dissociate" rather easily, and the further they moved from the small, flat center, the more likely they would be to slip out of control. The difference between marbles on a bowl and a mind operating outside the mid-levels of physical and mental balance is that the mind has self-rectifying abilities as well, which further complicate the picture.

If, for whatever reason, the physiological state varies too much from its narrow limits, or the arousal state goes too high or too low, then we can reasonably expect a loss of normal integrated function. The disruption of normal mental function will be experienced as the usual phenomena in any list of dissociative symptoms, just because that's what happens when a machine as complicated as the mind starts to spin apart. Thus, dissociation is a fact, but it is not a process, entity or phenomenon *sui generis*.

17-2. (d). Dispensing with dissociation. In the terms of my case, transient losses of concentration during low arousal (boredom) are common, but fantasies are the subject's response to boredom, and are not in the same class of phenomena. Children who are easily bored in school (such as the very bright) will tend to get a reputation as day-dreamers (or troublemakers); the correct response is to give them a more stimulating environment, not put them on drugs. A frightened person will start to develop a sense of unreality (depersonalization, derealization, time disturbances, etc.), so any condition associated with anxiety will show these phenomena. The list of DSM-IV diagnoses known to include dissociative phenomena includes every one of the anxiety states, plus every condition in which high arousal is common, meaning practically every abnormal mental state.

Furthermore, if we take the term Dissociation out of that particular textbook (or any book or paper on the subject of psychologically-determined dissociation) and replace it with 'anxiety,' we will not have reduced its information content; rather, we will have added to it by reducing confusion. Anxiety induces changes in normal mental function, that much was known to Euripides; we know highly anxious people become disorganized and develop odd experiences. Why, then, should we invoke another, unseen process to explain what we know anxiety does itself?

If we dispense with dissociation in psychiatry and replace it with the notion that deviations from ideal mental life have myriad causes, the most common of which is anxiety, then we will have done a very great service to our profession. Instead of seeing these diverse phenomena as the outcome of a single, unseen cause, we need to start to analyze them carefully, assigning them to the correct causative factor. In simple terms, we need to look at each case as an individual, scoring the 'dissociative' symptoms on two axes, the physical and the psychological (arousal). It is therefore not possible to state, on the basis of the symptoms alone, that a person necessarily experienced, say, childhood sexual contact, or violence, or anything. The early experiences cause the adult symptoms through the medium of an anxiety state, and shifting attention away from this (treatable) fact, to an unknown 'process,' is counter-therapeutic.

There is no such thing, process, entity or whatever of "dissociation." There is, however, a clearly delineated, step-by-step process by which normal mental function becomes uncoupled in a predictable, modular way under the influence of a huge range of factors, starting with one's own intention. There is also a wide range of normal functions, from the slightest sense of detachment in a boring meeting, through to the extreme (boys playing computer games, day-dreaming, men hunting, comforting voices, avoiding the horror of warfare or recurrent violence, etc.). However, much the same symptoms can also arise through physical illness or injury, which is where the medicine in psychiatry comes into its own. If that were not sufficiently complicated, the "dissociation syndrome" can be driven to new levels of complexity by the effects of anxiety, which can itself range from trivial to overwhelming. Through anxiety, the subject is pushed completely outside normal functional parameters. However, any other intense experience such as novelty, grief and rage can also do it, and we should not forget that old favorite, romantic love. Fortunately, this is a very abnormal state, and all sorts of strange things can happen during it, as Shakespeare knew full well.

For ordinary purposes, psychiatric texts can safely replace the word 'dissociation' with anxiety and everybody will be that much clearer about what is happening.

17–3. Eating Disorders

17-3 (a) Introducing anorexia nervosa. It would be a very considerable understatement to say that psychiatry has been obsessed with the very rare condition of anorexia nervosa, to the exclusion of having anything worthwhile to say about that increasingly common and deadly disorder, obesity. I suggest the fruitless psychiatric infatuation with anorexia has arisen from the optimistic belief that it looks like it should have a biological cause. Wasting diseases have always been part of general medicine. Why should psychiatry be any different? However, despite huge expenditure over the past fifty years, nothing consistent has ever been found. There is not one biological change in anorexia that is not also seen in enforced starvation. Furthermore, those who acquire the diagnosis (mostly adolescent females) are almost always free of any symptoms of formal mental illness.

The problem for any biological account of anorexia is finding a single brain lesion that can account for the totality of the features of this disorder, e.g., that it is becoming more common, that it strikes a particular age group, that these girls are so utterly insightless, that they are so stealthy in the ways they manage to lose weight, and so on. There are many wasting diseases, but none with such a peculiar combination of sociological and psychological features. A cognitive explanation, on the other hand, is simplicity itself: the patient has decided to lose weight, and will do anything and everything to achieve this goal. Of course, this simply shifts the matter to be explained back one step but that is preferable to invoking an unprovable brain disease. The question now becomes: Why should these girls want to starve themselves? There are two questions to be answered, why they start in the first place, and why they keep going.

17-3 (b) Explaining anorexia nervosa. Why start dieting? That is not a very profound question. Lots of people start dieting. Several times in my life, I have made the deliberate decision to lose weight, so I don't think there is anything strange about a person who decides to lose weight. Because I have never been technically overweight, I didn't do it for reasons of health. Therefore, I did it for reasons of vanity. Therefore, anybody else who loses weight for reasons of vanity is not insane. *QED.*

The cognitive explanation always starts with the least implausible explanation, and the idea of teenage girls losing weight for reasons of vanity is not counter-intuitive. Two well-known cognitive principles can provide an economical account for the phenomena of anorexia nervosa, discounting the future and sequential targeting. Let us propose that girls with low self-esteem are at least as likely to try to lose weight as girls with normal self-esteem. Further, let us propose that girls with rather rigid, self-involved and perfectionist personality traits are more likely to stick to a diet than impulsive, self-indulgent, disorganized or just plain dopey girls. So far, none of this breaches the bounds of commonsense. Actually, I don't have to explain why lots of girls start to diet, nor why some are successful. But why don't they stop when they reach their target? I suggest they don't stop because they have no specific target; that, along the way, the process of dieting breeds its own incentive such that losing weight becomes the unattainable end of a dream of perfection.

They start with the idea, "I am not a very attractive person." This is not novel. Lots of teenagers have this idea. Lots of boys have this idea, too. Some boys look at men with tattoos and say to themselves, "He has tattoos. He is popular. Therefore, if I had tattoos, I too would be popular." So they get one tattoo. It feels good so, after a while, they think, "One tattoo makes me feel good, so two tattoos should make me feel twice as good." So they get another tattoo, then another, until even the tattooist is struggling to find a bare bit of skin. Nobody calls them mentally ill; stupid, maybe, but not mentally ill. This is also true of people who have 300 studs through their faces, or who stretch their necks with thick copper rings until they can't take the rings off, or who bind their feet until they can no longer walk, and so on. They are not mentally ill.

Some other boys with low self-esteem look at well-built men and say to themselves, "He has lots of muscles and people say he is good-looking. Therefore, if I had lots of muscles, other people would think I am good-looking." So they start a program of body building, which involves grueling hours in a gym to the exclusion of normal social life, dangerous diets and, these days, dangerous drugs. Eventually, and at the risk of serious long-term damage to the health, including sudden death, this results in a grotesquely deformed body. Unless your name is Arnold, body-building will not result in fame, fortune, comfort, popularity or large genitalia, yet nobody calls body-builders mentally ill; at least, not to their faces.

Some other boys look at wealthy men and say to themselves, "He has lots of money. People respect him. Therefore, if I had lots of money, people would respect me, too." They work hard and make some money and it feels good, so they work harder and take chances and make some more, until they have a million dollars. But having one million dollars reminds them that there are lots of men with two million dollars, so they work harder and take more chances until, one day, they have two million dollars. But it isn't enough, they need more, they have to keep going. Nobody calls Mr. Gates mentally ill; he has probably been called most names in and out of the dictionary, but not that one.

A certain famous Australian cricketer had a very attractive wife. But there were other attractive women in the world, some of whom were a little pushy in their wish to meet him, so he met one. No doubt he enjoyed that, so he met another. One day, he announced he had met about one thousand of them but he has given no indication that even one thousand of them is enough. Nobody calls him mentally-ill; greedy, perhaps stupid, maybe even lucky, but not mentally ill. Or should I say, if having a thousand attractive women by the age of 35 counts as a mental illness, how many other men would like the same disease?

A woman feels she is not very pretty. She hears of an operation that can make her pretty, so she has it. It does indeed make her more attractive, so she has another. After 45 operations, she no longer looks pretty but she is unable to stop because now she fears looking unattractive.

All of this says that setting a goal, achieving it and trying for more is not *ipso facto* mental illness. It is usually called sequential targeting. I set myself a realistic target; because it is realistic, I achieve it. Having achieved it, the next target becomes attainable so, for no reason other than the fact that it is there and humans function better with goals, I make that my new target. Stamp collectors, car collectors, art connoisseurs, athletes (including sexual athletes), mountain climbers (especially mountain climbers), dictators, billionaires, all we are doing is following the restless human urge to keep going.

This explains why people keep going but it doesn't explain why they won't stop. I'm not sure that I have to explain this one because I might then have to explain why anybody worth $100 billion would want to destroy a miniscule competitor, or why a president with lots of weapons of mass destruction would want to destroy a tinpot dictator with no weapons of mass destruction. Some people are just not very good at saying, "Enough is enough," but they are not thereby mentally ill. Plenty of teenage girls can say, "Enough is enough," and they don't become anorexic. The few who can't see when enough is enough, who discount the risks, end up in trouble. It is quintessentially human to say: "Please, sir, I want more."

An unhappy teenage girl sees a model, and says to herself something like: "Models are attractive people. Models are thin. Therefore, if I were thin, I would be an attractive person." She might also have said: "That fat girl is not attractive. She is therefore unattractive because she is fat. I do not feel attractive, therefore I must be fat so, to feel attractive, I must lose weight." The options are very large and, because we are dealing with teenagers, the reasoning need not be watertight. All they have to do is convince themselves.

After a while, she loses some weight. It feels good. Nothing much else in her life feels good, so she loses some more. She may know of the risks of excessive dieting but she can convince herself they are too far in the future to bother with, or they won't happen to her, but these features (discounting the future), while common in teenagers, are not exclusive to them. Most politicians show a highly-developed capacity to focus on short-term wins and ignore future risks. Because she is not mentally ill, she knows not to let anybody realize what she is doing, so she conceals her activities by stealth and subterfuge. However, along the way, she changes from simply wanting to lose weight to fearing gaining weight, which is quite a different thing. Now, if she eats a normal meal, her level of fear builds up and up. Fear causes an unsettled feeling in the stomach but she mistakenly believes the food has caused an unsettled feeling in her stomach. She concludes that getting rid of the food will get rid of the unsettled feeling. Now she is caught in a self-reinforcing cycle of fear and self-loathing from which she cannot voluntarily escape. What once seemed like an exercise in feeling good has now become a totally different matter of fear reduction, and this is the reason she can't stop.

When people finally do realize what is going on and ask her to eat properly, they are asking her to do something she actively fears. However, she can't tell anybody she fears eating, just as a nervous teenage boy can't tell anybody he fears asking a girl out. It has to do with self-esteem: when the self-esteem is very low (which is why she started dieting in the first place), doing something that attracts contempt will push the self-esteem into self-loathing, which nobody can do voluntarily. When her frantic parents point to her reflection in a mirror and say, "This looks terrible," they are telling her what she doesn't dare admit. She has no choice but to tell them she is fat or to insist that she is still fat and keep going.

A biological explanation of anorexia would have to account for the simultaneous onset of a wide range of brain changes in a healthy person. It would also have to explain the passionate but diagnostic lack of insight of these patients. It seems vanishingly unlikely that so many changes could occur as separate and unrelated primary brain disorders; to make biological sense, they would have to be secondary to single, primary cause. There is, however, no *a priori* reason why a simple decision, a matter of mind, should not be that single, primary cause.

17-3 (c) Introducing morbid obesity. Somewhere along the line, the great Australian male became the Great Australian Myth. Even though the Outback is part of the national ethos, it is a fact that, after Singapore and Hong Kong, we are the most highly urbanized nation on earth. Sadly, this nation of tough cowboys and world-class sportsmen is now fatter than our mortal enemies, the English. 62% of Australian men are overweight but only 32% of them recognize that they are. Therefore, 30% of Australian men have a serious defect of insight, which puts them in the same class as anorexics. Up here in the Last Frontier of the Northern Territory, morbid obesity is alarmingly common. It is not at all uncommon to see people in their thirties who weigh 200kg (440lb). Obesity kills about 500 times as many people as anorexia nervosa, yet research papers on obesity hardly rate a mention in the psychiatric literature. This is a pity, because a small group of these people are motivated to gorge themselves wholly by an anxiety state, which means they are readily treated.

17-3 (d) Explaining (some) morbid obesity. These people experience intense symptoms of anxiety, mostly for social reasons. The actual reasons vary from one person to the next but are generally concerned with how other people will see them, how they will perform, and so on. There is nothing unusual about this. However, early in life, they learn that eating settles their "stomach nerves," so that is what they do.

These are the people who describe themselves as being "comfort eaters." Anything that makes them anxious will give them an intense sense of gastric upset; they differ only in how they respond to it. Most anxious people experience a churning stomach or "butterflies," or hollow, hungry, empty, gnawing or knotted feelings in the stomach, but they find that the mere sight of food makes them heave, so they avoid it. For whatever reason, the obese do not experience this reaction to food. Food, especially sweet or sticky, reduces their gastric disturbance so, whenever they become anxious, they eat. However, they soon run into a trap because their social fears are exaggerated by being obese. That is, being obese makes them anxious, and being anxious makes them eat, in a true vicious circle that leads to gargantuan obesity.

Just to complicate matters, many of them become secondarily anxious about having enough food to eat. Just as people who are dependent on drugs will start to panic at the thought of running out of drugs, so the morbidly obese also panic at the thought of not having enough food in the house. However, they won't admit this. Instead, they say: "I have a disease called obesity that makes me eat even when I don't want to. If the food is there, I have to eat it. I can't stop my cravings so if I don't have food, my disease will drive me mad." It's not a disease that drives them mad, it is their own fear that they will become overwhelmingly anxious and not have the antidote. It is the classic self-fulfilling prophecy of superstition: a person panics if he doesn't have the talisman he believes will stop him panicking.

Treating the anxiety state may result in a loss of weight where all else has failed. However, not all of them will be amenable to psychiatric intervention because they have spent their lives eating to avoid the unpalatable truth that they are anxious. Normally, they see anxiety as a moral failing and are reluctant to seek psychiatric attention or to reveal their symptoms. They will quite often sit sphinx-like in their chairs and deny flatly that they have ever experienced even the least symptoms of anxiety. The denial gives them away. Nobody is as calm as these people claim to be, but getting them to see it may prove impossible. They are not so dissimilar to alcoholics, who will admit they get the shakes from drinking, but will never concede they also get shaky when they haven't been drinking.

17-4. Addictions and Compulsive Behaviors

Unfortunately, these words have been hammered by the popular press for many years. People now claim to be addicted to running, to eating, even to sex, or to be compulsive gamblers, compulsive shoppers or compulsive liars, but all they mean is that they can't stop. The reason is simple: if they stop, they become unbearably anxious, so they choose to keep going.

The morphine user says: "I have a genetic chemical disease of the brain. I felt terrible every day of my life until I found morphine. Morphine is the specific drug to bring me back to normal. It puts you to sleep but it allows me to function like a normal person. If I can't get my fix, I get terrible withdrawals."

Persistent gamblers say: "When I'm sitting at the table, nothing else matters. I concentrate on the wheel or the numbers and all my troubles just fade away."

The committed runner will say: "When I'm running, there's only me and the pavement and the sky overhead. I get high but if I can't run, my endorphins go all over the place and I go into withdrawal."

There are many examples of what seems to be compulsive behavior, in which the individual describes a sense of being driven to do something that may be silly, expensive, fattening, dangerous, illegal or all five. The cognitive explanation for these types of behaviors is simplicity itself: the person has accidentally set up a self-fulfilling prediction, just the reverse of the phobia. The phobic person says: "If I do have a visitor/ see a frog/ offend someone, I will feel terrible." However, making this prediction frightens him, and his fear becomes the terrible feeling he didn't want. The person with so-called compulsive behavior says: "If I *don't* have drugs/ food/ running/ gambling etc., I will feel terrible." However, making this prediction frightens him, and his fear becomes the terrible feeling he didn't want.

It is common in people who use opiates. The user spends his life searching for drugs. He will say it is to prevent withdrawal but his problem is not opium withdrawal, it is pure fear. He is mortally afraid of what will happen to him if he doesn't have opiates. He knows, as surely as he knows the sun will set that day, that if he doesn't have opiates, he will feel terrible. He will call this withdrawal but, in fact, all his symptoms are consistent with a state of abject terror. He is terrified of how he will feel if he doesn't have opiates, and how he will feel just is terrified. That is to say, he has set up a self-fulfilling prediction. And the more often it happens, the worse he will feel.

This is true of many of what are called compulsive behaviors. The person is simply saying: "If I can't have/ do/ clean/ check X, I will feel terrible." But the further X seems from him, the more frightened he will become, which proves to him that he was right, he really does need X. He takes his sweating, shaking, pounding heart, churning stomach and dreadful feeling as proof of his belief that X is essential, that, without it, he can't function and nobody should have the right to deny him a peaceful life, it shouldn't be a crime because, if he can't have regular supplies of X, he becomes the victim and where's the justice in that? True, but he is the unwitting victim of his own fear.

This is why intravenous drug users often say that merely seeing a needle, or feeling the prick in their skin, gives them a "high." It is merely the same flood of relief that anybody would get if they thought that immediate reduction of a terrible feeling was at hand. That is, they feel relief at the prospect of relief, which is also a self-fulfilling prophecy. Unfortunately, one doesn't get much gratitude for pointing out these elementary truths.

Runners say much the same thing. When they are pounding the pavement, they feel a serenity that isn't available to them at any other time. If they can't go, they start to feel edgy and irritable, shaky and sweaty and so on, which just are the symptoms of anxiety. They have set up the prediction: "If I don't run, I will feel bad." Partly, this is due to an excessive concern about losing fitness (nobody loses fitness over a week), but mostly it is because, when they run, and only when they run, they are free souls.

Gamblers are very similar. They will say that, when they sit at the table or the poker machine, the outside world ceases to exist, they have no worries or concerns and they might as well be on the moon. Looking at the balls or cards or numbers, they become calm and focused and nothing else matters. Should we call this dissociation?

This explains why they keep going, but it doesn't explain why they start their so-called addictions or compulsions. Again, the cognitive answer is quite simple. Morphine is a very powerful tranquillizer. If a calm person takes it, he will soon go into a drugged, unresponsive state, if not actually to sleep. However, when an over-aroused person takes it, he will come back to normal, as shown by the Yerkes-Dodson curve. Morphine therefore appeals to people who are chronically over-aroused, or chronically anxious. Although they will normally not admit it, this is why they start taking the drug, and this is why they cannot stop. They know that, if they stop, they will revert to how they felt before they started, meaning terrible, and they fear feeling terrible. But the terrible feeling just is fear, so the trap closes on them.

When compulsive gamblers are not at the casino, they are tense and edgy, troubled by anxiety to the extent that life is frightening and miserable. However, when they take their minds off the larger world and focus on some numbers, all their worries fade away, so they have to keep going back. Normally, they will not admit they are anxious but the symptoms are there for anybody who takes the time to probe. Programs for compulsive gamblers that do not attend to the anxiety component will not succeed.

There are many reasons why people take up marathons but one would not expect comfort to be one of them. However, it is true of a proportion of compulsive runners that, when they tie on their shoes and hit the road, they feel a sense of liberation. It is the liberation of knowing that nothing and nobody can touch them, they are free of pressure, worry, decisions, aggression and so on, just as long as they are on the road. So they stay on the road, and get very angry at anybody (drivers, dog-owners, wives) who may try to push them off the road.

17–5. The Placebo Effect

17-5 (a). Introducing the Placebo Effect. Years ago, when I was working in southern Thailand, I was talking to a professor of chemistry at one of the universities about the value of traditional Thai medicine. Yes, he said, his cousin had developed osteomyelitis and the surgeons at the hospital wanted to take his leg off. The patient declined their offer and went to a traditional healer who worked on his leg until, in just three months, he was cured. "He still had his leg", the professor chortled, which proved that Thai medicine was at least as good as Western, if not better.

It might also prove, I replied, that the surgeons weren't very good practitioners of Western medicine, as they hadn't given conservative treatment a proper trial. "No," he retorted, "it was really that the patient had no confidence in Western medicine. He did not believe it could get him better, so his body failed to respond."

Now, to a Westerner, this seems rather silly. The patient's attitude does not determine whether the bugs in his bone will be killed by the particular antibiotic, nor will bits of dead bone (the sequestrum) be resorbed just because he meditates on them. Yet there is no doubt in any experienced practitioner's mind that the patient's expectations are a very powerful factor in his response to treatment. In fact, the individual's mental set is so powerful that huge drug trials have to be planned in such a way as to negate them. The positive effect created by the expectation that a treatment will be effective is called the placebo effect.

The word placebo comes from the thirteenth century Catholic vespers for the dead: "*Placebo Domino...*" "I shall please the Lord..." In the nineteenth century, and for the usual reasons of medical secrecy, it was filched to indicate a drug or substance given with the intention of pleasing the patient but with no intention or expectation that it would satisfy him by physiological means. It now means a substance given with the intention of evoking the particular response the patient expects. So if a person expects a tablet to cure his upset stomach, and he is given sugar pills that do just that, everybody is satisfied that he was making it all up and he should be treated very sternly to show him that medicine is not a game, thank you very much.

17-5 (b). Explaining the placebo effect. The notion that complaints of illness can be influenced by inactive substances or procedures is very important. In general medicine, the patient's preconceptions about the treatment can be extremely influential, and not just whether he takes his tablets or not. If he believes the treatment will work, he feels encouraged to wait until it has had a fair trial, i.e., he stops complaining about the disability, mainly because it no longer worries him so much. But it is more than just this: people do actually get better with sugar pills.

On a simple level, if a patient is convinced a tablet won't work, he won't take it. Different surveys indicate that only about 67% of the drugs prescribed in this country are actually consumed, which I would have thought an optimistic figure. I once told a man's wife to bring in all his drugs and she arrived with three full pillowcases.

The next factor is the effect of the drug upon anxiety. If a person is frightened about his illness, he will necessarily feel worse and complain more than somebody who isn't frightened. If he thinks he is getting an effective treatment, his anxiety level will drop, he will feel better and instead of complaining to the medical superintendent, will talk cheerfully to his neighbor or even encourage the others. That is, apparently objective measures of illness, such as pulse, muscle tension, gastric motility, complaints of pain, shortness of breath and the like will improve. He will be more cooperative with painful procedures, e.g., coughing or stretching exercises, and more inclined to wait while nature takes its course. A person who is not frightened of the near future automatically feels better than somebody who is, and that is part of the placebo effect.

However, it goes further. Some illnesses are directly influenced by higher centers. These include bowel dysfunction, asthma and epilepsy (an anxious person is inclined to hyperventilate, which destabilizes the epileptic focus). The research on biofeedback from about thirty years ago showed unexpected forms of higher control over autonomic dysfunction (unexpected by Western medicine). I expect we will continue to discover powerful forms of feedback control over many bodily functions.

Psychiatry differs from general medicine in that all the symptoms are subjective, and are not just influenced by the mental state, but are part of the mental state itself. Even in selected trials, antidepressants are only about 60% effective, compared with, say, antibiotics, which are almost 100% effective even in unconscious people. However, the placebo effect in psychiatry is approximately 40%, meaning the therapeutic efficacy of antidepressants is a dismal 20%. How can therapeutically ineffective substances have such a powerful effect? The answer is surely that the expectation of a better future just is the antithesis of both anxiety (it removes the threat of illness) and depression (despair means seeing no chance of recovery). Insofar as a person is suffering anxiety and depression (i.e., all except a few manic patients and a few cheerfully deluded schizophrenics), the expectation of improvement necessarily leads to improvement.

There is nothing magic about this; it is a merely a matter of redefining emotional states as the logical outcome of the belief system. The concept is only difficult to committed biological psychiatrists who believe in the unidirectional causation of emotional disturbances, i.e., that anxiety and depression are "caused" at the biochemical level, and that the mental contents have no effect upon the emotional state. It has to be said that they do not believe this for themselves, only for others. An emotionally stable biological psychiatrist (and aren't they all?) accepts without hesitation that his equability is due to superior moral equipment, and not just superior parents.

17-5 (c). A note on mass hysteria. Mass hysteria (mass psychogenic illness; mass sociogenic illness; outbreaks of multiple unexplained symptoms; deleted from DSM-IV) consists of sudden outbreaks of unexplained illness, usually in specific or closed groups of people, e.g., nurses in hospitals, soldiers, workers in restricted areas, students, etc.. The pattern is that one person will report sick, somebody will suggest an infective or toxic etiology then, suddenly, dozens of people working in the same area are collapsing with identical symptoms and there is a full-scale emergency. In these days of wall-to-wall television coverage of budgies falling out of trees, these heart-stopping dramas, with wailing ambulances, helicopters and brave emergency workers donning breathing apparatus, not to mention tearful girls being laid in swooning lines on the footpath, are the stuff of a bored television producer's dreams.

The explanation is simplicity itself: mass hysteria is the reverse of the placebo effect. By taking a placebo, a person induces the beneficial effects he expects. Mass hysteria is groups of people accidentally inducing in themselves the malign effects they fear.

The symptoms of any such outbreak just are the somatic and cognitive effects of anxiety, namely, sweating, tremor, weakness, racing heart, shortness of breath, dizzy sensations, churning stomach and nausea, dry mouth, choking sensations, blurred vision, flickering shadows, irritability, poor concentration, and so on. In various permutations and combinations, coupled with the latest Hollywood fad or alarmist toxic scare, time and time again, these few symptoms pop up in the headlines.

The mechanism is simply that anxiety is the most communicable of all emotions, perhaps because of an evolutionary advantage. If the focus of the anxiety is witches flitting around at sunset, then that is what groups of panicky nuns will see. If it is an arbovirus carried by insects biting lonely nurses in their chilly dormitories at night, then they will all develop muscle twitching, tremor, weakness, writhing movements, headaches and stiff neck. If it is toxic chemicals sprayed on groups of overwrought troops, then they will all develop tremor, palpitations, nausea, vomiting, rashes, forgetfulness and irritability. It doesn't matter what the focus, all that counts is that groups of excitable people think they might have caught it too. The thought of an unknown killer loose among them induces fear; fear induces bodily changes; bodily changes induce a medical evacuation; medical evacuation induces widespread panic among the mothers of the brave nurses/ soldiers/ workers, etc., and thence among politicians. The rest is history.

However, there is a sociological quirk that complicates the issue, that physicians would rather make a false positive diagnosis than false negative. In this, they are amply influenced and rewarded by politicians, newspapers and others. The eminent professor who takes the microphone and says, "We are closing in on the mysterious virus," will get heaps of publicity, a huge grant and invitations to lots of committees. Anybody who says, "Calm down, you're all panicking," will be blackballed. Sometimes there is a mysterious virus (HIV, HSE), but mostly there isn't, but the outbreaks are totally different anyway. Neither HIV nor HSE arrived in a factory, barracks or hospital one afternoon, and dead people do not figure in any outbreaks of mass hysteria, unless they are harmless old ladies burned at the stake.

17-6. Conclusion

The concept of the recursive properties of human emotion, especially anxiety, is central to each of these examples. It is central to any rational account of mental disorder. The evidence is that there is a powerful two-way connection between psyche and soma but I don't believe we have any more than the most superficial understanding of the power of the human mind to act upon the body. I am not suggesting in any way that there are "higher powers" or that there is anything supernatural about this. My theory is cast entirely within the realms of materialism, the doctrine that everything has a cause. There is nothing in the universe beyond matter and energy and the informational states that control them. This model does not rely on supernatural elements, nor does it forbid them, but it does say they aren't necessary.

All matter-energy equations in the human body are controlled; that much is given. There is nothing random about the way we stay alive. Our physical bodies are remarkable, but the mechanisms we share with chimps, rats and worms are quotidian. The mind, however, is something above and beyond the body, but not in any spiritual sense. It is an emergent quality, almost certainly shared to some extent by chimps and possibly dolphins, but it is amenable to rational enquiry.

The ultimate test of any theory of mind is that it explains mental disorder. I have used these small examples of quirks in psychiatry to demonstrate the scope of this biocognitive theory of mind. It seems to have very large explanatory scope; that its central thesis is still irrefutable should not be seen as a total disadvantage at this stage.

It might be suggested that I am making too much of anxiety, that I have merely taken one universal pseudo-explanation (chemical imbalance of the brain) and substituted another (anxiety), but I don't believe this is a valid criticism. What I have done is show that anxiety is a powerful mediating factor in a wide range of mental disorders just because of its recursive properties. More to the point, anxiety can be explained: it is not an explanatory dead-end.

In general, I have shown that diverse mental factors, current, remembered and not-so-remembered, act together to produce a state of hyper-arousal. This new, unstable state has both physical and psychological concomitants. These produce further disturbance followed by rapid and unconscious compensatory reactions; in turn, these interact with the new input to produce further changes, *ad infinitum*. Locked in self-reinforcing and self-perpetuating process, there can be only one possible outcome: mental breakdown.

Notes and References

Books:

Borst: Borst CV, Ed. *The Mind/Brain Identity Theory*. London: Macmillan, 1970.

Chalmers: Chalmers DJ. *The conscious mind: In search of a fundamental theory*. New York: Oxford University Press, 1996

Dennett Brainstorms. Dennett DC. Brainstorms: Philosophical Essays in Mind and Psychology. Hassocks, Sussex: Harvester Press, 1978.

Dennett *CS*: Dennett DC. *Consciousness Explained*. Little, Brown: New York, 1991. Page numbers refer to the 1993 Penguin edition.

Dennett *IS*: Dennett DC. *The intentional stance*. Cambridge, Mass: Bradford Books/MIT Press, 1989.

Dennett KM: Dennett DC. Kinds of Minds: Towards an Understanding of Consciousness. London: Phoenix Press, 1997.

DSM-IV: American Psychiatric Association. *Diagnostic and Statistical Manual IV*. Washington: APA, 1994

Kuhn: Kuhn TS. *The structure of scientific revolutions*. University of Chicago Press, 1962.

McKenzie: McKenzie BD. Behaviorism and the Limits of Scientific Method. London: RKP, 1977.

Popper and Eccles: Popper KR and Eccles JC. *The Self and its Brain*. New York: Springer Verlag, 1977.

Popper *C&R*: Popper KR. *Conjectures and Refutations*. London: Routledge and Kegan Paul, 1972.

Popper *LSD*: Popper KR. *The logic of scientific discovery*. London: Hutchinson, 1972.

Popper *OK*: Popper KR. *Objective Knowledge: an Evolutionary Approach*. Oxford University Press, 1972.

Skinner *AB*: Skinner BF. *About Behaviorism*. New York: Knopf, 1974. Page numbers refer to the Penguin edition, 1993.

Skinner *BFD*: Skinner BF. *Beyond Freedom and Dignity*. New York: Knopf, 1971. Page numbers refer to the Bantam Books edition, 1972.

Skinner *RBS*: Skinner BF. Why I am not a cognitive psychologist. In: *Reflections on behaviourism and society*. New York: Knopf, 1974.

Journals:

AGP: Archives of General Psychiatry.
AJP: American Journal of Psychiatry.
ANZJP: Australian and New Zealand Journal of Psychiatry.
AP: Australasian Psychiatry.
BJP: British Journal of Psychiatry.
PM: Psychological Medicine.
PR: Psychological Review.

Chapter 1

1. Berger PA and Brodie HK, Eds. Biological Psychiatry. Ch. 8 in: Arieti S, Ed. *American Handbook of Psychiatry.* New York: Basic Books, 1986

2. Trimble MR. *Biological Psychiatry.* Chichester: Wiley, 1988

3. Changeux J-P. *Neuronal Man: The Biology of Mind.* Oxford: University Press, 1985

4. Guze SB. Biological psychiatry: is there any other kind? *PM,* 1989; 19: 315-323.

5. Silove D. Biologism in psychiatry. *ANZJP,* 1990; 24: 461.

6. Guze SB. *Why Psychiatry is a Branch of Medicine.* New York: Oxford University Press, 1992

7. Eccles JC, in Popper and Eccles.

8. Lipowski ZJ. The integrative approach to psychiatry. *ANZJP* 1990; 24:470.

9. Smart JJC. Sensations and brain processes. Reprinted in Borst

10. Armstrong DM. *The Nature of Mind.* St Lucia: University of Queensland Press, 1980.

11. Place UT. Is consciousness a brain process? Reprinted in Borst.

12. Malcolm N. Scientific materialism and the identity theory. Reprinted in Borst.

13. Popper KR, in Popper and Eccles.

14. Churchland PM. *Matter and Consciousness.* Cambridge, Mass: Bradford Books/MIT Press, 1988.

15. Bullock A, Stallybrass O (Eds). *Fontana Dictionary of Modern Thought.* London: Fontana, 1977.

16. Audi R. *Cambridge Dictionary of Philosophy.* Cambridge: University Press, 1995.

17. Bennett MR, Hacker PMS. *Philosophical Foundations of Neuroscience.* Melbourne: Blackwell, 2003.

18. Hempel CG. *Philosophy of Natural Science.* Englewood Cliffs, NJ: Prentice Hall, 1966.

19. McLaren N. Chaos theory does not account for schizophrenia (correspondence). *ANZJP* 2006; 40: 816-17.

Chapter 2

1. Watson JB. Psychology as the behaviorist views it. *PR,* 1913; 20:158-177.

2. Pavlov IP. The reply of a physiologist to psychologists. *PR,* 1932; 39:91-127.

3. Skinner *BFD.*

4. Skinner *AB.*

5. Scriven M. A study of radical behaviorism. *University of Minnesota Studies in the Philosophy of Science,* Vol I, 1956.

6. Chomsky N. Review of Skinner's "Verbal Behavior." Language, 1959; 35:26-58.

7. McKenzie.

8. Dennett *Brainstorms.*

9. Kline R. Psychology Exposed, or: The Emperor's New Clothes. London: RKP, 1987.

10. Popper OK.

11. Efron R. The conditioned reflex: a meaningless concept. *Perspectives in Biology and Medicine*, 1966; 9: 488-514.

12. Yates AJ. The Theory and Practice of Behavior Therapy. New York: Wiley, 1972

13. Watson JB. The place of the conditioned reflex in psychology. *PR*, 1916; 23: 89-116.

14. Pavlov IP. *Lectures on Conditioned Reflexes*, Vol 2: Conditioned Reflexes and Psychiatry. New York: International Publishers, 1941

15. Eysenck HJ. Biological Dimensions of Personality. In: Pervin LA (Ed.). *Handbook of Personality: Theory and Research*. New York: Guilford Press, 1990

16. Eysenck HJ. *The Dynamics of Anxiety and Hysteria*. London: RKP, 1957

17. Peters RS. *The Concept of Motivation*, 2nd Ed. London: RKP, 1960.

18. Thomson R. *The Pelican History of Psychology*. Harmondsworth: Penguin Books, 1968.

19. Eysenck HJ. Introduction and General Features of the Model. In Eysenck HJ (Ed.). *A Model for Personality*. New York: Springer Verlag, 1981.

20. Popper and Eccles.

21. Eysenck HJ & Eysenck SBG. *Psychoticism as a Dimension of Personality*. London: Hodder and Stoughton, 1976.

22. Eysenck HJ. *Four ways five factors are not basic*. Personality and Individual Differences, 1992; 13: 667-673.

23. Eysenck HJ. Dimensions of personality: 16, 5 or 3? - Criteria for a taxonomic paradigm. *Personality and Individual Differences*, 1991; 12: 772-790.

24. McLaren N. A critical review of the biopsychosocial model. *ANZJP*, 1998; 32: 86-92.

25. Dennett KM.

26. Guze SB. Biological psychiatry: is there any other kind? *PM*, 1989; 19: 315-323.

27. Guze SB. *Why Psychiatry is a Branch of Medicine*. New York: Oxford University Press, 1992.

28. Swinburne R. Are mental events identical with brain events? *American Philosophical Quarterly*, 1982; 19:172-181.

29. McLaren N. Is mental disease just brain disease? The limits to biological psychiatry. *ANZJP*, 1992, 26: 270-276.

Chapter 3.

1. Ryle G. *The concept of mind*. Harmondsworth: Penguin University Books, 1973.

2. Dennett IS.

3. Popper *C&R*.

4. Slater E. The psychiatrist in search of a science II: Developments in the logic and sociology of science. *BJP*, 1973, 122: 625-636.

5. Masson JM. *The assault on truth: Freud's suppression of the seduction theory.* New York: Simon and Schuster/Pocket Books, 1998.

6. Bracken P. Science and psychoanalysis. *ANZJP*, 1987, 21: 137-139.

7. Eysenck HJ. Introduction and General Features of the Model. In Eysenck HJ (Ed.). *A Model for Personality.* New York: Springer Verlag, 1981

8. Popper *OK.*

9. Crews F. *Unauthorised Freud.* New York: Viking Penguin, 1999.

10. Sandler J, Dare C, Holder A. Frames of reference in psychoanalytic psychology III. A note on the basic assumptions. *British Journal of Medical Psychology*, 1972, 45: 143-147.

11. Freud A. *The ego and the mechanisms of defence.* New York: IUP, 1966.

12. Freud S. Introductory lectures on psycho-analysis. Quoted in Sandler J, Holder A, Dare C. Frames of reference in psychoanalytic psychology V. The topographical frame of reference; the organisation of the mental apparatus. *British Journal of Medical Psychology*, 1973, 46: 29-36.

13. Fenichel O. *The psychoanalytic theory of neurosis.* New York: Norton, 1945.

14. Alston WP. Logical status of psychoanalytic theories. In: Edwards P (Ed). *Encyclopedia of philosophy*, Vol VI. New York: MacMillan/Free Press, 1967.

15. Dennett *IS.*

16. Luria AR. *Higher cortical functions in man.* New York: Basic Books, 1980.

17. Lycan WG (Ed). *Mind and cognition.* Oxford: Blackwell, 1990.

18. Skinner *RBS.*

Chapter 4

1. Popper and Eccles.

2. Popper *LSD.*

3. Armstrong DM. In: Brazier MAB, (ed). *Brain and Mind.* CIBA Foundation Symposium No. 69 (New series) Excerpta Medica: Amsterdam, 1979.

4. Dennett *CE.*

5. Chalmers.

6. Dennett *Brainstorms.*

7. Skinner *AB.*

Chapter 5

1. Knight J. Psychiatry: eclecticism and empiricism. *AP* 1995: 3 407-410.

2. Pargiter R. Correspondence. *AP* 1996, 4: 151.

3. Kuhn.

4. Knight J. Correspondence. *AP* 1996, 4: 151.

5. McLaren N. See Ref. 29, Ch.2.

6 Rosenman S. American psychiatry: an unexpected, undesired and unplanned reform. *AP* 1996, 4: 118-121.

7. Abraham SF et al. The psychosexual histories of young women with bulimia. *ANZJP* 1985, 19: 72-76.

8. Chong SA, Choo HL. Smoking among Chinese patients with schizophrenia. *ANZJP* 1996, 30: 350-353.

9. McLaren N. Correspondence. *AP* 1996, 4: 30.

Chapter 6

1. Engel GL. A unified concept of health and disease. *Perspectives in Biology and Medicine* 1960; 3:459-485.
2. Engel GL. The need for a new medical model: a challenge for biomedicine. *Science* 1977; 196:129-136.
3. Engel GL. The care of the patient: art or science? *Johns Hopkins Medical Journal* 1977; 140:222-232.
4. Engel GL. The biopsychosocial model and the education of health professionals. *Annals of the New York Academy of Sciences* 1978; 310: 169-181.
5. Engel GL. The clinical application of the biopychosocial model. *AJP* 1980; 137:535-544.
6. Bertalanffy L von. *General systems theory.* Harmondsworth: Penguin, 1973.
7. Harre R. *The priniciples of scientific thinking.* London: Macmillan, 1970.
8. Lacey AR. *A dictionary of philosophy.* London: RKP, 1976.
9. Beer S. In: Bullock A, Stallybrass O, eds. *The Fontana Dictionary of Modern Thought.* London: Fontana/Collins, 1977.
10. Achinstein P. *The nature of explanation.* Oxford: University Press, 1983.
11. Leech G. *Semantics: the study of meaning,* 2nd ed. Harmondsworth: Pelican, 1981.
12. Popper *OK*
13. Dennett *Brainstorms.*
14. Ryan A. *The philosophy of the social sciences.* London: MacMillan, 1970.
15. Menninger K. *The vital balance.* New York: Viking, 1963.
16. Eisenberg L. Mindlessness and brainlessness in psychiatry. *BJP* 1986; 148:496-508.
17. Watson JB. Psychology as the behaviourist views it. *PR* 1913, 20: 158-77.
18. MacKenzie.
19. Howard C. The role of mental concepts in explaining neurotic behaviour. *BJP* 1977; 130:112-116.
20. Dennett *CE.*

Chapter 7

1. Livesley WJ. Trait and behavioural prototypes of personality disorder. *AJP* 1986; 143: 727-732.
2. Cloninger CR. A systematic method for clinical description and classification of personality variants. *AGP* 1987; 44: 573-588.
3. Livesley WJ. A systematic approach to the delineation of personality disorders. *AJP* 1987; 144: 772-777.
4. Widiger TA et al. A multidimensional scaling of the DSM-III personality disorders. *AGP* 1987; 44: 557-563.
5. Tyrer P, Casey P and Ferguson B. Personality disorder in perspective. *BJP* 1991; 159: 463-471.
6. DSM-IV.
7. Nurnberg HG, et al. The comorbidity of borderline personality disorder and other DSM-III-R axis II personality disorders. *AJP* 1991; 148: 1371-1377.

8. Dolan B, Evans C, Norton K. Multiple axis II diagnoses of personality disorder. *BJP* 1995; 166: 107-112.

9. Ellard J. personality disorder or the snark still at large. *AP* 1996;4:57-64.

10. Lacey AR. *Op cit.*

11. Ryle G. *op cit.*

12. Stumpf SE. *Socrates to Sartre: a history of philosophy.* 5th edition. New York: McGraw-Hill, 1993.

13. Parker G et al. Defining the personality disorders: description of an Australian database. *ANZJP* 1996; 30: 824-833.

14. Tyrer P. Comorbidity or consanguinity. *BJP* 1996; 168: 669-671.

15. Dennett *Brainstorms.*

16. Luria AR. *op cit.*

17. Eysenck HJ. Dimensions of personality: 16, 5 or 3? - Criteria for a taxonomic paradigm. *Journal of Individual Differences* 1991; 12: 773-790.

18. Eysenck HJ & Eysenck SBG. *Op cit.*

19. Eysenck HJ. Introduction and general features of the model, in Eysenck HJ (Ed). *A model for personality.* New York: Springer, 1981.

20. Eysenck HJ. Biological dimensions of personality. In Pervin LA (Ed). *Handbook of personality: theory and research.* New York: Guilford Press, 1990.

21. Cattell RB, Eber HW & Tatsuoka MM. *Handbook for the Sixteen Personality Factors Questionnaire.* Champaign, Ill: Institute for Personality and Ability Testing, 1970.

22. Norman WT. Toward an adequate taxonomy of personality attributes: replicated factor structure. *Journal of Abnormal and Social Psychology*, 1963; 66: 574-583.

23. McKenzie.

24. Kline R. *Psychology exposed.* London: RKP, 1988.

25. Watson JB. Psychology as the behaviourist views it. *PR* 20; 157-177, 1913.

Chapter 8

1. MacKenzie.

2. Brown JAC. *Freud and the neo-Freudians.* Harmondsworth: Penguin, 1964.

3. Bourne H. The insulin myth. *Lancet,* 1953, II: 964-968.

4. Sachdev P. Egas Moniz: a commemoration. *ANZJP*, 1999; 33: 463-466.

5. Kuhn.

6. Wilson J. The flight of the wild goose: the psychiatrist as a leader. *ANZJP* 2000: 34; 1-7.

7. RANZCP. *Position Statement No. 39* cited August 3rd, 2002. Available at www.ranzcp.org.au. This Statement on the College's official website carried the warning that it should not be viewed as official College policy. In fact, it has since been removed but nothing has replaced it.

8. Lachter B. "Chemical imbalance": a clinical *non sequitur. AP* 2001: 9: 311-315.

9. Harari E. Whose evidence? Lessons from the philosophy of science and the epistemology of psychiatry. *ANZJP* 2001: 35; 724-730.

10. Bloch S, Singh, BS (Eds). *Foundations of Clinical Psychiatry.* 2nd Edn., Melbourne: University Press, 2001.

11. Frances AJ, Egger HL. Whither psychiatric diagnosis? *ANZJP* 1999: 33; 161-165.

12. Engel PA, Engel AG. George L Engel 1913-1999: remembering his life and work: strengthening a father-son bond in a new time of grief. *ANZJP* 2002; 36: 443-448.

13. Taylor GJ. Mind-body-environment: George Engel's psychoanalytic approach to psychosomatic medicine. *ANZJP* 2002; 36: 448-457.

14. Singh BS. George Engel: a personal reminiscence. *ANZJP* 2002; 36: 467-471.

15. Smith GC, Strain JJ. George Engel's contribution to clinical psychiatry. *ANZJP* 2002; 36: 458-466.

16. Engel GL. A unified concept of health and disease. *Perspectives in biology and medicine* 1960: 3; 458-485.

17. Engel GL. The need for a new medical model: a challenge for biomedicine. *Science* 1977: 196; 128-136.

18. Engel GL. The care of the patient: science or art? *Johns Hopkins Medical Journal* 1977: 140; 222-232.

19. Engel GL. The biopsychosocial model and the education of health professionals. *Annals of the New York Academy of Sciences* 1978: 310; 168-181.

20. Engel GL. The clinical application of the biopsychosocial model. *AJP* 1980: 137; 534-544.

21. McLaren N. See Ref. 24, Ch.2.

22. Muir B. Comment on McLaren's critical review of the biopsychosocial model. *ANZJP* 1998: 32; 93-94.

23. Mullen PE. Comment on McLaren's critical review of the biopsychosocial model. *ANZJP* 1998: 32; 95-96.

24. Walters G, Bloch S. Publishing ethics in psychiatry. *ANZJP* 2001: 35; 28-35.

25. Bloch S. A call to authors: three solid reasons to publish in the *Journal.* *ANZJP* 2002; 36:1-2.

26. Bloch S. Editorial: A notable development. *ANZJP* 2002: 36; 289.

Chapter 9

1. Dennett DC. Current issues in the philosophy of mind. *American Philosophical Quarterly,* 1978; 15: 249-261.

2. Dennett *CE.*

3. Dennett *KN.*

4. Chalmers.

5. Audi R. *op cit.*

6. Dennett *IS.*

7. Dennett *Brainstorms.*

8. Bunge M. The mind-body problem in an evolutionary perspective. In: Brazier MAB (ed). *Brain and Mind.* CIBA Foundation Symposium 69 (new series). New York: Elsevier/North Holland, 1979.

Chapter 10

1. Chalmers.

2. Bunge M. *op cit.*

3. Reichard O. The mystery, majesty and the mythology of consciousness: Report and comment on the International Conference on 'Consciousness' held on 24-25 April 1999 at Kings College, London. In: *Newsletter of RANZCP Philosophy and Psychiatry Special Interest Grou*p, August, 1999.

4. Ryle G. *op cit.*

5. Dennett DC. Where Am I? Ch 17, in *Brainstorms*.

6. McLaren N. See Ref. 29, Ch.2.

7. Popper KR. In: Popper and Eccles.

A note on panpsychism: Chalmers wondered whether rocks might have some sort of consciousness just because they are organized and conceivably have input and output states (such as expanding during the heat of the day and contracting at night). I don't think this should be taken seriously. Organisation *per se* doesn't confer conscious experience or mental states on things, because experience is a *doing* within the organisation, a processing activity which manipulates the input to create something novel. If the structure is inert, as rock crystals are (that's what crystalline means), then nothing happens so the input and output states are "merely physical." They would no more lead to experience than would, say, moving the rock so that it faced north. I have no problems with the idea that consciousness arises through the manipulation of informational input states but the essential word here is "manipulation." That implies some organized structure to do the manipulating, but one thing crystals can't do is manipulate.

Chapter 11

1. Chalmers.

2. Ledoux J. *The emotional brain.* London: Weidenfeld and Nicolson, 1998.

3. Malenka RC, Nicoll RA. Long-term potentiation - a decade of progress? *Science* 1999, 285: 1870

4. Chomsky N. *Language and Mind.* New York: Harcourt Brace Jovanovich, 1972.

5. Dennett *CE.*

6. Popper and Eccles.

7. Popper *OK.*

Chapter 12

1. Kendler KS. Toward a philosophical structure for psychiatry. *AJP* 2005; 162:433-440.

2. Greenfield SA. Mind, brain and consciousness. *BJP*, 2002; 181:91-93.

3. Kuhn.

4. Audi R. *op cit*

5. Dennett *CE.*

6. Popper and Eccles.

7. Chalmers.

8. Dennett *Brainstorms.*

9. Turing AM. Computing machinery and intelligence. *Mind*; 59 (236): 433-54

10. Malenka RC, Nicoll RA. Long-term potentiation - a decade of progress? *Science* 1999, 285: 1870

Dennett referred to the Hungarian-born mathematician and logician, John von Neumann (1903-57). For more details of this little-known man's fascinating and productive life, see *Wikipedia*.

Chapter 14

Note 1: References to the seminal work by Yerkes and Dodson seem to have disappeared from most textbooks, both psychological and psychiatric. However, the resources are now available online, which is very helpful for those who (like me) don't have access to a university library. For a brief introduction, see the entry in *Wikipedia*. This can be accessed via the *Science* portal, then search *Reticular Formation* or *Reticular Activating System.*

The original paper by Yerkes and Dodson is listed in *Classics in the History of Psychology: an Internet Resource,* developed by Christopher D Green, York University, Toronto, Ontario.

The full reference is as follows:

Yerkes, Robert M, and Dodson, John D (1908): "The Relation of Strength of Stimulus to Rapidity of Habit Formation," *Journal of Comparative Neurology and Psychology*, 18: 459-482.

I have always been uneasy with the Yerkes-Dodson curve: Is it mere truism? That is, is it a genuinely novel discovery of something unexpected or does it merely graph a relationship that could not be otherwise? I lean to the latter, that it says something which could have been determined on first principles, without any experimentation whatsoever. Initially, I thought it may be simply a biological case of the Law of Diminishing Returns but that doesn't necessarily apply to cases where a change becomes destructive. More recently, I have decided it is in fact tautological since it is an example of "Too much is bad for you." In this case, it simply means that too much arousal is bad for you. Does that explain anything? No, nothing at all: too much of anything is bad for you, because that's what "too much" means. Of course, it also means that "not enough" is bad for you, as well, but not enough never worries grandmothers as much as too much. Oddly enough, going without has always been taken as a sign of moral superiority whereas too much is a deadly sin.

All biological systems operate within very narrowly defined parameters, and the human biological system is no different. We are so accustomed to these limits that we take them for granted but the body works very hard to keep us safe. Anything that pushes our systems outside those limits will result in malfunction, a governing principle that applies to complex internal functions just as it applies to ordinary biological systems. This principle applies to complex systems as well as the simple, but probably more so to arousal because it is itself absolutely fundamental to so many higher biological and psychological functions. Graphing any of these against a more basic parameter will result in the same distinctive curve. For example, graphing a motor performance such as playing the piano against serum potassium concentration will yield a similar curve.

Chapter 15

1. Doessel DP, Scheurer RW, Chant DC, Whiteford, HA. Changes in private sector electroconvulsive treatment in Australia. *ANZJP* 2006; 40:362-367.

2. McLaren N. Shrinking the Kimberley: Isolated psychiatry in Australia. *ANZJP* 1995; 29:199-206.

3. McLaren N. Only martyrs need apply: why psychiatrists should avoid isolated practice. *AP* 2003; 11: 456-459.

Index

Printed in the United States
129023LV00004B/8/A